D0207605

Process-Centered
Health Care Organizations

Suzanne P. Smith, EdD, RN, FAAN
Editor-in-Chief
Journal of Nursing Administration
Philadelphia, Pennsylvania

Dominick L. Flarey, PhD, MBA, RN,CS, CNAA, FACHE
President
Dominick L. Flarey & Associates, Inc.
Niles, Ohio
Editor-in-Chief
JONA's Healthcare Law, Ethics & Regulation
Philadelphia, Pennsylvania

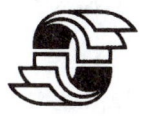

AN ASPEN PUBLICATION®
Aspen Publishers, Inc.
Gaithersburg, Maryland
1999

Library of Congress Cataloging-in-Publication Data

Process-centered health care organizations / [edited by] Suzanne P. Smith,
Dominick L. Flarey.
p. cm.
Includes bibliographical references and index.
ISBN 0-8342-1249-8
1. Health services administration. 2. Reengineering (Management).
3. Health services administration—Case studies. 4. Reengineering
(Management)—Case studies. I. Smith, Suzanne P. II. Flarey, Dominick L.
RA971.P764   1999
362.1'068—dc21   99-18270
CIP

Orders: (800) 638-8437
Customer Service: (800) 234-1660

About Aspen Publishers • For more than 35 years, Aspen has been a leading professional
publisher in a variety of disciplines. Aspen's vast information resources are available in both
print and electronic formats. We are committed to providing the highest quality information
available in the most appropriate format for our customers. Visit Aspen's Internet site for
more information resources, directories, articles, and a searchable version of Aspen's full
catalog, including the most recent publications: **http://www.aspenpublishers.com**
Aspen Publishers, Inc. • The hallmark of quality in publishing
Member of the worldwide Wolters Kluwer group.

Editorial Services: Denise H. Coursey
Library of Congress Catalog Card Number: 99-18270
ISBN: 0-8342-1249-8

Printed in the United States of America

1   2   3   4   5

Table of Contents

Contributors

Rella Adams, PhD, RN, CNAA
Senior Vice President, Nursing Services
Valley Baptist Medical Center
Harlingen, Texas

Maia Baker, MSN, RN
Administrative Director, Nursing
  Services
Valley Baptist Medical Center
Harlingen, Texas

Sherry D. Baker, MSN, RN
Director, Women's and Children's
  Services
Hillcrest Baptist Medical Center
Waco, Texas

**Edward L. Beard, Jr., MSN, RN,
  CNAA**
Vice President, Patient Services
Catawba Memorial Hospital
Hickory, North Carolina

Marjorie Beyers, PhD, RN, FAAN
Executive Director
American Organization of Nurse
  Executives
Chicago, Illinois

**Janice K. Bultema, MSN, RN,
  CNAA, NHA**
Executive Director, Transition
  Planning
Northwestern Memorial Hospital
Chicago, Illinois
Clinical Assistant Professor
Marcella Niehoff School of
  Nursing
Loyola University
Chicago, Illinois

Jo Anne Carrick, MSN, RN
Instructor
The Pennsylvania State University
Shenango Campus
Sharon, Pennsylvania

Marcia A. Colone, PhD, LCSW
Director, Case Management
Northwestern Memorial Hospital
Chicago, Illinois

Margrét Comack, MEd, BN
Director, Professional Practice
Toronto East General Hospital
Toronto, Ontario

Dorothy Counts, MA, RN, CPHQ
Clinical Resource Manager,
  Performance Improvement
Pennsylvania Hospital
Philadelphia, Pennsylvania

Markie Cowley, MSN, RN, CHE
Vice President, Patient Care and
  Nursing Services
Mission Hospital Regional Medical
  Center
Mission Viejo, California

Jill Donaldson, MSN, RN, CCRN
Surgical Outcomes Manager
Mission Hospital Regional Medical
  Center
Mission Viejo, California

Cyndy B. Dunlap, MPA, RN
Senior Vice President/Chief Nursing
  Officer
Hillcrest Baptist Medical Center
Waco, Texas

**Dominick L. Flarey, PhD, MBA,
  RN,CS, CNAA, FACHE**
President
Dominick L. Flarey & Associates,
  Inc.
Niles, Ohio
Editor-in-Chief
*JONA's Healthcare Law, Ethics &
  Regulation*
Philadelphia, Pennsylvania

**Paula S. Forté, PhD, MSN, RN,
  CNAA**
Director of Patient Services
Methodist Hospital, HealthSystem
  Minnesota
St. Louis Park, Minnesota
Adjunct Assistant Professor
University of Minnesota School of
  Nursing
Minneapolis, Minnesota

Lisa Freed, MSHA, RN
Administrative Director, Nursing
  Services
Valley Baptist Medical Center
Harlingen, Texas

**Anita Gottlieb, MA, RNP,
  CPHQ**
Quality Improvement Coordinator
Arkansas Children's Hospital
Little Rock, Arkansas

**Patti Higginbotham, RN, CPHQ,
  FNAHQ**
Vice President, Quality Management
Arkansas Children's Hospital
Little Rock, Arkansas

**Mary Lou Helfrich Jones, PhD, RN,
  CNAA**
Assistant Operating Officer, Women's
  Services
Duke University Health System
Durham, North Carolina

Bette Keeling, MSN, RN, CNAA
Nursing Coordinator
Hillcrest Baptist Medical Center
Waco, Texas

Curt Kretzinger, BSN, RN
Vice President, Patient Care
    Services
Heartland Health System
St. Joseph, Missouri

Maura MacPhee, MS, RN
Clinical Specialist
The Children's Hospital
Denver, Colorado

Jo Manion, MA, RN, CNAA, FAAN
Founder and Senior Consultant
Manion & Associates
Oviedo, Florida

**Magdalena A. Mateo, PhD, RN,
    FAAN**
Consultant
Boston, Massachusetts

Myra Mengwasser, MHA, RN
Partner
Ernst & Young, LLP
St. Louis, Missouri

**Mae Taylor Moss, MS, MSN, RN,
    FAAN**
President
Moss Management Inc.,
    International
Houston, Texas

Gail Paech, MScN, BScN
Former President and CEO
Toronto East General Hospital
Toronto, Ontario

Celine Peters, MN, RN
Director of Outcomes
    Management
Mission Hospital Regional Medical
    Center
Mission Viejo, California

Lana S. Peters, MHA, MBA, RN
Senior Consultant
Ernst & Young, LLP
St. Louis, Missouri

**Tim Porter-O'Grady, PhD, EdD,
    FAAN**
President
Tim Porter-O'Grady Associates, Inc.
Assistant Professor
Emory University
Atlanta, Georgia

Mary Pubentz, PharmD, RPh
Clinical Coordinator, Anticoagulation
    Clinic
Lutheran General Hospital–Advocate
    Health Care
Park Ridge, Illinois

Julie Schaffner, MSN, RN
Vice President of Operations
Lutheran General Hospital–Advocate
    Health Care
Park Ridge, Illinois

Kerry K. Seely, RN
Director, Acute Care Services
Hillcrest Baptist Medical Center
Waco, Texas

Suzanne P. Smith, EdD, RN, FAAN
Editor-in-Chief
Journal of Nursing Administration
Philadelphia, Pennsylvania

Hussein A. Tahan, MS, RN, CNA
Manager, Clinical Pathway Program
Mount Sinai Hospital
New York, New York
Adjunct Faculty
Case Management Programs
Pace University
Pleasantville, New York
College of Mount St. Vincent
Riverdale, New York

Janet Teeters, MS, RPh
Director of Operations, Pharmacy and
    Rehab Services
Lutheran General Hospital—
    Advocate Health Care
Park Ridge, Illinois

Karen Terry, MS, RN
Nurse Clinical Specialist
The Children's Hospital
Denver, Colorado

Linda D. Thompson, BSN, RN
Director, Medical-Surgical Services
Hillcrest Baptist Medical Center
Waco, Texas

Karen Vest, BSN, RN
Special Projects Coordinator
Valley Baptist Home Health
Harlingen, Texas

**Katherine W. Vestal, PhD, RN,
    FAAN, FACHE**
Partner
Ernst & Young, LLP
Dallas, Texas

**Phyllis M. Watson, PhD, MEd,
    RN**
Senior Vice President
Lakeland Regional Medical Center
Lakeland, Florida

Foreword

For the past few years, the health care industry has been undergoing a contentious revolution that has fed on conflict and uncertainty. Health care providers of all disciplines have seen their work, their roles, and their professional norms changed dramatically to meet the new agendas. While most would agree that many of the changes will benefit patients, the process of making transitions has been both challenging and painful.

In most health care organizations the focus has been on adapting care processes to meet managed care standards, drastically reducing costs through consolidation of services and reduction of staff, and adopting interdisciplinary teams to provide services. These changes are not necessarily bad; in fact, few would disagree that streamlining was necessary. However, the patchwork of improvements and the piecemeal approaches have often yielded further confusion, frustration, and fragmentation. It was easy to blame "reengineering" for the chaos, but, in truth, we must learn from our experiences and move on to the next generation of organizational improvement.

This book, *Process-Centered Health Care Organizations,* is intended to help health care organizations get to the next level of performance. We often lament that after all we have done to improve systems, they still are not optimal. That is true. So what can we do to keep making systems better?

Process-centered organizations require leaders who are process oriented. Process-oriented leaders have a mindset and knowledge base that will support process thinking, require process design and implementation, and measure results based on process outcomes. While this sounds easy, we all know that even the initial identification of critical processes in health care delivery is highly debatable. In fact, identifying the macroprocesses such as access, supported by specific microprocesses or care associated with specific disease entities, makes it possible for leaders to design solutions that meet both customer/client and organizational needs.

It is also useful to examine business processes in industries outside of health care. The sophistication of process-centered organizations, such as those that are Malcolm Baldrige winners, shows the depth and breadth of constantly improving processes. The Baldrige Award is now open to the health care industry, and those organizations that have embraced a process orientation may well be able to win this prestigious quality award.

There are some undeniable truths related to process-centered organizations. First, the process-centered concept and its operational imperatives must be embraced and consistently required by the leaders. Second, members of the staff and management must be given the knowledge and tools to design and implement processes across functional and political boundaries. Third, a culture must be established that has a low tolerance for outcomes that are measured and do not reflect excellence. And last, there must be a way to reward outstanding results, as well as consequences for those tolerating results that do not improve. Only then will the organization be able to move from mediocrity to excellence.

—Katherine W. Vestal, PhD, RN, FAAN, FACHE
Partner
Ernst & Young, LLP
Dallas, Texas

Preface

In 1993, reengineering gurus Michael Hammer and James Champy published *Reengineering the Corporation: A Manifesto for Business Revolution*. Defined as the radical redesign of an organization's processes, organization, and culture, reengineering has as its major goal a quantum leap in performance and the radical improvements that follow from entirely new work processes and structures. Following the book's release, reengineering became the hottest new management strategy in the business world, including health care.

However, while reengineering transformed health care organizations and allowed huge performance improvements, it left leaders and their employees with businesses they barely understood let alone knew how to manage. Very little of what health care leaders knew about managing task-oriented businesses applied to reengineered organizations with their new focus on core processes. Health care leaders discovered that they had to rethink "the kinds of work that people do, the jobs they hold, the skills they need, the ways in which their performance is measured and rewarded, the careers they follow, the roles managers play, the principles of strategy that enterprises follow."[1(p.xiii)] Likewise, leaders who chose the less radical path of redesign through total quality management also found that their organizational focus had shifted to processes.

To address the emerging concerns of reengineered and redesigned organizations that had become process-centered organizations, Hammer wrote *Beyond Reengineering*.[2] This book delineates the key components of and approaches to process-centered organizations, which, like the organizations themselves, will continually evolve. We have based this book on Hammer's basic concepts, which we believe can safely guide health care organizations in their quest to excel in their work and be ever responsive to changing environmental conditions. We strongly believe that nurse executives and nurse managers, as well as health care executives and managers, must learn and develop skills to lead process-centered organizations.

This book provides comprehensive theories, methodologies, and cutting-edge strategies for managing the process-centered organization; it also provides nurse executives, managers, and other health care providers with a comprehensive reference for approaching, implementing, and evaluating their own processes. The book is divided into two parts. Part I presents theories and methodologies relevant to managing a process-centered organization, and Part II presents a variety of process-focused case studies, ranging from patient care delivery to human relations management to role restructuring.

Our mission in producing this book was to provide health care leaders with an innovative reference that can be used to facilitate further transformations in the practice environment and in overall health care delivery. Health care professionals practice today in a time of great chaos and change. The mandate to change and transform health care delivery is real and ever present. A decade ago it was basically impossible to conceive of where the industry would be in terms of care delivery as we approach the new millennium. Many believed that by the year 2000 health care would be "fixed" and a period of "calm" would be realized. While we have made great strides in the quest for a new health care system, our jobs are not yet complete. Much more needs to be done and realized.

This book is one source of information and reference to guide health care leaders into the 21st century and to realize the transformations that are necessary to confront the issues of the new millennium. It is our hope that we have contributed to this journey in a proactive way through this work. Our public presentation of this book is accompanied by hope and faith in a new tomorrow that will bring a new and better health care delivery system for all.

Finally, we thank the contributing authors for taking the time to share their experiences and for helping advance our understanding of process-centered work and organizations. Their dedication and hard work demonstrates the type of commitment needed to further transform the health care delivery system. May we continue to learn and grow through the work they have contributed. We dedicate this book in loving memory to Muriel Smith and Virginia M. Flarey, whose lives were taken suddenly during this project, reminding us that life is precious and short and so we must live our dreams today.

Suzanne P. Smith, EdD, RN, FAAN
Dominick L. Flarey, PhD, MBA, RN,CS, CNAA, FACHE

REFERENCES

1. Hammer M, Champy J. *Reengineering the Corporation: A Manifesto for Business Revolution.* New York: HarperCollins Publishers; 1993.

2. Hammer M. *Beyond Reengineering: How the Process-Centered Organization Is Changing Our Work and Our Lives.* New York: Harper Business; 1996.

PART I

The Process-Centered Organization

CHAPTER 1

The New World of Health Care: Seeking Change and Improvement

Suzanne P. Smith, EdD, RN, FAAN
Dominick L. Flarey, PhD, MBA, RN,CS, CNAA, FACHE

Despite a decade of continued change and transformation of the health care system, chaos persists. Each day there is more need to continue the quest to develop a health care delivery system that meets the country's needs. Past problems continue to plague health care. Reimbursements are declining, staff morale is low, the number of uninsured continues to increase, and nothing is stable. Health care costs continue to rise despite innovations in care delivery such as patient-focused care, enabling technologies, and case management systems. Global downsizing, without the appropriate redesign of systems, also has been a threat to health care professionals. All of this drives health care professionals to wonder, "When will we get it right?" The fact that they ask this question at all is evidence enough that more radical change and transformation are needed.

How did health care professionals get in the predicament of needing to take dramatic, revolutionary, and radical measures to save their organizations? In retrospect, the harbingers of change are apparent. There were warning signs that, taken individually, seemed manageable. Now, however, it can be seen how seemingly discrete issues and problems related to health care were parts of the same picture—a malfunctioning system that is being treated with first aid instead of surgery. Despite the advances in health care, this scenario still exists.

This chapter presents a brief summation of the forces of change that have arisen over the past decade, as well as the need for more transformation. Much of this content is fact, but some is prediction. Regardless, the case remains strong for further radical change and overall transformation in the U.S. health care system.

Source: Reprinted from S. Smith Blancett and D.L. Flarey. Changing paradigms: the impetus to reengineer health care. In: Blancett SS, Flarey DL. *Reengineering Nursing and Health Care: The Handbook for Organizational Transformation.* Gaithersburg, MD: Aspen Publishers, Inc; 1995:3–14. Reprinted with permission.

THE CURRENT ENVIRONMENT

The key to understanding the path to further transformation of the health care system is to review the major issues in health care delivery. These issues include cost, structure, stakeholders, managed care, alliances, redesign, and quality. Each deserves an individual examination. This review leads into predictions for the future and allows a clearer definition of future challenges.

Cost

A critical factor that brought the health care system to the forefront of public and private scrutiny was its increasing share of the gross national product (GNP). General economic recession and inflation certainly had a part in spiraling health care costs. As costs for products, services, salaries, construction, unreimbursed care, and capital equipment increased, they were passed on to consumers, most often the government and insurance companies.

"In the United States, health care costs too much. Health care consumes 13.6 percent of our economy—compared with 9.7 percent for Canada, 10.2 percent for the nations of Western Europe, and 8.3 percent for Japan. Despite our appetite for leading edge drugs like t-PA, the additional $333 billion per year in economic share that we spend on health care in comparison to our traditional partners buys the United States the highest infant mortality rate and lowest life expectancy in the industrialized world."[1(p.3)] In light of these statistics and realities, approximately 41 million people in the United States have no health insurance coverage.[1]

An offshoot of the government's effort to curb expenses through reimbursement mechanisms was competition among providers. The health care industry's initial response was to get new equipment, new plants, and new services in an attempt to remain competitive and attract new business. These efforts to respond to decreasing margins and inpatient bed occupancy further contributed to the cost of doing business.

Competition has further increased health care costs. As organizations compete, they attempt to "outsmart" and "outdo" their community competitors. Such competition impedes the quest to contain costs. In fact, cost containment is really a fallacy. The ability to manage costs effectively is a challenge that continues to this day.

Downsizing was another strategy that taught organizations how to fail at transformation. Today it is realized that downsizing almost always results in poor-quality care. Poor-quality care in turn severely damages the system and the health care organization, as well as the community and the providers of care. Poor quality increases costs. This method of attempting to contain costs continues, however, despite the lessons being learned. As such, many health care organizations today struggle with quality issues as well as the need to further reduce costs. The pattern is circular, and many cannot find their way out.

Structure

The bureaucratic organizational structures of health care organizations also contributed to waste and economic inefficiency. Built on 19th-century principles, hierarchic organizational structures were "not designed to operate in today's highly competitive global markets, let alone take them successfully into the 21st century."[2(p.46)] Bureaucratic structures, with their focus on "specialization, uniform policies, standardized jobs, a career of promotions, impersonal relationships, and coordination from above,"[3(p.18)] work well with a passive labor force and a stable environment. These types of organizations are not good at perceiving and reacting to threats to their well-being. They stifle productivity and operational efficiency. The hospital also added a unique twist on the bureaucratic structure. "The 'business' of hospitals (caring for patients) was separated from the financial management of the enterprise,"[4(p.23)] which further encouraged a highly labor-intensive, highly segmented business.

Bureaucratic structures have also severely impeded innovation. Organizations are paralyzed in differing degrees from moving forward. Change becomes the enemy. Change breeds fear, skepticism, and unrest. As such, innovation is given low priority and placed on the "back burner." Without the freedom to innovate, organizations become static and slow, and, ultimately, they meet their demise.

It is now understood that innovation is one of the key solutions to the health care system's problems. Innovation requires changes in organizational structures as well as changes in the way organizations deal with their external environments. "Any given innovation requires customer and supplier partners to be implemented. And the more radical [and frequently more valuable] the innovation, the more deeply and broadly must other players, especially customers be involved. This places a premium on learning to manage a very wide community or network of organizations, in which all players share a vision about how to make the innovation happen."[5(p.211)] While mergers and acquisitions are causing organizations to come together, many such reorganizations fail because bureaucratic structures prevent this type of networking, and therefore innovation, from happening.

Stakeholders

Along with the imperative to decrease costs came changing public expectations. Better educated and informed consumers wanted a more active part in the management of their care. More consumers joined the ranks of the working poor or the uninsured, providing a stimulus for change. Unable to afford care, they use emergency departments for both primary and nonurgent care. In addition to increasing hospital costs for unreimbursed care, an ethical issue was raised in the public's eye as stories of mistreatment of these uninsured patients occurred. "We still suffer the national shame of having approximately 50 million uninsured citizens. Low-income citizens still do not have reasonable access to many necessary services."[6(pp.110–111)] The image of the health care institution was changing from concerned community caregiver to inept, fragmented, inefficient, and perhaps unethical provider.

Those with health insurance coverage often had their company-sponsored health care benefits decreased; consumers were directly paying larger percentages of their health care bills. Knowledge, coupled with increasing personal costs, led many consumers to begin questioning what they were getting for their health care dollar. They started demanding better service and better outcomes, in large part by lobbying their elected officials.

The work force was also changing. Better-educated workers felt entitled to find personal fulfillment and meaning from their jobs. The bureaucratic fragmentation of work processes into tasks and a hierarchic reporting system was not personally fulfilling or satisfying. We had "successful people producing results, but with no time in which to arrange themselves and change others."[7(p.29)] Administrators found the work environment and its structure challenged from within as well as without.

Another group of stakeholders no longer satisfied with a passive role in health care is the third-party payers—the government, business, and insurance companies. Through regulation and economic pressure, payers are assuming a significant and more overt influence on the delivery of health care services. Their influence comes from regulating and negotiating how much and what types of care will be reimbursed. The new paradigm has ushered in capitation as the preferred reimbursement system. This is the providers' response to their long-enduring dissatisfaction. They are demanding a new system of health care, one focused on prevention. "Capitation changes the focus of health care from treating illness to promoting wellness and prevention. In addition, capitation aligns physicians' and hospitals' economic interests and thus allows the two providers to work as a team in developing ways to enhance quality of care and reduce costs of care."[8(p.11)]

Managed Care

These and other factors led to a ground swell for health care reform. In 1992, President Clinton, along with numerous congressional candidates, was elected on a pledge to enact health care reform. His first-term actions forced Americans to face the fact that problems in the U.S. health care system had to be addressed. Exactly how became the turning point. The government and payers, feeling fee-for-service and prospective payment systems were not the answer, moved toward capitated payment systems. A major element of the Clinton Administration's plan for national reform rested on the concept of managed competition. Jack Hole, a physician and economist, stated that "under managed competition, most doctors and hospitals would join prepaid plans such as health-maintenance organizations that would compete for the business of large consumer groups. By rewarding doctors for prudent care and publicizing comparative medical results, this approach should help move medical care back to where most things that are done to patients actually improve their health. By drastically reducing waste, we can avoid or at least delay rationing."[9(pp.289–290)] Capitated payments and managed care mandate that health care institutions rethink their basic operation if they are to survive. Predications are that capitation may decrease inpatient utilization by 50 percent.[10(p.30)]

An integral part of capitated care for a designated population (an increasingly large part of institutions' revenue) is the mandate to identify and manage outcomes. Managed care buyers are selecting their provider institutions based on quality and effectiveness. This is one of the major challenges for health care organizations today: competing in the outcomes and quality arena. Capitation is also changing the traditional health care organization as we know it. The very concept of capitation mandates these changes for the organization to be successful. "Success under capitation will be characterized by: fewer hospitalizations, shortened hospital stays with improved efficiency of inpatient care, accelerated discharges from the hospital to other levels of care or the home through aggressive discharge planning and a truly coordinated continuum of care."[8(p.10)]

Alliances

There have been many institutional responses to competition and economic constraints. One major industry initiative is the formation of strategic partnerships, alliances, and networks. Health care institutions are establishing services and acquiring or partnering with others to provide a broad range of comprehensive services for specific patient populations under managed care. Physician-hospital groups are forming to integrate patient care services more adequately as well as to share the financial risks and rewards of a capitated system. Large health care corporations continue to buy and sell health care agencies with targeted services, seeking the right mix of services to excel in a rapidly changing environment. These changes have resulted in an explosion in the number of multiprovider networks and multihospital systems.

Redesign

The redesign of care delivery models was prompted by major institutional initiatives to control costs, improve patient satisfaction, and use resources efficiently. Encouraged by a multimillion-dollar project grant from the Robert Wood Johnson Foundation and the Pew Charitable Trust, hospitals started restructuring their systems in an effort to remain viable and responsive to many competing customers (government, physicians, staff, and payers). A major model of care delivery to emerge was patient-focused care, the main components of which were decentralization of key services to the unit level, delivery of care by teams (from a nurse partnered with a nursing assistant to interdisciplinary groups), and managed care measured by predefined expected outcomes during the course of an illness.

Quality

Total quality management (TQM) and quality improvement programs also emerged from pressure, first from external forces. The demand of third-party payers and consumers to know what they were getting for their health care dollar, limited resources, and the subsequent internal pressure to know and eliminate inefficient non–value-added work processes led to quality initiatives. Since teams are an integral part of a formal TQM program and most of the restructured systems used teams to deliver care, the critical role of frontline staff in making operations more efficient and effective became apparent. Staff development expanded beyond the acquisition of clinical skills to include team building, empowerment, delegation, budgeting, and governance.

THE FUTURE

While the initiatives discussed have certainly addressed some basic economic and delivery problems, the question is whether they are enough and will be adequate for the future. "Every day in hospitals across the country, CEOs and other senior managers sit at their desks and try to improve costs and service performance. They pull the 'levers' that they have been taught to pull to change the organization. But these levers do not seem to be connected to anything. Significant change continues to elude us. We reach out to new techniques like total quality management or continuous quality improvement, throw resources at them, and hope for the best."[11(p.21)]

What about the future? Are current initiatives and strategies for addressing issues related to limited and shrinking resources, quality imperatives, and a competitive environment sufficient to meet the needs of an uncertain future? Are we creating flexible approaches adaptable to whatever comes along or simply replacing an antiquated and static approach with an equally soon-to-be-outdated one?

The fact that health care leaders are ambivalent about reform and the degree of change they have to make in their institutions is seen in a recent report. The Health Care Forum Leadership Center queried health care opinion leaders on three future health care scenarios. The "Continued Growth/High Technology" scenario has health care consuming 17 percent of the GNP by 2001, with high technology proliferating but at a high cost; health care reform does not occur, patchwork managed care grows, as does medical indigence and unequal access. "Hard Times/Government Leadership" has a frugal universal access system with significant rationing of services based on cost benefit and outcomes research; heroic lifesaving measures decline; and researchers adopt a more frugal approach to innovation. Health care's percentage of the GNP declines to 11 percent by 2001.[12]

The third scenario is "New Civilization," in which "dramatic changes in science, technology, society and government hasten health care change. Care broadens its focus from the person to the community and the environment. National health reform favors managed care through a government/business partnership with discretion at the community level. This partnership would provide basic coverage for all with an emphasis on the continuum of care, health promotion and social HMOs. High tech and alternative therapies are common. Health care consumes 12 percent of the GNP in 2001."[12(pp.7–8)]

Interestingly, it was this third scenario that 87 percent of the leaders preferred; however, they thought it was the least likely to occur. Instead, they felt the reality would be "Hard Times/Government Leadership." This is an interesting paradox to consider. Our health care leaders can envision an ideal future, but they expect the worst. One has to suspect that this dual type of thinking probably exists in their organizational management as well. Many administrators show an "unwillingness to think rigorously and patiently about themselves or their ideas. . . . When leading an organization into the future, executives come to a fork in the road. As they come face-to-face with their organizations' needs to reinvent themselves, many executives hope for the best and opt for the prudent path of change."[3(p.19)]

Change is traumatic. Why put an organization and its people through radical change if simple adjustments will accomplish results? This attitude of not reacting quickly and doing nothing too dramatic seems to be borne out by an American Hospital Association (AHA) study.[13] The AHA reports that hospital actions taken in anticipation of what national health care reform might require has led to "controlling costs by managing better within fixed budgets, forming new partnerships with other providers and coming up with innovative solutions to community health problems."[13(p.1)] These efforts caused a decline in total hospital expenses. However, the AHA report points out that the decrease resulted from a decline in almost all measures of hospital use and a continuing shift from inpatient to outpatient services. So while health care executives have taken many initiatives to solve system problems related to economic delivery of care, initiatives that merely produce incremental improvements in the existing system might not be enough for the future.

How can one adapt to a future in which the only certainty is unpredictability, complexity, and turbulence coupled with scarce resources? If health care is to not only survive but prosper, all aspects of our organization have to change—structures, human resource procedures, information technology, and management and worker skills and attitudes. Management has to find ways to empower staff to design and adjust their work, its processes, and their organizational connections. Organizations have to change the education received by managers to stress the human side of the enterprise. And all participants have to learn how to cross organizational boundaries, whether they are interdisciplinary, interdepartmental, or intradepartmental.

What kind of organizational model can do all this? Perhaps the new organization of the future will be the intelligent organization, a market-based confederation of intrapreneurial teams that is structured to support and coordinate self-managing groups and teams.[3] The new architecture of the intelligent organization "lets people connect laterally, between specialties, geographies, or products, whether within or outside the boundaries of a particular organization. . . . [T]he intelligent organization creates clear visions of possible futures and acts quickly and effectively in a locally adaptive, yet coordinated way.[3(p.20)]

The intelligent organization has three essential ingredients: freedom of choice, responsibility for the whole, and limited corporate government. Freedom of choice is based on widespread sharing of information, which allows workers to make intelligent decisions. It implies that workers have freedom of speech, freedom of association, and the right to make contracts with each other and keep promises. It reinforces Drucker's contention that "knowledge is the only meaningful resource today [and that] knowledge employees cannot, in effect, be supervised."[14(p.14)] It upholds that

> We are entering a period that demands that we operate in such a way as to empower the incalculable assets of human intelligence and creativity. The major distinction, for example, between old and new methods lies not in the methods themselves, but in the ability to integrate human beings into meaningful work. The new world requires humans to function as essential information and idea resources, creating solutions we have never seen before. In this kind of situation, human labor is no longer a disposable commodity, but a unique creative resource, in

which an individual's development is as valuable as the organization's growth.[15(p.265)]

Responsibility for the whole is about leaders helping staff and teams achieve their highest potential so that they are integrated into and committed to the whole. It involves equality and diversity, voluntary learning networks, and democratic self-rule.

The final element, limited corporate government, acknowledges the fact that no central management team can design an organizational structure fluid enough to get the work done in the most efficient and effective manner. "It has to be done on the fly by the choices of all the people at work, people establishing the connections they need to get the work done. . . . [T]he primary role of the [corporate] center is to create the conditions that empower those doing the work to build systems to run their operations effectively."[3(p.21)]

The rate of change in health care is unprecedented. Driven by technological and economic forces, health care is being retooled and reshaped for the 21st century. The changes and challenges of the new health care world will differ markedly from those confronted in the past several decades. The authors believe that the following changes will drive the need for continued reengineering and the development of process-centered health care organizations.

Care Delivery

- Third-party payers will force a massive shift of care delivery away from the acute care setting and into the home, subacute care facilities, and outpatient centers.
- The hospital as we know it will become extinct. The largest delivery system will be home health care.
- In the next five years, the acute care inpatient census will be at least 50 percent of what it is today.
- Clinic services will be the second largest care delivery system. Many types of clinics will emerge offering communities a wide array of care services. Clinics will be strategically placed in malls, schools, and churches.
- By the year 2000, the average acute care length of stay will be three days.
- Hospitals will become triage centers with the primary objective of making rapid diagnoses and stabilizing patients. Most future inpatient units will be what are now known as critical status units; the typical medical-surgical units will be virtually empty.

- Obstetrical care will also shift from the acute care setting. Birthing centers will become vogue. Home births will flourish once again and be attended by nurse midwives, a back-to-the-future phenomenon.
- All but the most complex surgical procedures will be done in free-standing outpatient surgery centers where such procedures can be done more cost effectively.

Reimbursements

- The future will be a world of managed care. Local and regional networks of managed care providers will compete vigorously to be agents for patient care services. Health maintenance organizations and preferred provider organizations within a managed care framework will be commonplace.
- Fixed payment structures will prevail. Financial resources for care will be paid out in fixed rates regardless of the amount of care required. Capitation will thus be the major driving force for changes in medical and nursing practice patterns.

Physician Practice Patterns

- Physicians will be active participants in some type of integrated delivery system. The most popular will be physician-hospital organizations (PHOs), in which physicians and hospitals work together in strong partnerships to negotiate the delivery of care with managed care networks and mutually develop strategic plans for the delivery of high-quality, cost-effective care. Fixed-rate payment systems will force these partnerships and drive more and more changes in the way care is delivered, including the judicious use of resources.
- As the system continues to transform itself, fully integrated care delivery systems will emerge. There will be high levels of integration whereby physicians become employees of organizations and are contracted to provide a continuum of services. Private physician practices will be a rarity.

Physician Extenders

- In this new era, many nonphysician providers will emerge, such as nurse practitioners and nurse midwives. The government will fund and encourage the use of such providers in an ongoing effort to hold down health care costs.
- Reimbursement incentives will exist for organizations and group practices that use nonphysician providers.

Prevention

- The current focus on disease will shift to a focus on disease prevention, health promotion, and wellness.
- Many and varied health prevention programs will be developed. Nurses will play key roles in patient and public education, and many will practice in primary prevention practices. There will be great financial incentives for organizations and physician group practices to practice preventive medicine as healthy populations use less capitated dollars for care.

Practice Patterns

- Medical guidelines and protocols or pathways will be standard. These will be developed to assist the care team in delivering expedient and more efficient health care services. These pathways will become major financial initiatives in a capitated payment system, as length of stay and use of resources will be reduced.
- A major focus on quality and outcomes will prevail.
- Network payers will stringently monitor quality and outcomes. Organizations and practitioners who cannot meet these established standards will likely be excluded from managed care networks, PHOs, and other integrated delivery systems.
- The driving force for all care delivery will be based on nationally acceptable patient outcomes and quality indicators.

Continuum of Care

- Networks will mandate that providers offer a full continuum of services to patient populations.
- The driving force for the formation of group practices, integrated delivery systems, and organizational and system affiliations and mergers will be the overwhelming emphasis on a full continuum of care services.

Case Management Systems

- "Case management is the vehicle that nurses and other health care professionals will use to move health care delivery well into the next century."[16(p.465)] All specialties will have systems of case management, and all patients will be case managed to some degree.

- Case management will be the preferred delivery system because it emphasizes greater continuity of care, provides for more holistic and preventive care, and is focused on outcomes and outcomes management.[16]

EXECUTIVE PERCEPTIONS

As we move quickly toward the new millennium, it is interesting to note some current perceptions of priorities by hospital and managed care executives. The 1998 Hospitals & Health Networks Leadership Survey demonstrates the similarities in perceptions and priorities.[17] Both groups of executives were asked to rate 30 issues on a five-point scale in terms of importance for the near future. Here are their top five responses:

- Hospital executives
  1. controlling costs
  2. increasing patient satisfaction
  3. improving customer service
  4. physician and administration collaboration
  5. increasing market share
- Managed care executives
  1. improving customer service
  2. controlling costs
  3. information technology
  4. increasing patient satisfaction
  5. increasing market share

As can be seen, the responses of the two groups are similar. It appears that both types of providers are on the same page when it comes to future priorities. This is promising, and it is hoped that as time goes on there will be greater collaborative efforts between these providers in terms of goal attainment.

These priorities also need to be viewed in light of five of the most compelling factors that are affecting the health care industry today: changes in the reimbursement system, an aging patient population, the human immunodeficiency virus/acquired immune deficiency syndrome epidemic, advancing technology, and more educated patients as consumers of health care.[18] In assessing these factors, and in assimilating the executive priorities identified above, it becomes clear that the road ahead is paved with great challenges and complexities. Such great and lasting transformations will only be realized by organizations redesigning themselves into process-centered entities.

CONCLUSION

And so, the journey to re-create the health care delivery system begins. The following chapters present processes for work and systems reengineering as well as methodologies related to process-centered approaches to care delivery. It is evident that the transformations needed to meet the future challenges of health care can only be realized through radical internal changes in organizations. This book is a road map to that end.

REFERENCES

1. Kleinke JD. *Bleeding Edge: The Business of Health Care in the New Century.* Gaithersburg, MD: Aspen Publishers, Inc; 1998.
2. McManis GL. Reinventing the system. *Hosp & Health Networks.* 1993; 19:42, 44, 46, 48.
3. Brown T. The intelligent organization. *Industry Week.* 1994; 243(6):17–21.
4. Helppie RD. A time for reengineering. *Computers in Healthcare.* 1992; 10(1):22–24.
5. Boyett JH, Boyett JT. *The Guru Guide: The Best Ideas of the Top Management Thinkers.* New York: John Wiley & Sons Inc; 1998.
6. Reres M. *Managed Care: Managing the Process.* Glencoe, IL: National Professional Education Institute, Inc; 1996.
7. Bredin J. Parker's offense on defense. *Industry Week.* 1994; 243(8):29–30.
8. Kolb D, ed. *Assessing Organizational Readiness for Capitation.* Chicago: American Hospital Publishing Inc; 1996.
9. Eckholm E, ed. *Solving America's Health Care Crisis.* New York: Time Books; 1993.
10. Cerne F. Shaping up for capitation. *Hosp & Health Networks.* 1994; 68(7):28–37.
11. Lathrop J. *Restructuring Health Care: The Patient Focused Paradigm.* San Francisco: Jossey-Bass Publishers; 1993.
12. Curtin L. Sign of things to come. *Nurs Manage.* 1992; 23(7):7–8.
13. American Organization of Nurse Executives. Growth in hospital expenses slows as cost-cutting efforts reap dividends. *AONE News.* 1994; 3(1):1, 5.
14. Brown T. Peter Drucker: Managing in a post-capitalist marketplace. *Industry Week.* 1994; 243(1):13–18.
15. Land G, Jarman B. Moving beyond breakpoint. In: Ray M, Rinzler A, eds. *The New Paradigm in Business: Emerging Strategies for Leadership and Organizational Change.* New York: Jeremy P. Tarcher/Perigee Books; 1993.
16. Cesta T, Tahan H, Fink L. *The Case Manager's Survival Guide: Winning Strategies for Clinical Practice.* St. Louis: Mosby-Yearbook Inc; 1998.
17. Solovy A, Sunseri R. Leading the way. *Hosp & Health Networks.* 1998 August: 30–43.
18. Beckham JD. The vision thing. *Healthcare Forum.* 1994; 37:60–68.

CHAPTER 2

Reengineering: The Journey to a Process-Centered Organization

Dominick L. Flarey, PhD, MBA, RN,CS, CNAA, FACHE
Suzanne P. Smith, EdD, RN, FAAN

EDITORS' NOTE

Since this chapter was written several years ago, the value of reengineering for process improvement has been firmly established. An unexpected outcome of reengineering experiments was the new focus on core processes integral to an organization's existence. The value of reengineering as a first step on the journey to becoming a process-centered organization was realized. Reengineering cannot be displaced or ignored if an organization wants to truly transform itself into a process-centered one.

This chapter presents the authors' original work, "Reengineering: The Road Best Traveled," along with an updated section focused on life in organizations after reengineering. It provides a review of the concept and methodology of reengineering, coupled with newer information and insights into process-centered organizations.

The dogmas of the quiet past will not work in the turbulent future. As our cause is new, so must we think and act anew.

—Abraham Lincoln

"Despite a decade or more of restructuring and downsizing, many U.S. companies are still unprepared to operate in the 1990s."[1(p.104)] Businesses have failed to

---

Source: Adapted from D.L. Flarey and S. Smith Blancett. Reengineering: The Road Best Traveled in *Reengineering Nursing and Health Care: The Handbook for Organizational Transformation.* S. Smith Blancett and D.L. Flarey, eds., pp. 15–35 © 1995, Aspen Publishers, Inc; 1995.

keep pace with the rapid changes occurring in technology, customer needs, and quality service. Consequently, companies attempt to compete in today's turbulent environment while operating with archaic systems and processes. The result has been the demise of many large and small corporations. The business of health care is no exception.

Can business as we know it today survive? Is there a prescription for success? The answer is yes. The secret to revitalizing American business is reengineering. Reengineering is new. As the hottest trend in management today,[2,3] it is an intense method that focuses on the radical redesign of systems and processes to achieve quantum leaps in performance and defined outcomes. This chapter provides an in-depth discussion of the fundamentals of reengineering, as well as a methodology for operationalizing the concept. Case studies from industry are also presented.

THE REENGINEERING REVOLUTION

As with any emerging management trend, reengineering is being defined in endless ways. Despite its dilution, reengineering in the purest sense has been defined and operationalized. There is really only one concrete, far-reaching definition of reengineering. This definition was developed by the gurus of reengineering, Michael Hammer and James Champy. Thus, the substance of this book has been built on their working philosophy, definition, and concepts of reengineering.

Hammer and Champy define reengineering as "the fundamental rethinking and radical redesign of business processes to achieve dramatic improvements in critical, contemporary measures of performance, such as cost, quality, service, and speed."[4(p.32)] Reengineering is not about fixing processes; rather, it is about starting over from scratch.[4]

It is an innovative, far-reaching concept that touches every element of an organization. It is about reinvention—the recreation of processes, work, and systems. It directly impacts the very core of businesses and organizations. As such, reengineering drives major change, leading to radical transformation of the organization. When processes are reinvented, a rippling effect occurs. A few of the major organizational elements that are revitalized as a direct result of reengineering are:

1. governance and management structures
2. organizational culture and climate
3. quality initiatives
4. standards of work performance

5. compensation and benefit packages
6. labor relations
7. measurements of customer satisfaction
8. vendor relationships
9. employee recognition and reward
10. overall service delivery

The impacts on these elements are examined in detail throughout this book.

To fully understand and appreciate the concept of reengineering, it is necessary to examine its core features. "At the heart of reengineering is the notion of *discontinuous thinking*—of recognizing and breaking away from the outdated rules and fundamental assumptions that underlie operations."[1(p.107)] True reengineering means breaking with the past. It means that the old and often comfortable ways of doing things must be abandoned. It requires a radical shift in the way we think about work, our processes, our systems, and our entire business. This type of nonlinear thinking leads to change that is basic and irreversible. "The reason is that something happens in the mind; there is a new mind set, a new mental model, a new set of measures . . . the more nonlinear the change, the more irreversible it is. Top management recognizes that it is burning its bridges, and that there is no way back. But they have to understand that their bridges are probably burning anyway."[5(p.52)]

Reengineering then is a genesis in itself. It means asking this question, "If I were re-creating this company today, given what I know and given current technology, what would it look like? Reengineering a company means tossing aside old systems and starting over. It involves going back to the beginning and inventing a better way of doing work."[4(p.31)] Reengineering, then, is synonymous with reinvention. Reinvention is not about changing what exists; it is about creating what is not.[6] Reengineering is a process that gives us permission to be innovative, creative, and sometimes even a bit eccentric. It encourages us to tap our innermost skills and allows us, finally, to discard sacred cows and the traditional bureaucracies of the American corporation.

Another core feature of reengineering is its *cross-functional approach* to work.[2] Processes rarely operate independently, and systems certainly do not. The way in which businesses operate and work is accomplished is an interactive process. Processes and systems are in constant play with one another, and each significantly affects the ways in which the others operate. Reengineering, a global concept, impacts multiple business processes and, thus, multiple functional divisions. It focuses on reinventing these processes and systems in an integrated fashion, not in isolation.

Reengineering is also about *major, radical change*. It seeks quantum leaps in performance and outcomes. As a general rule, reengineering targets a 20 percent to 50 percent change in processes, with an equally planned transformation in costs, quality, timeliness, and satisfaction.[7] Thus, it is distinctly different from traditional total quality management and continuous quality improvement. In those methodologies, processes and systems are examined, and the focus is on "fixing" or making incremental improvements in them. Such initiatives are not as radical or bold as reengineering. This premise is substantiated by research data showing that traditional quality improvement programs generally result in changes of 2 percent to 5 percent.[7]

Another feature of reengineering is its *futuristic imperative*. True reengineering starts from the future and works backward.[2] It requires executives and managers to undergo an intense future-oriented analysis. It means having a vision of what could be, as well as specific goals and objectives for realizing the vision. It means rethinking what the business is[3] and what it must become for future success and viability. This concept of rethinking is vital to the success of any reengineering project. In order to "rethink" the business, reengineering focuses on defining desired outcomes and working backward to realize them.[8]

One essential feature for reengineering is that it must be a phenomenon that works from the top down to be successful.[2] Executive management must be fully committed to the concept and display a passion for transformation through reengineering. Reengineering requires the dedication of substantial amounts of fiscal and human resources, as well as time. It is not a quick-fix solution to old problems; it is about innovation and creation. Executives must understand the scope of reengineering and their need to reengineer the business. This philosophy and commitment must be sustained and communicated to everyone in the organization. Management support is critical to the overall reengineering process; it is a core feature. A reengineering initiative without ongoing, visible support from top management has no chance of success.

Exhibit 2–1 summarizes the core features and philosophies of reengineering. To reengineer successfully, it is essential that everyone involved in the project have a solid, fundamental understanding of these core elements. These elements also provide guidelines for ongoing assessment of whether or not reengineering is occurring. We recommend a frequent review of the elements throughout the reengineering process, along with an analysis of the total project. Adherence to the core features will help ensure that reengineering, not some other initiative, is being accomplished.

WHAT REENGINEERING IS NOT

Now that we have examined what reengineering is, it is necessary to reiterate what it is not. Such an examination will further clarify the core features and ele-

Exhibit 2–1 Core Features and Philosophy of Reengineering

1. *Radical change*—The focus is on radical change in processes and systems.
2. *Discontinuous thinking*—It involves a radical departure from dysfunctional ways of doing and thinking; it means breaking old assumptions and rules.
3. *Innovation*—The emphasis is on creativity and recreation, going where no one has gone before.
4. *Dramatic improvements*—The major imperative is realization of quantum leaps in defined outcomes, yielding dramatic not just incremental improvements in processes and systems.
5. *Start-from-scratch initiative*—The focus is on what can be, rather than what is.
6. *Genesis effect*—It is a birth, a new beginning, a time of creation.
7. *Cross-functional*—This is a synergistic process, crossing multiple functions and boundaries.
8. *Futuristic*—The emphasis is on future operations, not on the present or past, which demands visionary thinking and leadership.
9. *Driven from the top down*—This effort requires the absolute commitment and continuous support of top-level management to be successful.
10. *Organization focused*—All elements of the organization are readily involved and positively affected.

ments of reengineering. Careful attention must be given to what reengineering is not, because much misconception exists in the business world today. Many boast of reengineering efforts and projects, but in reality, few fulfill the definition of reengineering set forth in this chapter. Projects that are not reengineering do not reap the enormous gains and radical changes inherent in the methodology. Too often, executives and managers say they have reengineered and, when gains are small or nonexistent, develop a belief that reengineering does not work. This judgment is erroneous and often dissuades others from committing to the reengineering revolution. Reengineering is not about:

- accomplishing incremental or small-scale change
- reducing full-time equivalents (FTEs) to control costs
- switching vendors or changing products
- offering contests, slogans, or gimmicks
- providing quality improvement initiatives
- remodeling the physical plant
- restructuring the organization

- improving processes
- developing new services
- automating existing processes
- improving systems
- decreasing services
- marketing
- initiating mergers or joint ventures

Although many of these items may well be techniques or outcomes of reengineering, in and of themselves, they are not essential features. As mentioned previously, reengineering does impact the entire organization.

> Reengineering triggers changes of many kinds, not just of the business process itself. Job designs, organizational structures, management systems—anything associated with the process—must be refashioned in an integrated way. In other words, reengineering is a tremendous effort that mandates change in many areas of the organization.[1(p.112)]

The key to successful reengineering is to stay focused on the core features and elements of the process. The greatest mistake is to focus on the peripheral organizational elements. Confusion and frustration will generally result, and the overall objective of making radical changes and quantum leaps in performance will never be realized.

THE NEED TO REENGINEER

Why should organizations reengineer at all? Why invest heavily in the resources and time necessary to reengineer processes, systems, and organizations? Hammer and Champy[4] provide some insight into these questions by highlighting three major forces that have significant impact on the new business world.

The first major force is customers. Customers today are decidedly different from those of yesterday. Today's business customers have very unique needs and demand considerable individuality. They will go to great lengths to seek out companies who are very responsive to their needs and expectations. Making small improvements in service initiatives is not enough. Customers demand more. They are the central driving force today for businesses to reengineer their operations. Our environment today is consumer driven and will remain so well into the next century.

The second major force driving the imperative to reengineer is competition. Competition is widespread and constantly evolving. Today, many competitors focus on narrowly defined products and services with expert quality. Growing competition mandates that businesses reinvent themselves if they are to remain in the race.

The third force is change. While change is perceived as a constant, it is occurring in the new business world at accelerated rates. Over the past decade, people have become so accustomed to change that it is now viewed as a normal process. Becoming comfortable with change can be very damaging. Change today is occurring faster than people can comprehend it or keep pace with it. One striking example close to home is the rapid change occurring in health care. Driven by a national agenda for reform, this change is unparalleled by any other in current experience. Such change is causing health care organizations across the country to scramble for reengineering initiatives that will help ensure future viability.

When is the best time to reengineer? The answer is simple. The most appropriate time is when the organization is doing well and the required resources are readily available.[9] If reengineering is a last resort, chances are good that it will fail because reengineering is an all-or-nothing proposition.[1] It requires intense commitment and resources, as well as time. Reengineering cannot be accomplished in a day. Organizations on the brink of failure do not have the time or the capability to mobilize the required resources.

Consequently, reengineering must be planned for well in advance. It needs to be written into the organization's strategic plan[7] and planned for as a major initiative toward organizational transformation. It must become a routine management strategy. To survive into the next century, organizations must constantly reengineer their businesses. One method of incorporating reengineering into the constant, overall operations of the organization is to frequently address the following questions:

- What are our customer's needs, requirements, and expectations?
- What trends and changes are clearly affecting our business?
- What is the current environment of competition like?
- Which elements of our current processes and systems are not adding value?
- What is the future vision for this organization?
- What are the organizational goals and objectives for realizing the vision?
- How can current performance or products be reinvented or recreated?
- What radical changes can be made to ensure our future success?
- How flexible and fluid is the organization?
- How do we envision our future? Where do we want to be five years from now?
- What major paradigm shifts in the world are predicted to occur over the next decade, and how will they affect our business?

Frequently addressing these questions will most certainly lead organizations to many reengineering initiatives. These questions or imperatives focus heavily on a total re-creation of the organization. It is necessary, when reengineering, that we look at the effects of strategic processes on the organization as a whole.[9] "Many current business processes are based on decisions made by functional departments in an effort to optimize their own performance, with little attention to the impact on overall organizational effectiveness."[10(p.17)] Such thinking evolved from 200 years of industrial management.[4] Reengineering means breaking from this mind-set and moving away from the division of labor toward an integrated approach to organizational functioning.

The imperative for change throughout the organization is the key to future business success. Such change can be achieved through reengineering. Thus, the fundamental reason to reengineer is to blend the interactive components of the organization into a synergistic whole.[11] Once an integrated organizational system is created, it is structured around customers and the accomplishment of key strategic objectives rather than around functions and departments.[12] The greatest need to reengineer is to create an integrated organization that can respond quickly to customers and the constantly changing business environment. Thus, reengineering is a major change initiative. Through reengineering, a new infrastructure is created to accommodate continual change.[13]

THE NEED TO REENGINEER HEALTH CARE

There is no business today as complex as health care. The health care environment is changing at unprecedented speed. Unfortunately, health care organizations lag far behind other businesses in terms of their innovations, redesign, and ability to re-create themselves. The outcome has been the demise of many health care organizations over the past decade. If health care organizations cannot mobilize themselves for dramatic and radical change in the coming era, they will fail.

The need to reengineer in health care is paramount. To deal effectively with the coming global transformation of our health care system, all health care organizations will have to reengineer. Some major indicators for a rapid reengineering initiative are declining profits, customer dissatisfaction, and difficulty competing successfully for managed care contracts.[9] Health care organizations experiencing such difficulties have little time to begin a reengineering initiative.

In health care, the same industrial definition and concepts of reengineering apply as in other businesses. The definition of reengineering has been somewhat expanded for use in health care: "the radical redesign of the critical systems and processes used to produce, deliver, and support patient care in order to achieve dramatic improvements in organizational performance within a short period of time."[9(pp.28–30)] While the definition is really not different, it does place an emphasis on the delivery of care.

When reengineering in health care, it is important to focus on the major imperatives for successfully confronting the changing environment. "The mandates for health care providers are clear: develop organized, integrated systems of care; reduce waste and inefficiencies; focus on primary care and prevention; and improve quality and outcomes. In essence, we need to reinvent the delivery system."[12(p.42)] In reinventing the system, the major imperative for a reformed system is to build community health networks.[9] Reengineering is an excellent tool for this overwhelming challenge.

A METHODOLOGY FOR REENGINEERING

Several methodologies have been developed for reengineering.[4,7,14,15] All of them are organized, concrete, and proven to work. Their similarities are striking and their differences are few. The distinguishing feature among them is their degree of complexity. On the basis of the overwhelming imperatives to reengineer health care delivery, we have developed a methodology that is focused and can be easily applied to health care reengineering projects. The major distinguishing factor in our methodology is its concrete simplicity. This feature will allow health care organizations to reengineer with the speed necessary to survive the current health care revolution. When applied appropriately, it will provide for effective and successful reengineering of processes and organizational systems in health care. Our methodology consists of seven major steps:

1. internal and external assessment
2. visioning
3. planning
4. starting from scratch
5. testing
6. evaluating
7. revisiting

Internal and External Assessment

Before reengineering can happen, it is paramount that a comprehensive analysis of the organization's internal and external environment be undertaken. This analysis lays a solid foundation for the overall reengineering effort. Internal assessment means taking a long, hard, critical look at the organization. It means facing the realities of the evolution of the organization and its current status. It is often a painful process, but a necessary one if radical change is to occur. For successful reengineering, the assessment must be honest.

The assessment process must be a group effort of the organization's management team. Everyone must participate. It is imperative that executive management lead the assessment initiative to demonstrate the commitment that is essential to the reengineering effort. The most effective means to this goal is a management retreat, which further establishes the commitment by top-level executives and brings the management team together for a common cause and purpose. It also provides a social setting where participants can more freely interact and share their perceptions of the current internal environment.

The first task of internal assessment is to thoroughly assess the culture of the organization.[7] Some of the initial questions that must be answered in cultural assessment are:

- What is our current culture like?
- Is our culture a barrier to change?
- What are the values of the organization?
- How did our culture evolve?
- How did our organization get to where it is today?
- What are the organization's sacred cows?
- How do employees perceive the culture?
- What is the prevailing attitude of the employees toward the organization?
- How does our culture affect the way we lead?
- How does our culture affect the work life of the employees?
- How has our culture negatively affected the organization?
- Are people satisfied with the current culture?

Once the cultural assessment is complete, the team can begin a more in-depth diagnosis of the organization.

The best approach is through a diagnosis that generates a complete picture of how the organization really works. What assumptions are we making about our strategic position and customer needs that may no longer be valid? What functional units are most influential, and will they be as important in the future as they were in the past? What are the key systems that drive the business? What are the core competencies or skills of the enterprise? What are the shared values and idiosyncracies that comprise the organization's being? If explored in-depth, these types of questions generate responses that, taken together, paint a picture of how things really work.[6(p.106)]

The next step in the internal assessment of the organization is a focus on customers. Questions need to be answered:

- Who are our customers, and what are their needs?
- What do customers expect from us?[2]

- What is the status of customer satisfaction?
- How has the organization traditionally related to our customers?
- What are their perceptions of the organization?

Then the assessment must honestly identify what is dysfunctional in the organization. Questions that need answering include:

- What are the major dysfunctions in the organization?
- How has the dysfunction affected the organization's processes?
- In what way is the dysfunction slowing down the organization in achievement of its goals and objectives?

To complete the internal assessment, the following questions must also be answered by the management team:

- What is the current quality of our service?
- What is the overall leadership style?
- What are the strengths and weaknesses of our systems and processes?
- To what degree is the organization integrated?
- What is the degree of the division of labor?
- What is the financial status of the organization?
- What is our relationship with our medical staff?
- How do employees relate to one another?
- How is performance recognized and rewarded?
- How is performance measured?
- How is information communicated in the organization?
- What is the degree of employee satisfaction with the organization?
- What is the speed of our service delivery?
- What are our costs?
- What inefficiencies exist in the organization?
- What prevents the organization from moving forward?

Once all of the components of the internal assessment have been completed, a clear and compelling picture of the organization will emerge.

A comprehensive assessment of the external environment must also be completed. This evaluation is essential so that the management team can fully understand the nature of the health care business and the need to act quickly to confront the realities of our changing health care system. An external assessment must include answering the following compelling questions:

- What are the major changes occurring in our health care system?
- What is driving these changes?

- What is the role of government in health care reform?
- What is the federal reform agenda?
- What type of reform is occurring in our state government?
- Who are our competitors?
- What threats do our competitors pose to the organization?
- What do consumers want today in a health care system?
- What are our community's needs for health care services?
- Are these services meeting the community needs?
- In what ways are our competitors superior to us?
- What are our relationships with our vendors?
- How do our costs compare with those of other health care organizations?
- What is the image of the organization in the community?
- How does our medical staff perceive the organization?
- What is our relationship with payers?
- What external community services does our system offer?
- What is our length of stay or service like?
- How does our length of stay compare with other health care organizations?
- What are the outcomes of our recruitment efforts?
- What is the extent of our public relations efforts?
- Who supports our organization?
- What major external factors threaten the viability of the organization?

Completing the external environment assessment clarifies the need for the organization to undergo a total transformation through reengineering. It provides perspective on the opportunities, strengths, and weaknesses of the organization and the threats to its success, and it stimulates thought on how the organization must position itself for viability and future success.

Visioning

The internal and external assessments prepare the management team for the next major step in the reengineering process—visioning. The most important, difficult, and challenging aspect of this step is to be truly visionary, which requires the management team to tap their creative powers. Most health care organizations do not have a clear vision of what they want their new organization to look like after reengineering.

While visioning seems complex, it really is a simple concept. It involves imagination and creativity. Because this step is so essential to the reengineering process, a visioning retreat should be established for the purpose of bringing the management team together, with the overall objective of creating the new organization.

The first step in the visioning process is to accept the realities of the internal and external assessments. The team needs to thoroughly discuss its dissatisfaction with what currently exists and make a commitment to change the organization. The assessment phase clearly paves the way for visioning. It reminds the team of past mistakes and drives its thinking beyond the status quo.

The visioning session begins with the following question: If there were absolutely no obstacles or restraints, what would our organization look like? From here, the brainstorming begins. It is essential that the chief executive lead the visioning session to further support the concept that top management is fully committed to the reengineering initiative. It also places the chief executive in a new light, in the role of transformational leader.

Following the visioning session, the brainstorming material must be concisely developed into a vision statement for the new organization. It should read smoothly and should clearly identify the structure and characteristics of the new organization. Exhibit 2–2 presents a vision statement that was developed by a health care organization's management team under the leadership of one of the authors. This vision statement was developed in an overall process for organizational transformation through reengineering. The vision then is a clear picture of the future organization.

There are certain organizational imperatives for creation of the vision. The vision must be created by the entire management team, not just a choice few. This strategy will foster a real ownership by the team for the vision. The vision must be realistic, tangible, and not so far-fetched that it cannot come to fruition. Most important, the vision must be constantly and clearly communicated to everyone in the organization and to key players outside the organization, such as the community, vendors, and payers. The vision statement should be posted in easily accessible places throughout the organization.

The vision is the foundation for the transformation of the organization. It will never be realized, however, unless the employees believe in its promise. This can only happen when management is a role model and advocate for the vision. Communicating the vision is not enough; the management team must make it a visible, viable part of daily operations.

When the vision is created, important questions should be discussed.

Have you thought about your business thoroughly enough that, despite its complexities, you can explain how it hangs together and moves ahead in dynamic interaction with its environment? And there's another question, even more veiled in thinking about vision: Are you smart enough and wise enough to make sense out of this business and its marketplace?[16(p.62)]

Exhibit 2–2 Vision Statement for an Acute Care Osteopathic Hospital

The Medical Center will be a model organization known for providing holistic health care founded within the principles, teachings, and philosophy of osteopathic medicine. Our patients will receive the highest quality health care provided by a staff of physicians, administrators, professional nurses, and clinicians and by support staff committed to excellence in service delivery and continuous improvement. To establish a model organization, the members of the Medical Center Board, its physicians, administration, and staff associates will work together, unified under these guiding principles:

- *Respect for the individual*—Each staff associate, manager, and physician is regarded as the most valued resource of the Medical Center; individuals in the organization and each customer will be treated with respect and dignity.
- *Teamwork*—The organization will work synergistically as a place without walls or barriers to progress and change. All members of the organization will respect and value one another's ideas. Management and staff associates will work in partnership to drive the organization forward, unified, to face the challenges of today and the future.
- *Learning*—The organization will value learning and education to the highest degree, continue to support the programs established in osteopathic medicine, and establish and maintain programs that further the education and skill development of managers and staff associates.
- *Trust*—The foundation for every relationship between members of the organization is trust; in order to foster trust among staff, communication will be open and forthcoming.
- *Partnership and collaboration*—The organization will focus attention on working with the leadership of the surrounding communities to provide quality health care services for all those it serves and will seek out ventures with other health care providers that will extend opportunities for the organization to grow and expand the delivery of the specialized services of osteopathic medicine.
- *Continuous improvement*—The organization will support and foster change as a means to continue to improve the work environment and all aspects of its operations in the delivery of health care services.
- *Fiscal responsibility*—The organization will operate in a manner that maintains quality in service delivery while providing these services at a reasonable cost. All members of the organization will control the costs of operations and avoid misuse and waste. As a result of maintaining a sound fiscal base, the organization will secure the viability to continue to provide health care services to this community well into the future.

Without a strong, clear vision, the organization will remain stagnant, and transformation will not occur. Without vision, there is no future for the organization. The major advantages to visioning are:

- It clearly describes what the organization will become.
- It provides a road map for reengineering.
- It provides a compass for the organization in its transformation.
- It provides consensus in the organization.
- It defines what systems and processes need to be reengineered.

Planning

The next phase of the total reengineering initiative is planning. In this phase, the management team comes together and develops concrete, strategic plans for making the vision a reality. This phase, which focuses on what needs to be done to realize the vision, is difficult and challenging.

Planning must focus on four major imperatives for transformation and realization of the vision statement:

1. Increase the quality of all services delivered.
2. Dramatically improve the work environment for employees.
3. Increase customer satisfaction.
4. Develop efficient and effective processes that contribute to care delivery in a cost-effective way.

The planning session must be intense and must tap the skills and abilities of the management team, and the session must be led by top management. A new way of thinking must prevail. "When a company reinvents itself, it must alter the underlying assumptions and premises on which its decisions and actions are based."[6(p.98)] This is the time to face and relinquish the fear of change, to welcome change as a wonderful opportunity to become better. This is also a time for further identification of sacred cows. They must go; everything must seem possible.

The planning session begins by brainstorming what processes and systems need reengineering to transform the organization and realize the vision. As the session continues, the management team identifies what must be accomplished. These imperatives are then translated into major reengineering projects. From here, multifunctional teams are formed to tackle each reengineering project. A team leader is elected, and team members volunteer to participate.

Then, the teams need to meet in small planning groups and begin writing the project plan. The goals and objectives of the project must be established. This team session includes planning for recruitment of staff members to join the teams. The team should identify any constraints that will exist and develop a plan to overcome them. An initial budget should be developed on the basis of resources required for the project. A timetable for the project should also be developed at this time. A project can take from a few months to four years, with the typical project taking 9 to 12 months.[9]

A facilitator should be chosen for each team. In addition, executive management must commit to sponsoring a team-building seminar for the project team members. The rewards of such an effort will surely outweigh the costs.

Project teams are resource intensive. They must meet frequently, and executive management must commit to providing them with the human and fiscal resources necessary for reengineering. All teams should meet together once a month to share their progress.

Starting from Scratch

The very core of reengineering is found in the phase of starting from scratch. The previous phases lay the foundation for this critical point in the process. In this phase, actual reengineering of processes occurs. This phase is the most time intensive of all the steps in the reengineering initiative, the most challenging, and the most enjoyable. Hammer and Champy[4] advocate one tool for process reengineering: a blank sheet of paper.

Once processes have been identified for change, the reengineering team must re-create the process, not simply attempt to improve it. If improvement is what you want, then improvement is what you will get. However, if dramatic change with outcomes of speed, quality, efficiency, and effectiveness is the desired outcome, then the process must be reengineered.

Reengineered processes need to look very different from traditional ones[4] because reengineering is about radical change and dramatic improvements, innovation,[3] and re-creation. To reengineer, the teams go to the drawing board, start with a blank sheet, and totally re-create the process.

To assist in process reengineering, the following guidelines should be adhered to:

- Delete everything that does not add value; this is the essence of reengineering.[3]
- Let no organizational facet be immune to change or elimination.
- Be innovative—break all assumptions.[3]

- Focus on the breadth of the process.[14]
- Innovate mental work, and do not replicate physical work.[17]
- Focus on total customer satisfaction.[11]
- Coordinate the management of change into the new process.[18]
- Focus on the objectives of process reengineering.[19]
- Re-create processes so that workers make the decisions.[4]
- Remodel the work flow to streamline the business operations.[15]
- Incorporate automation, which is a key enabler in process reengineering.
- Design work into process teams.[4]
- Focus on keeping the process simple.
- Cut out all redundancy in the new process.
- Implement quality initiatives in the new process.[20]
- Set up the process for ongoing, continual improvements.[20]
- Define desired outcomes of the new process.
- Draw a flowchart for the new process.
- Redesign the work of the new process.
- Constantly add value to the process.
- Destroy the division of labor in the process.
- Redesign many jobs into one.[4]
- Challenge the process as it is being created, and constantly rethink it.

Learning to reengineer processes comes by doing. There is no secret formula or magical trick to it. The guidelines above will be helpful in the re-creation of processes. Another major imperative to focus on while reengineering processes is the development of goals. Exhibit 2–3 presents the 12 major goals of the reengineering of health care systems. These goals should be used as an additional support to process reengineering and the overall organizational transformation initiative. These defined goals provide further structure for the reengineering of processes and of the organization.

Testing

Once teams have completed the creation of new processes, the testing phase can begin. In this phase, a performance model of the newly reengineered process is developed.[7] The model is presented to the staff most involved. Education, training, and motivation for the new process are led by the project team. All staff education should include problem cause-and-effect analysis, rudimentary statistical process control, and group problem-solving techniques.[21] Further plans are developed for the implementation of the new process; these include automation and physical redesign of facilities, as appropriate.

Exhibit 2–3 Goals for Reengineering

1. *Synergy*—a focus on integration of systems and processes so that the whole will be greater than the sum of its parts, with all systems and processes working together in harmony
2. *Organizational transformation*—realization of a radically changed and transformed organization through reengineering, with the organizational imperatives for transformation driving the reengineering effort
3. *Change*—prevalence of change throughout the project, with change expected, planned, and managed
4. *Success*—organizational success now and in the future
5. *Reconfiguration*—the ability of the organization to successfully downsize without compromising quality, to become "lean and mean"
6. *Partnerships*—development and thriving of partnerships with customers, vendors, and payers
7. *Efficiency*—emphasis on timely delivery of services
8. *Effectiveness*—care delivery resulting in excellent clinical outcomes, with a primary objective of quality patient care
9. *Role redesign*—redesign of the role of management to that of transformational leader
10. *Competitiveness*—emphasis on being highly competitive in the marketplace, especially in managed care
11. *Systems thinking*—functioning of the organization as an open, interactive system rather than in specialized isolated divisions
12. *Knowledge*—a focus on cultivation of knowledge, producing an organization where constant learning is promoted and valued

Time frames for testing the process innovation must also be established. They should be realistic and not rushed. Staff must be afforded ample opportunity to buy into the new process and make it work. One of the major reasons for failure of reengineering projects is that the organization was not ready to make a commitment to the time and energy required to test the new process.[7]

Reengineering is an organized response to change,[18] so some resistance is to be expected. Resistance can be minimized by ongoing communication, staff involvement in team ad hoc committees, and education about change and how to deal with it. The testing process requires much time. Employees must become desensitized to the magnitude of change, not necessarily to the new process. The management and reengineering team can assist in this change process by demonstrating their commitment to the new process and/or system and by demonstrating that it is highly valued by the organization. The prevailing attitude must be that constant stimulation through new goals and process configurations fuels the fires of creativity and productivity.

Evaluation

The implementation evaluation is the next phase of the project. In this phase, the reengineering team and the employees systematically evaluate the new processes over a defined time frame. To assist in the evaluation process, it is necessary to define outcomes for the project. Exhibit 2–4 presents broad-based outcomes that can be established for any reengineering project in health care. These outcomes should then be concisely analyzed against the realized outcomes of the project. Specific outcomes for each newly developed process must also be established.

Exhibit 2–4 Outcomes for Reengineering

1. *Transformation*—evidence of radical change in processes, systems, and within the organization, with changes positive, transformational, and measurable
2. *Simplicity*—simplified processes and systems, with complexities of former processes nonexistent
3. *Cost reductions*—demonstrable reductions in overall and specific costs, as a result of process innovation
4. *Cultural transformation*—re-creation of the culture of the organization, with change no longer feared or a barrier to innovation
5. *Quality*—enhancement of the quality of all services delivered by the organization, with measurable improvements in quality
6. *Expediency*—improved time of response to the customer as a predominant element of the organization, with services delivered in a realistic and timely fashion
7. *Satisfaction*—increase in overall satisfaction of all identified customers of the organization, with improvement in satisfaction over time
8. *Increased market share*—establishment of a competitive organization, with increased market share in the community and improved ability to acquire managed care network contracts
9. *Focus on customer*—complete dedication of the organization to providing service to customers
10. *Viability*—establishment of the organization as strong, financially sound, and well on its way to future success

Evaluation must be carefully planned and ongoing. Critical indicators must be developed and measured frequently. The evaluation phase is enjoyable, as the organization begins to realize the fruits of its labor. The reengineering project must also be evaluated against the vision statement. Is the vision becoming a reality? If reengineering was done correctly and with commitment and support of the management team, it will be easy to see the vision unfold.

Revisiting

The last phase of the initiative is to periodically revisit the reengineering process. As change continues in the health care environment, the methodology for reengineering must constantly be revisited. As change occurs, environments are affected, and the need for more internal change becomes manifest. Our health care system will never be static; it will constantly evolve. As it evolves, the organization must be positioned for more change. The reengineering process is the strategy that can be used to drive needed change in the future.

CASE STUDIES

To fully appreciate the scope and depth of reengineering, it is helpful to examine case studies. Reengineering is new, so few case studies have been published. Most of these cases have been from industry rather than from health care, because reengineering has its birth in general industry. The following is a very brief synopsis of noteworthy cases from industries that have successfully reengineered.

An excellent case study of effective reengineering in the IBM Credit Corporation was presented by Hammer and Champy.[4] Prior to reengineering of the processes for this organization, the process for client application for credit to final approval was composed of five major steps, with many different employees involved. It generally took from six days to two weeks to approve an application. The duration of this process was unacceptable to customers and gave them ample time to obtain financing elsewhere. When the corporation examined the process, it found that the actual application approval process took only 90 minutes.

Management soon realized that the problem was not the required tasks or the people doing the work; instead, it was the process that was inefficient and causing them to lose market share. The management team set out to reinvent the process. In its re-creation, or reengineering, the corporation replaced specialists with generalists. Instead of the application being sent to five or six specialists for piecemeal task completion, one generalist now processes the entire application.

The outcomes were very impressive. Evaluation of the reengineered process showed that application process time was reduced to four hours, the number of positions was reduced, and the number of processed applications increased over 100-fold. This is an excellent example of process innovation with far-reaching outcomes. The core elements of this reengineering process were speed, simplicity, cost reductions, and customer satisfaction.

Hammer and Champy[4] provide us with another example of successful reengineering—Ford Motor Company. Ford's accounts payable department employed 500 people prior to reengineering. To reduce costs and downsize the operation, Ford initiated a reengineering project. The procurement process, which included accounts payable, purchasing, and receiving, was eventually targeted for reengineering. The old process was extremely complex, was redundant with unnecessary checks and balances, and involved a slow, time-consuming system overloaded with forms and papers and many people processing receivables in a piecemeal fashion.

Ford reengineered the procurement process, and the change and outcomes were radical. The new process is simple. The authorization for payment of receivables is accomplished at the receiving dock through automation when products are received. Ford broke all of its traditional rules and assumptions. The outcome of the re-created process is speed and dramatic cost savings. Ford now has only 125 people in its vendor payment process.

Another excellent example from industry is that of GTE.[2] When it reengineered, GTE looked at its telephone operations business. These particular operations accounted for the majority of the company's annual revenues. An organizational analysis indicated that GTE needed to enhance its customer service. Reengineering took place on the basis of the new assumption that customers want one-stop shopping—"one number to fix an erratic dial tone, question a bill, sign up for call waiting, or all three, at any time of the day."[2(pp.41–42)]

In its reengineering initiative, the company created a customer care center and piloted it. The project encompassed a massive physical redesign and automation of processes to link up the various services. New software was developed to allow operators free access to databases so they can handle all of the customer requests. In the reengineering process, GTE eliminated enormous amounts of work, and the pilot studies showed a 30 percent increase in productivity.

The reengineering in health care is just beginning. In Part II of this book, many dynamic case studies from pioneering health care organizations and businesses that have successfully reengineered are presented. As reengineering becomes more common and studies of reengineering are published and reviewed, it will become apparent that reengineering is not just a new fad, but rather, a solid methodology for driving radical, needed change in health care delivery.

LIFE AFTER REENGINEERING

Life after reengineering is interesting. Many believed that such an environment could exist only as an idealistic thought. However, transformed health care organizations are reaping the rewards of years of reengineering and further transforming themselves into process-centered organizations. The post-reengineering phenomenon is growing fast and will continue to expand well into the next century.

Michael Hammer,[22] in his recently published book, *Beyond Reengineering*, explains in great detail the next paradigm for organizations that have successfully reengineered. He calls such organizations Process-Centered Organizations and explains that any and all organizations that hope to survive and thrive in the next century must become process centered.

Hammer describes the theory of this new type of organization in this way: "process centering, more than anything else, means that people—all people—in the company recognize and focus on their processes."[22(p.9)] A simple-enough description, but in reality, it is a monumental task. What Hammer describes is a new post-reengineering organization that is defined by its processes. No longer does the organization operate within bureaucratic structures amidst poor integration and fragmented approaches to operations; rather, such organizations define themselves by their processes.

The era of reengineering began the movement to process-centered approaches for organizational transformations. Organizations learned that all the work of the organization can be appropriately classed within a major process. As health care was reengineered, the magnitude and importance of identifying the core processes became more clear. Just what types of processes were identified in health care? Some of the major ones common to most health care organizations today are

- the process of care delivery
- medication administration
- admission of a client to the care setting
- discharge of the client to other levels of care
- patient care documentation
- patient teaching/education
- the nursing process
- documentation of patient outcomes
- billing for health care services
- compliance with regulations and laws
- order entry for diagnostics
- patient transportation
- wellness/prevention education and practices

- credentialing of health care providers
- management of variances to pathways

These can all be considered core processes. If we look back in time, we see that this list comprises most of the major process transformations that have been undertaken in health care during the reengineering era. Organizations have made dramatic transformations in the overall care delivery process through innovations and reengineering of older processes. Outcomes of this era include:

- newer patient-focused delivery systems that are more fully integrated and less fragmented
- newer multidisciplinary path–based care processes that focus on the whole patient and care management of populations
- a paradigm shift away from models of disease to models of wellness and prevention
- the introduction of new, more innovative technologies and automations to expedite and create more user-friendly processes for clients such as speedier admissions and discharges
- new methods of patient care documentation that are more focused and streamlined, providing greater levels of communication about clients
- models of care that intimately involve partnerships between providers and clients and their families
- a shift to a focus on outcomes at all levels of care delivery and organizational operations
- more effective billing methods that are automated, expeditious, and user friendly for staff and clients
- more sophisticated processes for care provider credentialing, ensuring more secure and better investigative methods for properly assessing competency

One only has to stop and think about the last decade of health care transformation to readily see the great strides made through reengineering. In this new era of process centering that has arisen from reengineering, we are just beginning to realize the potential for further transformations and stellar outcomes in the near future.

THE PROCESS-CENTERED ORGANIZATION

Yes, life is good after reengineering. In this new life, all members of the organization can see the benefits of process reengineering and begin to think and act in terms of strengthening and further reengineering core processes. As we learned in the early days of reengineering, becoming a process-centered organization is a journey and not a destination. Organizations must, on a regular basis, continue to reevaluate their processes and pursue continued total quality improvement and reengineering. This is mandatory as the health care environment continues to change at a rapid speed; it is the only way we can meet the demands of new and evolving systems.

While many organizations have successfully reengineered, many have failed. This is also true in health care. Many health care organizations have become truly process centered, many are on their way to becoming so, and many have had no success in reengineering. Unfortunately, a number of health care organizations have failed to apply the principles and methods of reengineering, and so today they lag significantly behind in their ability to transform themselves. Such outcomes may be due to a lack of understanding of what reengineering is, a lack of motivation to learn how to reengineer, organizational paralysis due to fear of change, or an unwillingness to provide the support and resources needed to successfully reengineer.

The lack or absence of reengineering efforts in health care organizations is creating many hardships across the country. In some sense, it may be too late for many. On the other hand, those organizations that have been committed to reengineering are moving fast and keeping up with the demands of the ever-changing health care environment. They accepted the challenges of the past decade and are now reaping the rewards of their efforts.

What does a process-centered organization look like today? The answer is relatively simple if the organization has assimilated the principles of reengineering appropriately. It is an organization in which processes reign. Everything the organization does and its methods of operation center around core processes. Leaders today manage processes, not departments. Work is seen as a process rather than as a task-oriented, piecemeal endeavor. Everyone is involved in processes, and the work is performed in an organized and cohesive fashion. All staff understand the processes and their role in them. There is a great deal of multidisciplinary integration—many different people coming together as a team to practice and participate in a process rather than perform a department's work. Barriers have been removed. For health care organizations, boundaries, kingdoms, and segments of care no longer exist. All involved in the process are focused on the process. Their participation is one in which they see themselves as partnered with many different people and specialties. They do not practice solo anymore. They practice in a more fully integrated environment. No longer is care highly fragmented. Rather, care is coordinated in a multidisciplinary environment.

The concept of the process-centered organization can be illustrated by an examination of how a core process might look today. For example, in the core process of admission of a patient to a care setting, one process-centered scenario might be as follows:

- In the new organization, there is no admitting department. Clients enter the system via the emergency department or via automated links from community care offices and clinics with the care organization's automated systems.
- Upon arrival, a registered nurse (RN) and an admissions specialist work with the client together. The RN begins establishing rapport with the client and assessing the client. The admissions specialist speaks with the client, verifies admissions data needed, reviews general consent, and reviews payer information with the client. Clients are physically in their room on the patient care unit. The admissions specialist enters admissions data on the client using a bedside terminal. The admissions specialist has also been effectively cross-trained as a benefits specialist and works with the client regarding benefits and payer contract issues. The admissions specialist sees the whole process of admission as one of assessment, data collection and entry, and investigation and teaching regarding benefits.

In this scenario, the process of admission is a shared process. It is not done in piecemeal ways. It is integrated with the involvement of the RN, the client, the family, and the admissions/benefits specialist. The process has been designed around the client's needs. It is more focused, more expeditious, and more comfortable for the client; it allows family involvement and more privacy; and it serves also as an assessment phase and benefits examination phase. This core process has been reengineered to meet the client's needs, as well as the needs of the staff and the organization for a more efficient and effective process. The admissions process has been dramatically transformed. It looks very different from the pre-reengineering days. Admission of a client is now seen as a core process.

A process-centered organization takes great strides to identify all of its processes. Once they are identified, it makes a commitment to transforming the processes on a regular basis. It also commits to providing the appropriate support and resources needed to realize quantum leaps in process reengineering and design. It provides the necessary leadership to move processes forward and keep its employees focused on processes rather than departments. It supports an integrated, multidisciplinary approach to its operations and identifies its operations by way of processes. Once this has been accomplished, the organization continues to change, transform, and reengineer the core processes to meet changes in the external and internal environments. Such reengineering of core processes becomes cyclic. Again, it is a journey, not a destination.

CONCLUSION

Process-centered approaches and process-centered organizations allow more far-reaching innovations and transformations. The concept allows organizations to move ahead in the quest to make their mission and philosophy for patient care come alive. The authors believe that the successful health care organization of tomorrow will be the process-centered one. They see this transition to a process-centered philosophy and operation as essential to health care organizations' future survival. Health care organizations and health care delivery are complex. They also exist within a highly complex and changing environment. The authors echo Michael Hammer's belief that to thrive in the 21st century, health care organizations must become process centered.

The following chapters serve as a road map for organizations and readers who are embarking on the journey to become process centered. Part I of this book provides in-depth theories and concepts related to becoming process centered. Part II lets readers experience varying degrees of process centering from organizations that have been successful in their quest to become process centered. The goal is to provide you with information and insights on how this journey might unfold for you.

REFERENCES

1. Hammer M. Reengineering work: Don't automate, obliterate. *Harvard Business Rev.* 1990; 68(4):104–112.
2. Stewart TA. Reengineering: The hot new management tool. *Fortune.* 1993; 128(4):41–48.
3. Coan T. Start-from-scratch thinking: The prerequisite for reengineering. Presented at the annual conference of the American Organization of Nurse Executives; April 11, 1994.
4. Hammer M, Champy J. *Reengineering the Corporation: A Manifesto for Business Revolution.* New York: Harper Business; 1993.
5. Sheridan JH. The huntmaster's solution. *Industry Week.* 1994; 243(5):49, 50, 52.
6. Goss T, Pascale R, Athos A. The reinvention roller coaster: Risking the present for a powerful future. *Harvard Business Rev.* 1993; 71(November/December):97–108.
7. Wachel W. Reengineering: Beyond incremental change. *Healthcare Executive.* 1994; 9(July/August):18–21.
8. Easton R. Reengineering health information management: The first steps. *J AHIMA.* 1992; 63(6):50–57.
9. Bergman R. Reengineering health care. *Hosp Health Networks.* 1994; 68(3):28–36.
10. Tonges M, Lawrenz E. Reengineering: The work redesign-technology link. *J Nurs Adm.* 1993; 23(10):15–22.
11. Lowenthal J. Reengineering the organization: A step-by-step approach to corporate revitalization. Part I. *Qual Prog.* 1994; 27(1):93–95.

12. McManis GL. Reinventing the system. *Hosp Health Networks.* 1993; 62(19):42–46.

13. Morris D, Brandon J. Reengineering the hospital: Making change work for you. *Comput Healthcare.* 1991; 12(11):59–64.

14. Hall G, Rosenthal J, Wade J. How to make reengineering really work. *Harvard Business Rev.* 1993; 71(6):119–131.

15. Morris D. You may be a target for business reengineering. *Comput Healthcare.* 1991; 12(3): 31–32.

16. Beckham JD. The vision thing. *Healthcare Forum.* 1994; 37:60–68.

17. Duck JD. Managing change: The art of balancing. *Harvard Business Rev.* 1993; 71(6): 109–118.

18. Morris D, Brandon J. Reengineering: More than meets the eye. *Comput Healthcare.* 1992; 13(11):52–54.

19. Helppie RD. A time for reengineering. *Comput Healthcare.* 1992; 13(1):22–24.

20. Greising D. Quality: How to make it pay. *Businessweek.* 1994; 3384:54–59.

21. Bernd DL, Reed MM. Reengineering women's health services. *Healthcare Forum.* 1994; 1: 63–67.

22. Hammer M. *Beyond Reengineering: How the Process-Centered Organization Is Changing Our Work and Our Lives.* New York: Harper Business; 1996.

CHAPTER 3

From Structure to Culture: A Journey of Transformation

Margrét Comack, MEd, BN
Gail Paech, MScN, BScN
Tim Porter-O'Grady, PhD, EdD, FAAN

Toronto East General Hospital (TEGH) is a 400-bed community teaching hospital located in south central Ontario, Canada. Prior to reorganization, the hospital featured a traditional hierarchical organizational structure, with functions organized around departments and services. While significant downsizing had occurred in previous years, the roles and work processes had not changed significantly, except for the fact that individual responsibility had expanded and processes had become more complex. System redesign was initiated in the fall of 1995. The intent of the redesign process was to improve business effectiveness and to reorganize processes and roles around population-based services. A major change in structure and leadership roles does not necessarily lead to change in individual behaviors at the point of service. The development of a culture that would support the strategic goals of patient-focused care, point-of-service decision making and partnership soon became a priority. This chapter describes the journey of cultural transformation that began with the implementation of a revised organizational structure in September 1996.

The design and implementation of the new organizational structure (Figure 3–1) was a nine-month process that involved hundreds of staff and physicians. Once the structure and roles were defined, it became clear that the real work of change was at the point of service. A significant amount of effort was then focused on the design and development of process improvements that would enhance professional practice and quality of care, improve work processes, and strengthen relationships.

Acknowledgments: The authors wish to acknowledge the commitment and support that the staff and physicians at Toronto East General Hospital demonstrated during the change processes described in this chapter. The journey toward a healthy work culture and a patient-focused system continues because of their dedication to searching for more effective ways to practice and work together.

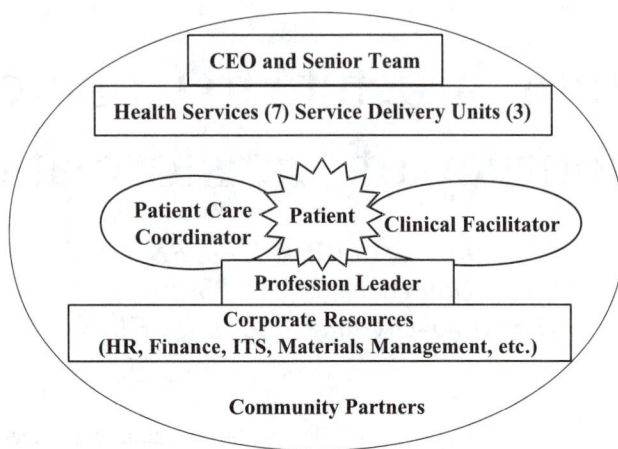

Figure 3–1 Organizational Structure: Toronto East General Hospital

BACKGROUND

The organizational redesign was based on the principles of product-line management. A unique feature of this particular design strategy is the intention to focus on specific services and markets[1] and the designation of a product champion who has responsibility to promote the product inside and outside the organization.[2] The hospital was reconfigured into seven population-based health services and three service delivery units, which provided support such as laboratory and diagnostic imaging, as well as pre-, peri-, and postoperative and emergency services to all patient populations.

Leadership roles for each of these services were developed using a framework that articulated the desirable qualities for leadership in the new system. Traditional qualities of effective managers have been described along the lines of directing, controlling, and coordinating. In shifting to a new culture, the requisite qualities for leaders were defined as

- energetic
- results oriented
- innovative and problem solving
- pattern recognition and systems development abilities
- ability to manage complex adaptive systems

- interpersonal conflict resolution skills
- negotiation skills
- scenario-planning skills

Individuals were invited to participate in a series of workshop sessions in which they were observed and assessed against the desired qualities and asked to complete a series of psychometric assessments that measured personal attributes and talents. The 10 leaders for the services were selected based on the results of this assessment process.

New Roles

Roles for each service were developed to support both staff development and patient care (Exhibit 3–1). The clinical facilitator role provides learning support and resource to the interdisciplinary staff within each service. The patient care coordinator provides clinical coordination at the patient care level on a day-to-day basis. An expectation for all staff to be more self-directed and autonomous was an underlying principle of the redesign process.

Since each of the professional departments and the associated roles of director and supervisor were deleted, a process to define the accountability for professional practice was initiated. This helped to clarify the essential elements of professional practice with respect to those issues that were independent and those that were interdependent, thereby requiring collaboration with the service leader.[3]

Exhibit 3–1 Roles and Responsibilities

Roles	*Old Paradigm*	*New Paradigm*
Patient Care Coordinator	Control of clinical area	Day-to-day coordination of care
Clinical Facilitator	Educator, teacher	Resource for self-directed learning
Profession Leader	Director, manager	Professional leadership located with staff
Health Service Leader	Manager, controller of tasks	Coordinator of decision making at point of service
Vice President	Authoritarian, boss	Coach, mentor

A role of profession leader was defined, and each professional group selected an individual to assume this role as a portion of his or her full-time equivalent. This meant that leadership for each profession was located within the staff.

At the senior management level, the vice president role was reframed to incorporate more of a coaching function as opposed to the traditional hierarchical "power over" relationship. At the core of these changes was a belief that individuals should be accountable for outcomes within the scope of their role and that relationships between all staff ought to support the strategic directives of the hospital, the health service, and patients and families.

A process was initiated for physicians to develop a plan for determining how they would integrate with the new organizational structure. This resulted in the development of a role for a medical director for each service. It was also helpful in clarifying physician accountability with respect to quality of care and administration. The tension related to perceived power shifts as a result of the reorganization subsequently emerged as a serious issue of control between the physician group and the hospital's senior administration and board of governors. Health care managers and physicians have been in a century-long conflict over the perceived takeover of medical practice.[4] The issue in creating integrated health systems is not a balance of power but rather the emergence of collegiality as a fundamental organizing principle. A process to develop satisfactory relationships (Exhibit 3–2) to integrate the physicians' role in the management structure of the hospital has been initiated; however, more work is required to achieve a solution to this challenge.

Implementation Issues

The implementation planning phase for the new organizational structure was accomplished over a two-month period. Traditional roles of manager, supervisor, and director within the professional departments and patient care areas were de-

---

Exhibit 3–2 Relationship with Physicians

Traditional	*Desired*
• Authority based	• Partnership
• Balance of power	• Collegiality
• Linear	• Pluralistic
• Tolerance	• Shared values
• Individual entrepreneurship	• Integration, trust, and sharing

leted, and staff were relocated into new reporting relationships within the health services. Clinical areas were reconfigured to locate the patient populations consistent with the new design, and modifications were made to geographic areas to support care requirements. Within three months of the announcement of the new structure and new leaders, the entire system had been reshaped. Chaos and uncertainty for staff, as well as for those individuals who assumed new roles and responsibilities, were a strong theme. In addition, many people who were unsuccessful in attaining new roles left the organization prior to the implementation date. A feeling of loss as well as significant change in work relationships was evident.

"In a world of emergence, new systems appear out of nowhere. The forms they assume originate from the dynamic processes set in motion by information, relationships and identity."[5(p.87)]

Leaders must think of tasks as a field of work that needs to be accomplished rather than as being structured by roles.[6] When supervising moment to moment ceases, creativity and energy flow from employees who are able to connect their sense of self with what the organization is doing. People need to understand the organization's purpose so that they can use their own creativity to accomplish that purpose. The leaders need to create the time and space for order to emerge and to help people focus on results.

Creating a system in which people are able to function in more effective ways and in which patients and their families experience a more meaningful quality experience meant that the work of change shifted to the point of service. Changing the structure was the first phase; the most significant phase has been creating the environment in which staff could achieve the primary goals of patient-focused care, point-of-service decision making, and partnership (Exhibit 3–3).

Exhibit 3–3 Transforming the Culture

Old Paradigm	*New Paradigm*
• Hierarchy	• Partnership
• Provider focus	• Patient focus
• Medical "fix it" model	• Health/wholeness
• Episodic care	• Continuum of care
• Institutional service (routines and rituals)	• Professional service (mutual goal setting)

Shared Governance

The concept of shared governance was adopted as a strategy to assist the services to develop as effective product lines by enabling the partnerships to focus on patients in a more meaningful way and by locating accountability and decision making closer to the point of care. Shared governance is an organizational concept that provides a framework for horizontal integration of the system[7] and for locating accountability at the place where decisions are most appropriately made.[8] People need to focus on and be accountable for outcomes. The concept of shared governance is a major influence in empowering people to recognize the power inherent in a role and in ensuring that defined outcomes are achieved. In addition, this framework assists the system to structure around the patient and not the provider.

Shared governance is supported by the following four principles,[8] which became useful in effecting the changes in the system:

1. *Accountability.* Each individual in a given role has a stake in defined outcomes.
2. *Equity.* Each individual's role is understood and is based on relationships, not status.
3. *Ownership.* All individuals are invested in the defined intent of the system.
4. *Partnership.* Relationships create the horizontal linkages that make the system effective.

With the intensity of such major system transformation, the four guiding principles of accountability, equity, ownership, and partnership assisted people to carve out new futures and to live the change as it was happening.

SYSTEM TRANSFORMATION

"Organizations could accomplish so much more if they relied on the passion evoked when we connect to others, purpose to purpose."[5(p.63)]

The three major goals of system redesign—point-of-service decision making, patient-focused care, and partnership—provided a global focus for all of the initiatives, which unfolded in unique ways within each of the health services, service delivery units, and some of the corporate support areas such as pharmacy and environmental services. While generic expectations for outcomes related to these goals were defined, each of the services was encouraged to customize the design and implementation of strategies according to its unique issues. While not mutually exclusive, the goals provide a framework for organizing the many activities that evolved as the change process moved throughout the organization.

Point-of-Service Decision Making

The goal of point-of-service decision making is to create the roles and relationships that sustain ownership and accountability.[8] Realizing that the majority of decisions in the organization relate to direct care or the coordination of care and that "decisions always belong at the place closest to where they are implemented,"[8(p.51)] a vision to achieve 90 percent of decision making at the point of care was defined. Shared governance structures within each of the health services and service delivery units were designed and included a governing council and subcouncils that focus on particular issues unique to the service, for example, policy and practice, quality improvement, resource utilization, human resources, and ethics.

Service-Based Councils

Membership of each group included all levels of staff and physicians and also community representatives or former patients. In addition, staff members were encouraged to assume leadership roles as chairs of the subcouncils. Since all professional staff had recently been reallocated from their traditional department or clinical unit structure to a health service or service delivery unit, the new councils provided forums for building relationships around common concerns or issues that were service specific or patient focused. In addition, the council format created opportunities for staff to develop new partnerships and to work together in ways that supported achieving the best possible outcomes.[7–9] Another benefit was the fact that small group work is thought to assist survivors of major downsizing projects to connect by creating a small community around a common purpose and providing a framework for personal and collective growth in the new system.[10]

Building a sense of shared values and a common purpose were incentives for each of the service areas to create mission and vision statements as a first priority in getting organized. A variety of approaches were used to assist people to work together in accomplishing this.[11] Within each of the service areas, a process was undertaken to explore values and beliefs and to create mission and vision statements unique to the service but consistent with the values and direction of the organization.

"The manner in which the people in the setting gather is the heartbeat of a healthy systems design."[9(p.65)]

Benefits and Burdens

One of the early realizations in the implementation of council structures was that this was a significant change for staff who were accustomed to working at the direct care and patient care team level. The ability to consider issues that reflected a concern for the effectiveness of the service within the larger system or external community was a new experience and required a learning process. Within some services, and also at a system level, workshops were provided on a variety of issues such as performance management, labor relations, utilization, and financial management.

A huge issue for direct care providers was the time required for scheduled meetings or related activities. For nurses, the issue was compounded by their shift schedule and the difficulty in getting away, or being away, from their direct care responsibilities during a scheduled shift. Solutions to this problem involved scheduling meetings less frequently and for longer times so that nurses were either freed from the direct care assignment for a period of time or paid to come in on scheduled off-duty times. For the other professional staff, the additional meeting time often meant a longer day in order to meet the expectations for direct care. Creative strategies to enable staff to participate effectively in the shared governance structures are ongoing.

An immediate benefit of the design of service-based councils was the fact that physicians realized the importance of their involvement in the decision-making process that occurred at these meetings. Partnerships with the physician group in each service were enhanced by their participation in the service-based councils and working groups. An ongoing challenge is the clarification of the role of the medical director in each service. The role is designed to provide administrative support to the service leader with respect to medical matters and coleadership on issues pertaining to the effectiveness of the health service. Operationalizing this on a day-to-day basis has been more or less successful, depending on the nature of the service or the personal leadership styles of the individuals involved. Both the physicians and service leaders would agree that they are still struggling to clarify the expectations of the medical director role and their contribution to the service and the hospital system with respect to the administrative processes.

The four principles of partnership, ownership, equity, and accountability provided the framework for design and focus as the councils developed their work processes. Inclusive decision-making processes and a focus on outcomes created the environment for effective point-of-service decision making. Accountability, decisional authority, and locus of control for many issues continue to be a challenge in the new structure. At the service level, most staff are very effective in managing the business issues. Some wonderful examples of how staff have worked together to improve processes or have planned change in a variety of ways has been a source of great hope for the leaders.

SYSTEM INTEGRATION

At the system level, where issues affect or are affected by more than two services, the process and structure for creating horizontal linkages has been a management and design challenge. System integration was identified as a gap in the early phase of the implementation of the new structure, and several attempts to create a process to meet this need were attempted[12] but found to be ineffective.

One year after the system was redesigned, a multistakeholder group was formed to address this challenge. The decision structure task group was composed of staff, facilitators, leaders, and physicians. A consultant supported the process. The group spent six months designing a system-level structure that included three councils with mandates to provide leadership and integration on matters related to operations, quality of care and practice, and executive management. The framework for this system-level structure followed a theoretical model.[8(p.35–68)] Membership was designed to create a variety of perspectives at each council and to provide cross-representation such that issues that overlapped more than one council's mandate could be dealt with appropriately. The designation of physician members for each of the three councils continues to challenge the traditional medical staff roles of service chiefs and department heads. What is required on each council is the physician perspective with regard to either quality of care or administrative processes. Who the representatives will be and how this will unfold are currently in a planning phase. The proposed system-level council structure is presently on hold because leadership changes have occurred at the senior management and board of governors level of the hospital.

A survey of staff that had been completed in the early phase of developing the system-level councils determined that the issues that challenged most staff one year after implementation were related to who decides what, where, and when. In addition, some of the traditional processes for signing authority and approval were still in place, making it impossible for staff to activate some of the decisions that were now within their scope of accountability.

ACCOUNTABILITY FRAMEWORK

The decision structure task group developed a framework for accountability and locus of control in an effort to clarify the location for decisional authority throughout all levels in the organization. The framework was an attempt to articulate accountability by group and individual role against the hospital's strategic directives and included the board of governors, system-level councils, service-based councils, care teams, and staff. A grid was designed to describe accountability of chairpersons and members of each of the system and service councils in an effort to focus the group process and make more effective use of time in meeting the groups' mandate and decisional goals. The tools were designed to focus the councils' activities on decision-making processes and discourage the typical rambling discussions that often occur in group gatherings, as well as to clarify performance expectations of individuals who participated in the shared governance councils.[9,13] In other words, it would not be acceptable to simply show up for meetings unprepared or unable to participate effectively in meeting the group's mandate.

Shifting from a job-oriented and task-based approach to work to one that focuses people on their accountability for outcomes has been challenging to operationalize. While individuals now participate effectively in the service-based councils, the shift to an accountability-based system at the point of care remains a challenge. For many staff who work in fast-paced, complex environments, it is more comfortable to stay in the task-based mode and to depend on others, such as leaders or facilitators. Shifting to a mode in which they must be less process focused and more knowledgeable,[14] accountable for specific required outcomes, is a major change.

It is not surprising that this remains the greatest challenge, particularly for some groups of nurses who have been buried for decades under a militaristic hierarchy of authority and control. As the economic imperative of health reform demands a faster and more complex pace of work, staff are increasingly challenged to examine traditional routines and rituals that may have served them well in the past but may not be either meaningful or necessary in the present.

The accountability framework holds some promise as a tool that could assist staff to operationalize the expectations of the new system and to integrate the desired behaviors into the performance management and development process.

PATIENT-FOCUSED CARE

The redesigned system challenged staff in every dimension of work—not only in their relationships with each other but also in the ways in which they work with patients and families. Health care professionals are accustomed to "doing for" or "doing to" people as they enter the health system. In a patient-focused approach, mutuality drives the coordination of care and is an ongoing process that seeks out what is important to the person receiving care.[15] Learning to really *be with* patients and families while coping with the pace and complexity of the hospital environment continues to challenge staff.

It is not surprising to note that what patients and families want from a health care experience is not necessarily what providers think they want.[16] People seeking health services want to be treated as unique individuals and not as body parts or disease entities. Health is about the wholeness of the person and is described as body, mind, and spirit in balance.[15] Shifting to a culture that values and respects patients' preferences, supports a more holistic approach to people, and reflects a concern for health and not just the medical diagnosis is a major transition for most care providers.

Patients are normally satisfied with the technical aspects of their care, but in the care process, their individuality is lost and their personal needs are not met.[17] Patient-focused care is an approach that consciously adopts the perspective of the person receiving the care and aims to establish mutual goals that meet the person's unique needs. A conceptual framework that describes seven dimensions of patient-centered care was developed by the Picker Institute to support an evaluation process for health care systems. The dimensions provided the context for operationalizing patient-focused care at TEGH. The dimensions are as follows:

1. respect for patient's values, preferences, and expressed needs
2. coordination and integration of care
3. information, communication, and education
4. physical comfort
5. emotional support and alleviation of fear and anxiety
6. involvement of family and friends
7. transition and continuity

PROFESSIONAL PRACTICE MODEL

A model for professional practice that incorporated the values and beliefs of patient-focused care was designed (Figure 3–2). The purpose of the professional practice model is to articulate the complexity of the practice paradigm and to provide a framework for clarifying accountability within the scope of each discipline's unique service. Physicians were not involved in this process, choosing to manage medical practice issues within their own quality management processes.

The first component of the model was designed on the basis of how an individual learns.[18] Learning can be grouped into three major domains: cognitive or knowledge, psychomotor or skill, and affective or personal qualities. The affective domain is that invisible layer of practice that includes the provider's critical thinking, clinical judgment,[19] and human capacity for caring.[20]

The affective domain in this model is the area of greatest challenge in defining ownership and accountability. A significant effort has been initiated to assist staff at all levels to explore attitudes, beliefs, and assumptions and to change behaviors so that the intention of focusing on what really matters to patients and families can be achieved. The other interesting component to this process is honoring and

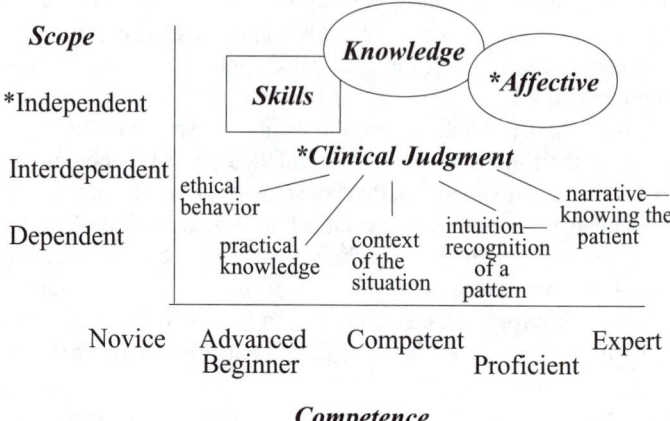

Figure 3–2   Professional Practice

valuing those expert practice patterns that are largely invisible and not documented. The area of ongoing challenge continues to be in this domain as the journey continues toward a culture where people experience meaningful care and service.

The second component of the model focused on competence. The provider, with these three domains of knowing or being, functions in a five-level range of competence from novice to expert.[21] Since many staff had been relocated to new clinical areas, the level of their skill and ability to practice could shift along this competency range depending on their individual learning needs. The third major component of this model is the scope of professional practice, which includes the following three categories of services for which providers are accountable[15]:

1. *Delegated*—services that enhance the health of the person and require a physician's order
2. *Interdependent*—services that enhance health by assessing, monitoring, detecting, and preventing physiological complications associated with certain health situations or treatment plans
3. *Independent*—services that enhance health by assessing, monitoring, detecting, diagnosing, and treating the human response to health or situations

The model provides the basis for continuing work to clarify the scope of practice for each discipline through the development of standards and the professional documentation system.

Standards of Practice

Recent legislative changes in the province of Ontario define an expectation that each professional college or association provides standards and strategies to ensure that its registrants are practicing at a competent level. A shift to locate accountability for competence with the registrants was consistent with the TEGH goal for self-directed autonomous and accountable providers. Standards of practice have historically been used to describe expectations for practice or patient care. They are principles or norms that guide professional behaviors.[22] The profession leaders at TEGH developed a generic framework for standards of practice that defined three categories:

1. *Patient-focused care*—incorporates the defined principles and dimensions of patient-focused care
2. *Professional practice*—articulates the process of practice for each discipline
3. *Professional accountability*—describes ethical behavior, legal accountability, safety, competence, and partnership with others

A generic matrix was designed that included descriptive statements about the standard in each of the three categories. To make the standards reflect the reality of the practice setting at TEGH, indicators and evaluation criteria were developed. The indicators are descriptions of behaviors that support the standard, and the evaluation criteria are the expected outcomes (Exhibit 3–4). The intent of this process was to break down the guidelines into operational directions and to articulate accountability for outcomes.

Each professional group developed its own standard of practice document using the generic framework and the content of their college or association standards. Once the generic practice standards document was developed, some groups created more specific indicators to reflect the unique practice expectations of specific patient populations, such as critical, mental health, and maternal newborn care. The intention of the framework was to provide a tool that would support performance management and development and enable staff to be self-directed. The document also supported a peer review process and realistic performance review by a leader who did not have the same professional background as the particular staff person.

Staff are currently in the process of testing the professional practice standards documents as a basis for the performance management process. Modifications by professional group or patient care area will enrich the process and make it a more effective tool.

Exhibit 3–4 Professional Practice Standards

Nursing Practice	Standards Related to Professional Practice	
Standard	**Indicator**	**Evaluation**
Assessment: Each nurse assesses the individual utilizing a planned and organized process.	• Based on the individual's condition, each nurse exercises clinical judgment in assessing the individual upon admission and on a continuing basis. • Documentation of the admission assessment is initiated as soon as possible and completed within eight hours.	• Compliance with the standard is measured through planned and systematic activities at the Health Service, Service Delivery Unit, and hospital levels. • Documentation in the individual's record includes: → an initial focused assessment on the individual's arrival to the unit → overall assessment and patient history is completed within eight hours → evidence of ongoing assessment • Documentation of assessment is completed according to College of Nurses and the Health Service and Service Delivery Unit guidelines.
Each nurse assesses the individual utilizing a planned and organized process.	• Subjective and objective data are continually collected and analyzed, in keeping with the nurse's scope of practice, to determine nursing diagnosis. • The subjective and objective database encompasses body, mind, and spiritual components; the individual's perception of health, and goals and expectations related to health.	• Documentation demonstrates use of a variety of data collection and communication techniques, such as: → Interviewing → Consulting → Auscultating → Percussing → Palpating → Observing → Inspecting → Monitoring → Measuring → Asking → Listening → Accepting → Giving recognition → Encouraging → Providing description → Seeking clarification → Touching

The expectation for staff to shift their thinking and practice patterns to an approach that demonstrates patient-focused care and the complexity of their accountability for demonstrating competency are daunting. In addition, access to information, supplies, and equipment is impeded by numerous system processes as well as traditional practice patterns and rituals. Currently, a major project to automate the information system within the hospital is under way. This has created an opportunity to redesign the professional documentation process based on the values and beliefs of patient-focused care and to provide more integrated and meaningful patient information.

Professional Documentation

The future design process for professional documentation is a conceptual challenge. The goal is to create a system that is based in a health framework, focuses on the uniqueness of the person, and integrates professional information such that duplication and repetition are avoided. Designing the functional components and information fields to incorporate each discipline's scope of practice and professional accountability means that not only the tasks or interventions but also the assessment, plan of care, patient education, and relationship to outcomes must be included.

The documentation system and the process improvements are providing an effective leverage point for changing old patterns of thinking and behavior. A group of staff has been assigned to the computerization project named "Gateway to the New Millennium," and a future state design team that includes all professional disciplines has been formed to support the planning requirements for the new documentation system. This project, more than anything else, is creating the opportunity for dialogue about values and what matters for each discipline, and the early implementation of some components of the project has generated excitement and hope from the small gains that have been achieved thus far.

PARTNERSHIP

"Systems are relationships that we observe as structures, but these relationships can't be structured. The dense web of a system develops as individuals explore their need to be together. In this way, people create the structures for accomplishing the work of the organization."[5(p.83)]

As the system shifted from the traditional hierarchical model to one based on horizontal structures, the emphasis on relationships and the need to create more effective working partnerships was evident. The relationships of hierarchical structures are transactional and focus on tasks and time, problems and crisis thinking, and connecting people around judgmental interactions.[15] Transactional relationships ensure that rituals, patterns, and routines are accomplished. The new paradigm that locates decisions at the point of service requires a culture and relationships built around shared mission and vision. Partnership is a mental model that describes relationships that nourish others; that connect people as higher human beings; that join people's hearts, hands, and minds; and that create opportunities to make humanness more visible.

Most people are creative, meaning-seeking beings who are searching for relationships and places where possibilities can be explored.[5] The changes to the organizational structure and roles at TEGH were designed to facilitate more effective work processes and decision making. As the work of organizing staff within the newly created service areas proceeded, strategies designed to promote this concept of partnership were initiated. This continues to be the hardest and most challenging work because it is not about simple change but about personal transformation. People are accustomed to and comfortable with the power and authority traditionally associated with jobs and positions in the organization. However, this kind of culture isolates people and focuses on getting things done and doing them as told. Creating new roles in which people are seen as equal and in which collective wisdom is valued is a major transition. Nourishing relationships connect people at the invisible level and are ignited by a common mission.[23] Just as the mission of health care is about ensuring not only a functioning body but a functioning soul, the relationships required in the new culture require a wisdom for being together differently.

"The twenty first century will be anything but business as usual. Institutions must now balance the need to make a living with the natural ability to change. They must also honor the souls of the individuals who work for them and the great soul of the natural world from which they take their resources."[24(p.11)]

Partnership Workshop

Partnership workshops were held for staff within four months of the change to the new organizational structure. This was a two-day process led by external colleagues. The workshop was designed to teach staff about the principles of partnership and to uncover some expectations that different groups might have, with the goal of being able to work together in more effective ways. For example, what kinds of things did staff need to see from the senior management team or leaders that would assure them that the values would be lived out in the day-to-day reality of the work setting? Similarly, the values, beliefs, and expectations that leaders now held for the staff were shared in a role-playing and skit format. A unique feature of this workshop was that it brought all levels of staff (direct and nondirect care staff) together as equal players.

The partnership workshop occurred just as the service-based groups completed mission and vision statements and prior to the implementation of the service-based council structures. While the number of staff who experienced the workshop was small in comparison to the total number of staff, small groups of people began the journey of living out the principles of partnership. This established role models for others and created momentum as the implementation process continued.

Dialogue as a Strategy

Healthy relationships do not just happen. In a setting such as TEGH, where people have worked together for long periods of time, a rearrangement of the structure and the leadership roles does not necessarily lead to the shift in thinking and behavior that previously has been described. The way in which people connect with each other, through conversation, discussion, and even body language, has a significant effect on the nature of the work relationships. Through a contract with the Clinical Practice Model Resource Centre, TEGH staff became aware of an approach that many organizations have adopted to enable people to develop healthy work relationships.

Dialogue is an ancient art practiced by primitive societies and experienced in the modern world largely by accident. Communication is generally characterized by two kinds of discourse, both important, but especially powerful in their synergy.[25] Discussion is characterized by a sustained emphasis on winning or having one's views accepted by the group. Dialogue is a process in which all individuals gain insights that could not be achieved individually. Complex issues are explored from many points of view through the practice of concrete skills: advocacy, inquiry, listening, and silence. People participate in developing a pool of common meaning by suspending assumptions and exploring experience and thought, a process that enables individuals to move beyond their original viewpoint.

A dialogue workshop was held soon after the new structure was implemented. More than 150 staff members attended this one-day event, which was didactic and experiential in design. Within two months of this workshop, weekly practice sessions were established for all staff in the organization to attend. On average, 10–12 staff members from all areas and levels of the organization attended each practice session. The process was introduced to educate individuals who had not attended the workshop, and the one-hour session focused on a statement or a question that was not work related, such as the following:

- Are we human beings or human doings?
- Must each of us be the change we want to see?
- What is it about the work that we do that arouses our passion?

During the session, the following skills are practiced:

- advocacy or speaking from "I"
- inquiry or checking out assumptions to explore background information
- listening intently without judging or assuming
- silence

Silence is the most difficult skill to practice because most people are so accustomed to talking. It is often in the few moments of silence that individuals experience personal insights that generate significant learning.

As well as the weekly sessions, staff groups in various areas initiated the practice of dialogue skills in their regular team meetings or planned dialogue sessions that mirrored the process of the hospitalwide sessions. The intention of these sessions was to help people to understand how their thinking patterns affected their relationships with each other and to learn how to be together in a different way. In creating a healthier work culture and the rich relationships that are essential to partnership, dialogue skills help individuals to communicate in more respectful and meaningful ways.[26] Some of the benefits that staff experienced as a result of dialogue practice sessions were evidenced by more listening and fewer interruptions during staff discussions and better problem resolution between individuals, especially between individuals in different clinical areas. There is a general feeling that the pace of the meetings has slowed down, allowing individuals to be heard, and that the contributions that come from discussion on difficult issues are more likely to be heard now than previously. Dialogue practice sessions have become a safe place for people to share thoughts and experiences and to learn to respect and value each other in a much deeper way. Relationships have been enriched as a result of this process, and the journey of creating more effective partnerships has been very rewarding.

EVALUATION

The evaluation of the changes in structure, process, and roles has occurred in formal and informal ways during the two years following implementation of the redesign. Within service areas, the structures of the service-based councils have been modified to reflect the needs of the areas or to create more effective partnerships between individuals or groups. For example, one service area that had formed its subcouncils based on issues, as opposed to geographic area, has now chosen to redesign the groups according to geographic area. It appears to be more meaningful for this particular service if individuals who work directly with each other on a particular clinical area are allowed to form their own subcouncil to manage their unit-specific issues. In another service, the governance structure has been redesigned to include more people in the subcouncils and fewer on the main governance council.

The roles of leader and clinical facilitator have evolved to reflect the unique needs of the services that they support. The clinical facilitator role was originally designed as a temporary role, and it is now clear that staff support for professional development within the service areas is ongoing. The patient care coordinator role was originally designed as a temporary role that individuals could assume for defined periods. In some areas this works well; in others, a permanent appointment has been necessary to provide consistency and continuity for the day-to-day operations of the clinical area.

The professional leader role continues with individual providers sharing the accountabilities in a variety of ways. The major source of challenge has been in dealing with the issues that require collaboration between service leader and profession leader, for example, appropriate allocation of staff by full-time equivalent to service areas, vacation relief, and workload adjustments when a provider has accountability in more than one service. The issues have been resolved through involvement of whole professional groups working in collaboration with the appropriate service leaders and by shifting responsibility for coming up with solutions to the professional staff members themselves.

The challenge of horizontal integration of the system continues. Problem solving and decision making are more effective than in the early implementation phase because the partnership between individuals is more effective. However, managing broad system-level issues continues to be a challenge, particularly as it affects or requires physician involvement.

An evaluation framework has been designed to reflect the data collected for the balanced scorecard and to incorporate the work on cultural transformation (Figure 3–3). The balanced scorecard is a matrix format that measures organizational success against the hospital's strategic directives. Since patient-focused care is the first strategic directive, the measurement and evaluation of how this is being achieved is an ongoing challenge. An approach that included both qualitative and quantitative methods was designed to explore and describe patients' and providers' experience of quality.[27] The Picker Institute[16] was contracted to conduct a survey of discharged patients in the fall of 1996. The purpose of this was to gather information related to patients' perceptions of how well their needs were met during their experience of hospitalization. Findings indicate that there are issues to be addressed in each dimension of those things that really matter to patients.[16] A patient focused quality task force has been initiated to address the issues identified in the Picker Institute survey and to coordinate a process for ongoing staff development with regard to patient-focused care.

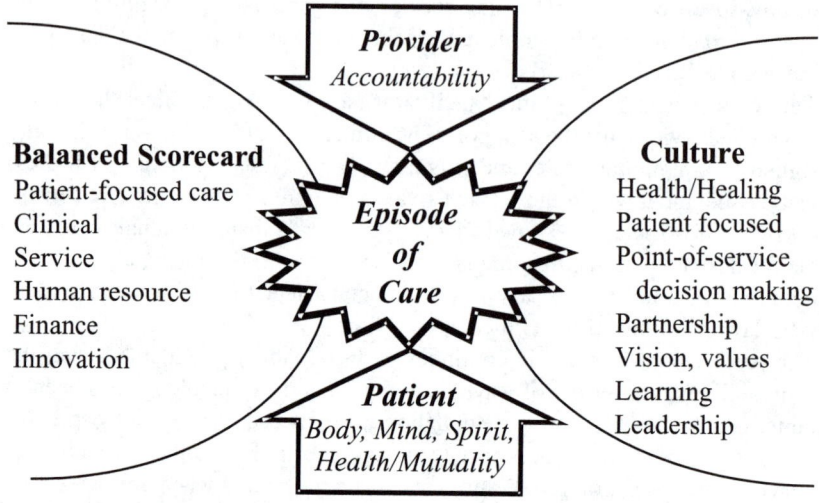

Figure 3–3 Cultural Transformation

CONCLUSION

The change processes that staff and physicians at TEGH experienced have been considerable. At this point, there are defined areas of success and obvious areas that remain a challenge. The organizational structure and roles have been effective in creating services based on patient population needs. The devolution of professional departments and the assignment of staff to interdisciplinary teams within the services have broken down barriers and created partnerships closer to the patient care areas. The integration of physicians within the service-based structures has been more or less effective and in some areas requires further refinement. The general condition of staff at the point of service varies from service to service. In some cases there is momentum and enthusiasm for the new direction and the added responsibility that shared governance has provided. In other situations, staff morale is low and individuals feel burdened with the increasing complexity of care requirements and the additional accountability that shared governance implies.

The establishment of the seven health services and three service delivery units has added to a silo effect in the organization. Integration at the system level, that is, the implementation of structures that create horizontal linkages, is a required next step. The greatest challenge that lies ahead is defining a meaningful partnership with physicians at the system level. In addition, the transition to a medical staff structure that clarifies accountability, ownership, equity, and partnership among the board of governors, the senior administration, and the system-level structures is in the early stages. It may be that the very architecture of the hospital system is incompatible with a mutually satisfactory arrangement between physicians and health care providers.[4] In creating integrated health systems, the nucleus should be the interdisciplinary group and patient-focused practice. The politics of hospital-based systems and traditional patterns and practices continue to have a stronghold on the change process.

Shifting the culture to one in which individuals value partnership and patient-focused care will be an ongoing journey. While there was considerable effort directed toward staff development throughout the process of transition and implementation, it was not enough. Staff would say that they feel isolated from leaders and often on their own with the challenges of managing the everyday issues. The traditional hierarchy provided a safety net of managers and supervisors who were available to assist with or solve problems. With those roles deleted, staff are now required to be more accountable and responsible for finding solutions and managing issues that emerge in their everyday practice. This has been hard for some staff who have worked for decades in traditional systems. For others, it has unearthed tremendous leadership capacity. The learning process should never be short-changed, and the reality of being able to walk the talk of the new paradigm is personal work at every level.

The work of change is located primarily in two places now: at the system level with integration of the physicians and design of the horizontal linkages, and at the point of service. The hospital is currently orienting a new board of governors and searching for a new chief executive officer. In addition, work will be initiated in clarifying decisional authority and accountability at the governance level of the hospital.

The findings of the recent survey by the Picker Institute have provided concrete evidence for moving ahead with the work toward a patient-focused care system. The patient focused quality task force includes staff, physicians, and community representatives, and its mandate is to define priorities, benchmarks, evaluation processes, and a learning plan to ensure that the needs and wishes of patients are incorporated into the next phase of system development.

In planning for the future, the mission, vision, and values of the hospital will be reviewed and strategic directives developed that are consistent with the internal changes as well as the external influences affecting health care in this province. One thing clear to all staff is that the activities they have engaged in during the past three years have awakened a passion for a very different way of working together. While some things may never change, the quality of the relationships staff have with each other and with patients and families has improved and provides the motivation for continuing to believe that the effort was, and continues to be, worthwhile.

"It is the ability to keep finding solutions that is important; any one solution is temporary. There are no permanently right answers. The capacity to keep changing, to find what works now, is what keeps any organism alive."[5(p.13)]

REFERENCES

1. Zelman WN, Parham DL. Strategic, operational, and marketing concerns of product-line management in health care. *Health Care Manage Rev.* 1990; 15(1):29–35.

2. Bowers MR, Taylor JA. Product line management in hospitals: An exploratory study of managing change. *Hosp and Health Serv Adm.* 1990; 35(3):365–375.

3. Comack M, Brady J, Porter-O'Grady T. Professional practice: A framework for transition to a new culture. *J Nurs Adm.* 1997; 27(12):32–41.

4. Goldsmith JC. Driving the nitroglycerine truck. *Healthcare Forum J.* 1993; 36(2):36–44.

5. Wheatley MJ, Kellner-Rogers M. *A Simpler Way.* San Francisco: Berrett-Koehler Publishers; 1996.

6. Wheatley M. How leaders can create adaptive, energetic organizations. *Health Prog.* 1995 (January-February): 14–15.

7. Porter-O'Grady T. *The Leadership Revolution in Health Care.* Gaithersburg, MD: Aspen Publishers, Inc.; 1995.

8. Porter-O'Grady T, Hawkins M, Parker M. *Whole Systems Shared Governance.* Gaithersburg, MD: Aspen Publishers, Inc.; 1997.

9. Wesorick B, Shiparski L, Troseth M, Wyngarden K. *Partnership Council Field Book— Strategies and Tools for Co-Creating a Healthy Workplace.* Grand Rapids, MI: Practice Field Publishing; 1997.

10. Bumbaugh M. Moving beyond survival after downsizing. *Nurs Manage.* 1998; 29(2):30–33.

11. Senge P, Kleiner A, Roberts C, Ross R, Smith B. *The Fifth Discipline Field Book.* New York: Currency Doubleday; 1994.

12. Aikman P, Andress I, Goodfellow C, LaBelle N, Porter-O'Grady T. System integration: A necessity. *J Nurs Admin.* 1998; 28(2):28–34.

13. Kayser T. *Mining Group Gold—How To Cash in on the Collaborative Brain Power of a Group.* El Segundo, CA: Serif Publishing; 1990.

14. Drucker P. *Post-Capitalist Society.* New York: HarperCollins Publishers; 1994.

15. Wesorik B. *A Journey from Old to New Thinking.* Grandville, MI: Grandville Publishing; 1995.

16. Gerteis M. What patients really want. *Health Manage Q.* 1993; 15(3):2–6.

17. Gerteis M, Edgman-Levitan S, Daley J, Delbanco T, eds. *Through the Patient's Eyes.* San Francisco: Jossey-Bass Publishers; 1993.

18. Bloom B. *Taxonomy of Educational Objectives: Handbook 1, Cognitive Domain.* New York: David Mackay; 1956.

19. Benner P, Tanner C, Chesla C. *Expertise in Nursing Practice—Caring, Clinical Judgment, and Ethics.* New York: Springer Publishing; 1996.

20. Roach M. *Caring from the Heart—The Convergence of Caring and Spirituality.* Mahwah, NJ: Paulist Press; 1997.

21. Benner P. *From Novice to Expert—Excellence and Power in Clinical Nursing Practice.* Menlo Park, CA: Addison-Wesley Publishing; 1994.

22. Kirk R, Hoesing H. *The Nurses' Guide to Common Sense Quality Management.* West Dundie, IL: S-N Publications; 1991.

23. Wesorik B. *The Closing and Opening of a Millennium: A Journey from Old to New Relationships in the Work Setting.* Grand Rapids, MI: Practice Field Publishing; 1996.

24. Whyte D. *The Heart Aroused: Poetry and the Preservation of the Soul in Corporate America.* New York: Doubleday; 1994.

25. Senge P. *The Fifth Discipline—The Art and Practice of the Learning Organization.* New York: Currency Doubleday; 1994.

26. Wesorick B, Shiparski L. *Can the Human Being Thrive in the Work Place? — Dialogue as a Strategy of Hope.* Grand Rapids, MI: Practice Field Publishing; 1997.

27. Andress I, Comack M. Creating a caring culture: An evaluation framework. *RN Journal* (in press).

CHAPTER 4

Process Reengineering: Strategies for Analysis, Redesign, and Refinement

Jo Anne Carrick, MSN, RN

Logical, creative, and complex, all at the same time, has often been the way reengineering has been described. This phenomenon is a paradox to some degree, since reengineering aims to simplify work processes, not complicate them. Where the challenge and complexity lie is in organizing the reengineering effort, understanding business processes, unleashing the creativity of the reengineering team, and managing the organizational changes required to execute the reengineering plan. Once an organization embraces reengineering, all work activities are geared toward managing the processes that are central to the core of their business operations. In process-centered organizations, all people in the organization recognize and focus on their processes. This chapter describes methods used to identify the core business processes in health care as well as how to identify and analyze processes for change.

BUSINESS PROCESSES IN HEALTH CARE

Over the years, as health care became highly specialized, many of the jobs people performed were oriented to a single task or function. Using methods developed for another era, waste, delays, bottlenecks, and problems contributed to the high costs of health care. Small departments and elaborate hierarchies prevailed. To varying degrees, the current processes were never engineered to begin with; they just evolved.

Clearly, in initial reengineering efforts of health care organizations, experience was limited. Many organizations initiated continuous quality improvement programs and used the concept of patient-focused care. In these efforts, layers of management were eliminated, and highly specialized single-function jobs were reconfigured to create cross-functional roles.[1] Several aspects of this redesign were quite radical and different. Imagine a hospital without nurses' stations or one where patients are admitted directly to the unit where care is provided, whether it is short term (i.e., same-day surgery) or long term (one to several days), thus eliminating the admissions department. In this design, duties once performed by phlebotomists, electrocardiogram technicians, intravenous therapy teams, respiratory therapy technicians, or unit secretaries are completed by staff who are cross-trained and multifunctional.

Some consider this concept an outcome of reengineering patient care in the hospital setting, but others argue that patient-centered care is only an initial attempt to do limited reengineering.[1] Despite the controversy and limited data on the cost benefits of patient-centered care, these changes certainly drew health care leaders to identify and focus on the core business processes that were used to provide patient care. As business processes improved and organizations became process centered, reengineering and process improvement now focused on the global processes and the subprocesses used to achieve product and service outputs. For health care providers, the key elements centered on the care delivery model as the basis for patient care.

CORE BUSINESS PROCESSES IN HEALTH CARE

In health care there are six fundamental elements of patient care that create the core business processes. From these key elements, all the subprocesses can be identified. It is these processes that influence the structure and function of any health care organization. When reengineering or continuous quality improvement is used to improve processes, some of these subprocesses are eliminated, improved through process analysis (total quality management), or reengineered. In process-centered organizations, these core business processes create the primary focus of managers and workers alike. They are the focal point of what is done to provide patient care, whereas the processes dictate how it is to be done.

The fundamental elements of patient care, the care delivery model, are illustrated in Exhibit 4–1. These elements required to provide patient care are not described by departments or functions but are more global in nature. This challenges us to view care in a more conceptual manner. Element 1 consists of the processes required for patients to gain entry and subsequently exit the system. The next high-level process, element 2, is to create a record of the event or encounter. This record encompasses both past and present data and serves to represent the entire patient record database. It is one of the unique elements of the care delivery model that interconnects with all the other five elements.

Elements 3 and 4 encompass the activities necessary to identify problems and diagnose illnesses. From these elements flow the treatment plan and implementation (element 5). Element 6 relates to the ongoing monitoring and evaluation of

Exhibit 4-1 Patient Care Delivery Model

Patient
The process starts with the patient needing health care.

	Processes	*Subprocesses*
Element 1	Care Acquisition	Entry and exit in the health care system
Element 2	Patient Record	Create and maintain a record of the encounter(s)
Element 3	Test and Examination	Perform an examination, assessment, professional evaluation, and technical diagnostic evaluation (invasive and noninvasive)
Element 4	Diagnosis	Issue a judgment/diagnosis, identify treatment care requirements, and issue care directives
Element 5	Treatment	Provide treatment, prevention, palliation (administration of therapeutic substances, invasive and noninvasive procedures)
Element 6	Monitor, Evaluate, and Revise	Monitor and evaluate patient outcomes and care, revise plan of care, plan to meet short-term and long-term care needs, and facilitate the acquisition of resources

Infrastructure
The processes that support and facilitate the members of the organization to perform the care delivery elements

Source: Reprinted from J.S. Maehling, Process Reengineering: Strategies for Analysis and Redesign in *Reengineering Nursing and Health Care: The Handbook for Organizational Transformation,* S. Smith Blancett and D.L. Flarey, eds., p. 64, © 1995, Aspen Publishers, Inc.

---

the patient and the care provided. The last element includes planning to meet short-term and long-term care needs and facilitating the acquisition of resources to meet those needs. Surrounding these elements are the processes that create the infrastructure and support the execution of the care. Examples of support processes would include housing and feeding patients and producing bills for services.

Using the concept of process mapping applied to these care elements, health care organizations can identify basic business processes. Within these limited basic processes are the numerous subprocesses that are performed to conduct one's business. Embedded in the care delivery model are subprocesses, tasks, or functions that are performed to accomplish the primary element. Exhibit 4–2 shows the care delivery model elements and their subprocesses. It illustrates the nature of the many types of work and processes performed in providing patient care.

For example, to complete a diagnostic evaluation, a test may be performed. Subprocesses and tasks would include scheduling the test, transporting the patient, obtaining physician interpretations, producing the report, and communicating the results. Numerous subprocesses, tasks, and functions can be included within the elements.

Using the care delivery model, health care organizations will be able to accomplish the first task of reengineering and achieve the first element of becoming a process-centered organization, that is, recognizing and naming all of its processes.[2] Then, through reengineering and continuous quality improvement, these subprocesses will be improved, reengineered, or eliminated. Again focusing on the major elements of the care delivery model, leaders of health care can use this as a framework to identify business strategy and direction. It allows for a method to clearly communicate to employees the major focus of the organization and the employees' role in accomplishing the outputs of processes. It is the basis for identifying key measures of process performance and for the ongoing management of the processes. As a result, all elements of process centering can be accomplished.

MANAGEMENT STRUCTURE

In process-centered organizations, traditional organizational charts become a thing of the past. Now process owners are responsible for the design of the processes: creating and maintaining the design and making sure that processes are organized in efficient and productive ways.[2] Not directly involved with the people of the organization, process owners' specific job is to link, facilitate, and enable those who actually do the work. Coaches then are required to focus on the people of the organization and to "assess the present and future demands for workers with particular skills, develop the supply of skilled individuals, allocate resources, guide and mentor employees, and intervene to help resolve performance problems."[2] In health care, a process owner could be an individual with a broad business and clinical background, where necessary. The process coaches are those individuals with specific expertise in the specific process, such as a nurse for clinical areas or a laboratory technologist for processes related to laboratory processes.

Exhibit 4–2 Subprocesses of the Care Delivery Model

	Element 1	Element 2	Element 3	Element 4	Element 5	Element 6	
Infrastructure **Support Processes**	Entry and exit in the health care system	Create historical and current patient information database and record of encounter	Perform an exam, assessment, professional and technical diagnostic evaluation	Issue a judgment or diagnosis Identify treatment care requirements Issue care directives	Provide treatment, prevention, palliation	Perform ongoing monitoring, evaluation, revision of plan of care Plan to meet short-term and long-term care needs and facilitate acquisition of resources to meet needs	**Infrastructure** **Support Processes**
Clean and Maintain the Environment	Admission process	Initiate and maintain current encounter data input	Schedule tests Perform tests	Issue physician orders	Schedule and perform surgical procedures	Perform daily monitoring and evaluation of patient and care	**Facility Maintenance** **Staff Education, Orientation, and Training**
Prepare and Deliver Food to Patients	Emergency department triage and registration	Store and maintain past medical records	Notify and perform consultation	Order transcription	Administer therapeutic agents (medications, IVs, radiation)	Plan discharges	**Communications Processes among Staff (Report, Meetings, Memos)**

continues

Exhibit 4–2 continued

	Element 1	Element 2	Element 3	Element 4	Element 5	Element 6	Communications processes among staff (report, meetings, memos)
Human Resources Management, Hiring, Employee Relations	Outpatient registration	Retrieve past medical records	Perform tests	Assist other professions ordering care and treatments for patients	Perform rehabilitative therapies (physical, occupational, and speech)	Perform utilization and peer review	
Performance Evaluations, Salary Administration	Short stay and same day surgery registration	Code encounters for payment	Report test findings	Communicate diagnosis	Health teaching, health promotion	Assist long-term care placement	
	Discharge from services	Transcribe dictated encounter events	Obtain tissue and blood samples for exam	Obtain patient treatment preference and consent	Provide respiratory therapy		
	Bill and Collect Payment for Services	**Management of Fiscal Affairs, Budget, and Planning**		**Transport Patients**	**Order, Deliver, and Receive Supplies**		**Scheduling Staff**

Source: Reprinted from J.S. Maehling, Process Reengineering: Strategies for Analysis and Redesign in *Reengineering Nursing and Health Care: The Handbook for Organizational Transformation*, S. Smith Blancett and D.L. Flarey, eds., pp. 66–67, © 1995, Aspen Publishers, Inc.

Applying this management structure to the care delivery model and its elements, process owners can be identified to manage the major elements, and coaches would include those managers involved directly with the employees performing the work. As an example, one of the elements of the care delivery model is care acquisition. This is defined as the entry and exit into the health care system. Within this element are subprocesses that include admission and discharge registration and emergency department triage and registration. Now, in the time of managed care, certification and precertification for admission or diagnostic and surgical procedures are also required during entry to the health care system. Other subprocesses in this element of care could include outreach, referral, and marketing programs that seek to attract and identify patients appropriate to utilize the organization's services.

The process owner in this example would globally manage the subprocesses within this element while coaches would guide employees within the various departments to accomplish the tasks and outputs of the specific processes. The process owner could be a director within the organization who has the business and clinical background to understand all of the factors that influence the registration process. This individual must also be at the level of administrative authority to implement the necessary changes that would be required to manage the process in a global manner.

With the process owner overseeing the process throughout the organization, a process such as registration into the system could be streamlined and consistent among all departments even though the process could occur in multiple places. In addition, the process owner would be better able to identify opportunities to connect processes such as outreach intake of patient information and the registration process. Thus, process owners can identify opportunities and work directly with the coaches and the quality improvement and reengineering teams to target their activities so that they will be most beneficial to the organization.

IDENTIFYING REENGINEERING OPPORTUNITIES

In their book *Reengineering the Corporation,* Hammer and Champy identify three factors that can be used to determine priority for deciding which processes to target for reengineering: dysfunction, impact, and feasibility.[3] While this is not a specific formula for all reengineering projects, it can be used as a guide for process owners and reengineering teams trying to make choices. These principles for identifying reengineering opportunities still apply in process-centered organizations. However, some additional strategies may be considered.

Initial reengineering efforts may have greatly improved the design and execution of day-to-day business processes. In fact, processes may have improved so much that a process itself may have become the business' product or specialized service. An example of this would be a health care organization streamlining its care of patients with chest pain to such a degree that the organization can advertise this streamlined care as a product. It can promote the use of its service because of its efficiency and quality outcomes.

As organizations direct their business strategies to extend the reengineering effort, they may desire to intensify their processes, that is, improve them to better serve the customer. Other efforts may include fashioning strategies to extend, augment, convert, innovate, and diversify processes.[2] Exhibit 4–3 lists these strategies, their definitions, and examples of how they can be applied to health care. All of these objectives will aid in the identification of reengineering and process improvement opportunities.

UNDERSTANDING PROCESS REQUIREMENTS

As processes are targeted for change, reengineering teams must not rush to the design table. The next step is to clearly understand the current processes and then move forward to their reinvention. Teams will need to ask important questions about the core elements and their subprocesses:

- What is required to receive or admit a patient into a program or facility?
- How many tasks and people does it take to perform this function?
- What are the current costs?
- What is the quality of care, and how much time does it take to achieve the output?
- Do the steps in the process add value to the output, or does the entire process and its output add value for the customer?
- Is this process still necessary for the business strategy? Should it be eliminated? Do new processes need to be created?
- How is information technology being used?

To search for answers to these questions and to organize team activities so that process requirements can be understood, the initial step is to document the process. Perhaps the process is well documented from previous reengineering and continuous quality improvement efforts. It is important, though, that this documentation portrays the overall picture of what happens, including what is done, who does it, and other relevant aspects (e.g., forms and equipment) of the process. Performance measures, time elements, problems, bottlenecks, and issues that surround the process must be identified next. These must be identified to determine the financial benefit of the proposed changes.

Once processes are clearly documented, two key questions are asked: (1) What are the assumptions? (2) What steps are required? At this point, the team must

Exhibit 4–3 Identifying Reengineering Opportunities

	Category	*Definition*	*Example*
Reengineering	Dysfunction	Fragmented, redundant processes	Processes that have regular delays or bottlenecks or that require multiple approvals
	Impact	Benefit the organization greatly by financial gains, increasing market share, increasing customer satisfaction	Decreasing length of stay and the cost of care
	Feasibility	Has the highest likelihood of success in the reengineering effort	Change will not require extensive financial and staff resources
Process-Centered Business Strategies	Intensification	Improving processes to better serve customers	Decreasing emergency department waiting time from the current 30 minutes to 15 minutes
	Extension	Using strong processes to enter new markets	Expanding behavioral health programs to include specialties in adolescent and geriatric care
	Augmentation	Expanding processes to provide additional services to customers	Centralizing scheduling so that patients only have to call once for appointments to various service providers
	Conversion	Taking a process that you perform well and performing it as a service for other companies	Serving as a referral lab to perform tests that are not done cost effectively by other organizations
	Innovation	Applying processes that you perform well to create and deliver different goods or services	Extend patient case management to new patient populations
	Diversification	Creating new processes to deliver new goods and services	Enter into new markets to start providing care for new patient populations (e.g., performing surgical specialty services for neurosurgical patients)

Source: "Identifying Reengineering Opportunities" from BEYOND REENGINEERING by MICHAEL HAMMER. Copyright © 1996 by Michael Hammer. Reprinted by permission of HarperCollins Publishers, Inc.

search for the reasons why things are done in a particular way. With further probing, the team will begin to uncover the critical outputs of the process studied and its true purpose, which will set the stage for the creative design of the new process. Often the true requirement for a process is as simple as paying the bill, performing the treatment, obtaining the blood sample, communicating the order, or changing the level of intensity of care the patient now requires. However, the extensive processes involved in accomplishing these key outputs are elaborate. As the reengineering team looks further into the process, a search should ensue for the assumptions embedded in the current processes, clarification of process requirements, and a determination of whether tasks add or do not add value to the output of the process. This analysis will reveal that assumptions often lead people to believe that things must be done in a particular way. When the requirements are examined, the desired outcome becomes apparent. It then becomes clear that it was assumed, not validated, that the elaborate tasks are required to accomplish the desired outcome.

Uncovering the necessary requirements of key processes moves the reengineering team into the creative process of identifying a new approach. It also allows the team to consider new approaches to reach business strategies of process-centered organizations. While identifying assumptions and requirements of processes, reengineering teams can explore what the new requirements will be when the organization wants to merge or extend the output of this process to other entities within the organization. Exhibit 4–4 illustrates how this analysis is done for the transfer of patients to referral centers. The first step is to list the process tasks, and then identify the assumptions that justify performing the process task. When the requirements are identified, the question of whether the task adds value or not can be answered. If this process is to be extended to another entity within the organization, the next question to explore is what the requirements are for this process task in this new environment. From here, the teams can begin to identify problems and issues that will influence the design of the process so that it can work in the organization in a global manner.

In the next phase, teams achieve breakthroughs by striving to think differently in their design approaches. They must also focus heavily on considering technology as a key enabler to the new design and seek alternatives that simplify processes and make them more cost effective.

CONCLUSION

In summary, the methods described are strategies recommended for process reengineering, improving current processes, and conceptual methods for identifying core business processes for organizations to center their focus. As always,

Exhibit 4–4 Identifying Assumptions and Requirements

Process Tasks	Assumptions	Requirements	Adds Value?	Requirements for New Sites
1. Patient is identified as appropriate case for transfer to referral center.	Physician, nurse, or social worker must initiate this process, analyze the case, and search for the right center.	A decision must be made on what care is needed and what center provides the services that match the care required. One individual can coordinate this process.	Yes Yes	Will need the decision to be made by a case manager in cooperation with the physician
2. Centers appropriate for patient needs are explored.	There are several that match this patient's needs. The centers will accept the patient in a timely basis. The patient and family will agree on the center that is recommended.	All options are explored in relation to cost and quality, and the patient is given a choice in the decision.	Yes	May need to add additional sites to accommodate patients in the new location
3. Family is approached with recommendations.	Physician, nurse, or social worker must initiate this step.	Must have informed consent by family and active involvement in the decision.	Yes	No different requirements
4. Family visits the center.	Family will do this independently.	Family must take initiative to visit centers and take an active role in the decision-making process.	Yes	No different requirements
5. Application forms are completed.	Papers must be filed after family makes the decision.	Centers need patient information and verification of payment prior to admission.	Yes/no—Perhaps this step can be streamlined in step two when searching for the appropriate center. Opportunity for automation is identified here.	Will need to maximize the transfer of patient information when transfers occur

process reengineering is no easy task. It does not, however, have to be laborious and extensive, and it does not take years to achieve dramatic improvements. It requires a management structure to create the focus for managers and staff to center all of their attention on the key elements of the products and services they provide. Once everyone is centered on these work activities, the opportunity for improvement and optimum productivity can be achieved. The organization can then move forward to the far-reaching goals of its mission and direction.

REFERENCES

1. Bergman R. Reengineering health care. *Hosp Health Networks.* 1994; 68(4):28–36.
2. Hammer M. *Beyond Reengineering: How the Process-Centered Organization Is Changing Our Work and Our Lives.* New York: Harper Business; 1996.
3. Hammer M, Champy J. *Reengineering the Corporation: A Manifest for Business Revolution.* New York: Harper Business; 1993.

CHAPTER 5

Chaos or Transformation? Managing the Process of Innovation

Jo Manion, MA, RN, CNAA, FAAN

To successfully navigate the chaos of the new millennium, the health care organization must be able to tap into the creative potential of its employees. Health care organizations today face a critical choice: Innovate and change or expect to be replaced by organizations that do. It is the choice between chaos and transformation.

Creativity and innovation are hallmarks of the most successful health care organizations in the country today. Successful innovation is not magic or something that just happens when the synergy is right. Organizations with a track record of successful innovation have discovered that innovation must be managed. Innovation management is a developmental process, a process of becoming that does not happen overnight.

These successful organizations have established an internal climate that supports entrepreneurial activity and goes beyond paying lip service to the idea of innovation and employee intrapreneurship. They recognize that innovation must be systematic, organized, and managed rather than sporadic, incidental, and accidental. Innovation is expected and encouraged in the organization, and seen as part of the work to be done rather than something that happens in addition to the "real work" of the staff.[1]

Source: Reprinted with permission from J. Manion, Chaos or transformation? Managing the process of innovation. *Journal of Nursing Administration,* Vol. 23, No. 5, pp. 41–48, © 1993, J.B. Lippincott Company.

Acknowledgments: The author thanks Diane Miller, BSN, MAOL, RN, and Sharon Cox, MSN, RN, consultants with Creative Nursing Management, for "sharing the light" and helping others understand a new framework for managing the change; and Nancy Post, of Post Enterprises in Philadelphia, Pennsylvania, for the tremendous work she has done in helping others understand the importance of balancing energy in their lives personally and professionally, and for the practical application of these principles to an organization.

Health care innovation and empowerment are closely related. Individuals must be empowered before innovation will occur on a systematic basis. However, not all individuals who are empowered in their daily practice accept responsibility for innovation. In some cases, the individual may not have the specific skills needed, or the traditional, bureaucratic system they are in has too many barriers to innovation.

Some of the most effective innovations are developed by people who know the organization at its core. Health care workers form the core of any health care organization and are in a position to be essential innovators. Take nurses, for example: Nurses are at the point of patient care delivery. Nurses have a generalist background that results in an understanding of the broad spectrum of needs exhibited by the client and family. On the other hand, creativity, the skills of intrapreneurship, and the management of change have not been part of nurses' formal education nor, in many instances, part of their socialization into the workplace. Most nurses have been socialized to the nursing role in a bureaucratic, hierarchic organization whose structure alone intimidates the novice innovator. Each of the health care disciplines has its own advantages and disadvantages when it comes to being innovatively orientated.

Innovation is the key to transformation of the health care organization and the health care system. While creativity is thinking up new ideas or putting things together in a new way, innovation is the implementation of the new or creative idea. Innovation implies that something has changed as a result of the creativity. The innovation may be a new product or service or a new way of doing something. It may be as small as a simple change in the department or as major as the development of an entirely new service or the redesign of work flow between departments. Managers and executives experience more success in their roles if their staff are skillful implementers of new ideas, and a specific process model can be helpful.

THE FIVE PHASES OF INNOVATION

The five stages for managing innovation are based on an energy model adapted for organizations by Nancy Post, an organizational development consultant.[2,3] The framework has also been used for managing change in an organization.[4,5] The five stages or phases are preparation, movement, team creativity, new reality, and integration. During the preparation phase, major concerns to be managed are the mission and purpose and certain resource allocation issues. During the second stage, structural issues such as decision making, authority levels, planning, and organizational structure are considerations. Team creativity, the third phase, involves overall coordination and cooperation, priority setting, networking, climate setting, and internal communications. During the phase of the new reality, productivity and maintenance of the change are key considerations. Integration, the final phase, requires attention to quality control and evaluative efforts.

Assessing performance in managing these developmental phases is a critical first step for any organization or department seeking to improve its skill at innovation management. The assessment tool in Exhibit 5–1 can be useful in such an assessment. The items are organized in groups of 10, with each group relating to one phase of innovation management. Questions 1 through 10 relate to phase 1, questions 11 through 20 relate to phase 2, and so on. Scores of 10 or less for each cluster of 10 items indicate areas of needed work. Specific interventions will be discussed for each phase.

The five phases can be used as a balance model as well as a developmental model. The key elements in each phase must be considered fully. If any of the five phases are weak, there will be an imbalance in the system, which will impact the effectiveness of innovation management in the organization. Likewise, if there is an overemphasis on the characteristics of any phase, there will be imbalance and difficulties in the system. For instance, the mission of the department as it relates to innovation and expectations for innovation from staff must balance with the resources available or there will be dissonance; similarly, a work group that is always planning but never reaches a decision is out of balance.

This model is also a developmental model and as such is sequential in nature (Figure 5–1).[6] Following these steps in sequence can help the leader manage the process of innovation. It is also an interactive and dynamic model. The primary issues of each phase are identified, and although it is recommended that they be considered sequentially, the issues of one phase can also appear and are appropriate to consider throughout the entire cycle. For example, although evaluation is a key element of the final phase, evaluation must also occur during the entire process, not just at the end.

Phase 1: Preparation

In the first phase, preparation, the two major issues of purpose and allocation of resources must be considered and managed. This phase is the foundation of the process. It is primarily leader driven and is often the responsibility of the executive and the team of internal leaders. Clear lines of responsibility should be identified and decisions made about appropriate levels of authority.

Simply put, innovation must be an important element of the organization's mission and a part of the everyday language before it will be accepted as a value. The leaders within the organization need to have and share a clear picture of how the organization will look and how the people within it will behave if innovation is a priority. The relationship of innovation to patient care and customer service must be clearly stated and demonstrated. Not only will it be important for members of

Exhibit 5–1 What's Your IQ (Innovation Quotient)?

Directions: Answer with the same environment in mind for each question. For example, complete the questionnaire thinking of the entire organization, the department, or a specific work group. Don't answer one question thinking of a single department and the next item thinking of the entire organization. Answer by circling Y for yes, N for no, and S for sometimes to indicate the frequency.

Y   S   N   1. Does the mission statement or statement of purpose include any reference to employee creativity and innovation?

Y   S   N   2. Do job descriptions or role expectations include the expectation for individual innovation or support of innovation?

Y   S   N   3. Do the annual goals include implementation of innovative ideas or strategies that increase employee creativity or innovation?

Y   S   N   4. Are the people who are always questioning the status quo and looking for a better way encouraged and seen as "creative types"?

Y   S   N   5. Is there a lot of energy and enthusiasm for change?

Y   S   N   6. Do employees have ready access to funding for innovative projects?

Y   S   N   7. Are mentors and sponsors available in the organization for the novice innovator?

Y   S   N   8. Do staff and managers have time during their normal workweek to work on innovations and creative projects?

Y   S   N   9. Do individual managers have control over funding so low-cost projects can be funded without a lot of rigamarole?

Y   S   N   10. Are resources shared between departments and work groups?

Y   S   N   11. Is time taken to actually plan for innovation (as opposed to moving very quickly from identifying the need to actual implementation)?

Y   S   N   12. Is there an established process for managing change and innovation that internal leaders understand and are expected to use?

Y   S   N   13. Is a formal proposal format or business plan required before an innovative idea is considered for implementation?

continues

Exhibit 5–1 continued

Y S N 14. Do all members of the department know what the expected format is?

Y S N 15. Is there flexibility in how the plan unfolds? (Or are people held to the specifics of the plan, i.e., the time frames, expenditures projected, process used?)

Y S N 16. Do the staff have easy access to the executive leadership team without having to go through multiple layers of management?

Y S N 17. Are plans developed before decisions are made?

Y S N 18. Are there established, agreed-upon time frames for completion of projects?

Y S N 19. Are levels of authority clearly identified for project teams and committees?

Y S N 20. Does the organization have a clearly articulated vision that includes an innovative environment and appreciation of creative ideas?

Y S N 21. Do problems actually get solved in the organization so that staff are not dealing with the same problems they dealt with years ago?

Y S N 22. Is there a spirit of cooperation in the organization? Can an innovator find others to cooperate in implementation?

Y S N 23. Do individual innovators retain control over their innovation as it is implemented rather than the idea being passed over to a manager or project director to actually implement?

Y S N 24. Is the general climate in the organization supportive, encouraging, and seeking of change and innovation?

Y S N 25. Is there a high level of trust in the organization between work groups, units, departments, managers, and clinical staff?

Y S N 26. Are the priorities established, resources assessed, and progress made on the important and major change projects underway rather than expending time and energy in an excessive number of projects at one time?

Y S N 27. Is the majority of the management within the organization stable and effective rather than involved in crisis management, continually "putting out fires" and feeling burned out?

continues

Exhibit 5–1 continued

Y   S   N   28. Are employees and managers skilled in creativity techniques such as storyboards, attribute analysis, brainstorming, and mind mapping?

Y   S   N   29. Can an individual innovator easily pull together a team of people from other departments and work groups to work together on a project?

Y   S   N   30. Are people comfortable with mistake making rather than seeing mistakes as something to be feared and avoided?

Y   S   N   31. Do people in the work group, department, or organization support each other rather than engaging in a significant amount of blaming, bickering, and backbiting?

Y   S   N   32. Are people in the organization encouraged to take care of themselves?

Y   S   N   33. Do people in the organization feel that they can set limits, say no to assignments and requests, and not become involved in a particular change project?

Y   S   N   34. Are managers and leaders well centered with a healthy balance of energy rather than feeling burned out and out of balance?

Y   S   N   35. Are workaholic behavior and perfectionism discouraged?

Y   S   N   36. Is the environment in the organization basically stable and secure rather than an environment of great anxiety, high flux, and chaos?

Y   S   N   37. Are there mechanisms in place that give long-term support to changes and innovations that are implemented?

Y   S   N   38. Is there recognition and support that productivity increases occur only after the change is well established rather than immediately?

Y   S   N   39. Are experienced coaches available for novice innovators?

Y   S   N   40. Are there specific interventions planned and implemented to nurture people during change and major innovation?

Y   S   N   41. Are the values of the organization or work group clearly articulated, with a clear connection between quality and innovation?

continues

Exhibit 5–1 continued

Y S N   42. Can employees articulate the values of the organization, and are the values articulated consistent with what is being practiced? (For example, while innovation and creativity may be articulated as important, in actual practice there is no allocation of resources to support it.)

Y S N   43. Are employees and leaders in the organization inspired to become involved as innovators rather than being exhausted with the day-to-day work demands?

Y S N   44. When new responsibilities and tasks are accepted, are current responsibilities and tasks modified?

Y S N   45. Are managers and leaders skilled at managing change and the emotions involved to reduce the chaos and turmoil that typically occur when something changes? Is it acceptable to express negative feelings about change (or is this seen and dealt with as resistance)?

Y S N   46. Are people in the organization receptive to and excited about change rather than "fed up" with change and the "promise that things will be better after this, but they never are"?

Y S N   47. Is there a specific evaluation process to determine whether or not, or in what ways, the change has been beneficial?

Y S N   48. Are mistakes freely shared and seen as opportunities for everyone to learn?

Y S N   49. Do people feel comfortable about eliminating the unnecessary (or is it difficult to let go of things from the past, including people or ways of doing things)?

Y S N   50. Do people look forward to the future and change rather than continually lamenting over the "good old days," the way things were before the merger, before the change?

Scoring Directions: Each Y is 2 points, each S is 1 point, and each N is 0 points. Total the number of points.

Interpretation: If the total score is 70–100, the environment is supportive of innovation; if the total score is 50–70, the environment is somewhat supportive of innovation; if the score is below 50, the environment is a barrier to innovation.

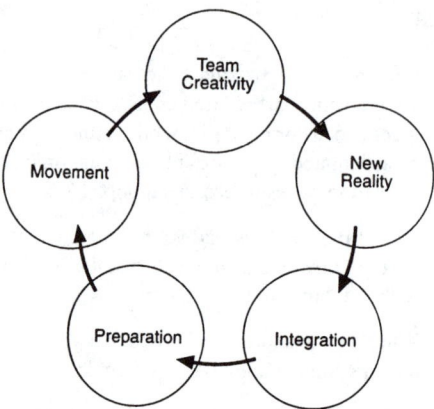

Figure 5–1 A Five-Phase Innovation Management Process

---

the leadership team to speak the language of innovation, they must communicate the expectation for innovation to the staff. This can be further emphasized by inclusion in the organization's and department's annual goals, performance appraisal process, and position descriptions.

The complementary issue of this first phase is allocation of resources, including human and material resources. Adequate resources must be available if innovation is an expected part of the work of the organization. These resources include time, access to other people, funding, and personal development time. It is difficult for people to work on innovative projects wholeheartedly if they must also carry a full work schedule. Although an enthusiastic staff member will be committed enough to do so, it is an abuse of the human resources of the organization to expect this additional commitment on a long-term or continuing basis. People will be "used up" quickly. Mentors and sponsors must be available in the organization or department for the innovator. Resources openly shared between departments and work groups will increase the environmental support for innovation.

In some instances, human resources need further development. Leaders and clinical and support staff should be carefully assessed to determine the need for educational opportunities. Managers should be prepared for their roles as innovation managers. Individual innovators need programs or opportunities that focus on innovation and the skill development needed by a successful innovator. All members of the organization benefit from general programs focusing on the need for innovation, essential skills, and their role in supporting fellow staff members who are innovators.

People need to hear this message repeatedly and observe actual behaviors and structural changes that support innovation before they will internalize the message that innovation is desirable and expected. The vision and day-to-day language must be congruent with the behavior of leaders. In some instances, changes in the structure of the organization may be needed. Dissonance is created if executives, managers, and leaders continually espouse the need for innovation, but staff have no access to funding for innovative ideas, new ideas can be implemented only after a tedious and difficult approval process, or the creative individual who is always searching for a new and better way is seen and treated as a troublemaker and one to be controlled. Leadership behavior must be congruent with the message being delivered.

Phase 2: Movement

Once the foundation is solidified, the leaders are clear about their purpose, the purpose has been consistently communicated, and resources are in place, staff will begin to experience actual support for innovation. The second phase, movement, is next in sequence. During this phase, the structural elements supporting innovation throughout the organization need to be established. A vision of how innovation will be carried out in the organization and how it will result in changes is critical. If the vision is clear, the structure needed to support that vision follows. The two aspects of this phase are planning and decision making.

Planning for a structure that supports innovation in the department is critical. Executive leadership facilitates this planning with participation and input from all levels within the organization. A process for evaluating new ideas, gaining approval, and arranging funding must be established. Two separate structures may be needed: one for large projects that involve integral changes in the organization and actual funding and a simpler process for ideas with less impact and a lesser need for resource allocation. One approach being used today is the establishment of a center for innovation within the organization. This provides a structure for building a financial support base, generating revenue, and receiving gifts. Establishing a specific process for seeking innovative ideas from staff members and guidelines for approval and funding decisions is part of the work of a center and supports the work of innovation throughout the system.

Potential innovators often need skill development in the planning function. Some innovative projects are approved with very little planning because they involve a small number of people and do not require additional funding. Formal business planning, however, may be necessary for large projects that have significant ramifications in the department and organization or require extensive resource commitment. Innovators need support and encouragement in learning how to develop a business plan. Support from other departments, such as finance or marketing, may be needed. Planning for staff to have access to these resources will be important.

The complementary issue of this phase is decision making, and it is closely intertwined with planning. Once the planning is done, decisions must be made. In some organizations, this is clearly out of balance. Much time is spent in planning, but plans are never carried out because actual decisions are not made. Once innovation-supporting structural changes are determined, assignment of responsibility is necessary. How will the process be initiated? Who will be responsible? How will levels of authority be decided? Realistic time frames need to be established for each element of the plan and for communicating the plan to staff.

As planning is completed, the need for further education and skill development for both managers and staff will become obvious. Planning skills often need to be developed or improved. In addition, there must be recognition that innovation planning is a process, not an end. By its very nature, innovation does not unfold as planned, and thus there must be support, not just tolerance, for ambiguity, making mistakes, and plan revision. Visioning and strategizing are key skills for innovators in addition to the basic skills of group leadership, meeting effectiveness, and consensus decision making.

A potentially unexpected reaction from staff and managers that may surface during this phase is anger. Although it may not be significant or widespread, it may be present. When a structure and process that support innovation are established in a department, the very creative individual may see them as stifling rather than liberating. Managers and leaders who have been supportive of the concept of innovation may feel irritated when they realize that successful management of innovation will take time and skill, that it doesn't just happen. They may need to develop new and different skills. It will be important to see beyond initial resistance and evaluate whether the structure established supports innovators or stifles their work. Too much structure can inhibit creativity.

Phase 3: Team Creativity

Once the foundation and structural issues have been dealt with, during the third phase things begin to come together. This phase is described as team creativity, or maturation, as the innovators within the organization actually begin using the structure that has been established. The issues of priority setting, climate developing, coordination, cooperation, team building and networking, and internal communications must be considered. Each of these issues is an important key, and lack of attention to any one will result in a system out of balance.

Priority setting is easier if the structure for evaluating and approving projects is effective. A formal structure assists in identifying the projects that will be supported in the organization during the year. In almost every department, however, there will be many other changes and projects being implemented simultaneously. A major concern most organizations are experiencing is the need to fix everything yesterday. Unfortunately, an organization or department that is engaged in too many projects may be reducing the likelihood that any are managed well. Determining the sequencing of major projects in the system can be difficult, especially when other important projects are added because of external demands. Priority setting is the difficult task of determining what is most important to accomplish with the resources available. It does not mean doing everything that needs to be done but rather making the difficult choices among those things that could be done. This requires extreme honesty by executives and leadership teams and a willingness to refuse implementation of projects for which there are no support resources.

Establishing a climate conducive to innovation is a key managerial role. Managers must be prepared and educated about the different elements of climate and group culture and accept responsibility for the climate within their work group. Managers who see their role as a catalyst are needed: They release the energy of innovators within the staff. The response to mistakes made is a major element related to climate. If the system or the individuals within the system have a punitive or blaming response to mistakes made, the environment will impede and stifle innovation. Do staff members feel comfortable about making mistakes, and do they understand that the making of mistakes is inevitable? Or do staff members want an environment where they do not make mistakes? When mistakes are accepted as part of work life and as lessons to be learned, people are more likely to be risk takers and successful innovators.

During this phase, attention must be given to the coordination of efforts to prevent duplication. Roles and responsibilities must be clearly identified and boundaries established. Levels of authority and access to resources must be discussed before the innovator receives approval and begins work on a project. Too often, the limits and boundaries are not discussed until conflicts or problems occur. Cooperation must be obtained from coworkers, project team members, and potentially from other departments, depending on the project or innovation. Executives and managers may need to "pave the way" or "open the door" for the innovator to obtain needed cooperation from other departments in the organization. Executives and managers who state expectations of cooperation and act as role models will help innovators work intradepartmentally in finding others to cooperate with the project.

Working effectively with a group or a project team is an important skill for many innovators. Although an individual innovator may need extensive coaching to be successful in this area, it is often more productive than pulling the project from the person who had the idea and assigning it to someone in the department who has already developed these skills. Each situation will need to be evaluated separately. Staff members may need to learn how to lead meetings, manage group process, and use consensus decision making. Many project teams are more effective with members from multiple disciplines and support departments in the organization. Access to specialists between departments is important. Members of the project team may need training in practical creativity techniques, such as game playing, brainstorming, mind mapping, storyboards, and attribute analysis.

Communication is the last key issue of this phase. If effective innovation is to occur, staff members need access to information. This includes information about the organization and trends in health care and in their discipline. Truly amazing innovations can occur when members of the department understand the big picture and the major challenges the organization is facing. Open communication between all layers of the organization is critical. Key messages often need to be repeated as many as 10 times through a variety of methods. Usually, the fewer the layers of organizational structure, the more open the communication becomes.

Members of all departments need to learn and use direct communication skills with each other. Negotiation skills are critical for innovators. People in the organization are expected to manage their relationships in a healthy and productive manner. This is not a typical pattern of behavior in most health care organizations and departments, and many times it must first be shown by the leaders before it is used by staff members.

Phase 4: New Reality

The fourth phase is the new reality. The key issues relate to stabilizing the environment, maintaining the direction that has been set, and actually producing results from the innovative projects and changes that have occurred. A common error made in innovation management is expecting productivity improvements or gains too early in the cycle. In projects where there are expected productivity gains, it may be months before the gains are realized, and productivity measures should not be prematurely used as a measure or indicator of success.

Stabilizing the change or innovation is an important step and should be considered carefully. Ways to anchor the change must be sought. This can be done by formalizing a structure or process that was used in trial, or by formally communicating the improvement or new service to the entire organization. Establish methods of rewarding and recognizing the innovator and project team. Rewards may come through increased learning and skill development, increased access to funding for future projects and educational support, or actual monetary rewards. Recognition can be through sharing of successes at staff meetings, through department or organization newsletters, or through specific celebration ceremonies. External opportunities for recognition and applause are wonderfully reinforcing for project team members. Support in publishing successes is another way of rewarding and recognizing innovators.

Productivity will be highest when managers and staff members are well centered, with a healthy balance of energy. During periods of intense change and innovation in a department or organization, people can overexpend their reserves of energy, leading to overall decreases in productivity. Encouraging self-care and paying attention to the self-care needs of managers and staff are critical in an organization that innovates successfully. Although innovation is hard work, it can be energizing for many people. There is a tendency to not pay attention to replenishment needs. Successful innovation managers recognize that change work takes a great deal of energy, and sometimes time frames need to be modified, the frequency of meetings decreased, or extended periods away from the work encouraged. The result will be increased productivity and creativity.

Phase 5: Integration

The final phase of the developmental cycle is integration or closure. The key issues in this stage relate to evaluative functions and quality. This phase is often overlooked or undervalued, and yet it is critical for future successes in the system. Although evaluation is an important process throughout this developmental cycle, at this phase it is a key issue. The innovation should be measured for its beneficence and effectiveness. During the planning phase, key indicators of success were developed. The process used to develop or implement the innovation is evaluated. Key questions should include the following: What did we learn? What would we do differently? Is there anything we can stop doing? Cultivate an attitude within the organization that these questions are a normal part of the process. Never let the evaluation process be construed as placing blame.

The quality of the innovation and the implementation process is the critical issue at this stage. How would the process be changed the next time? What are the lessons learned? In addition, the relationship between the innovation and quality of patient care should be clear and used as an indicator of success. The innovation may be only indirectly related to patient care, but the implementation of creative ideas implies that something is better as a result of the new idea.

An important leadership function during this phase is to take the time to go through closure. Too often a project or innovation is completed without formal closure. Closure can occur in the form of celebrations or events. These can be held even if the project or intended innovation was a failure. There are lessons to be learned and successes in the most dismal of failures. In almost every instance, innovations occur as the result of the efforts of many people in the organization. It is important to focus on the success or the process rather than the individual whose idea it was in the beginning. Recognizing and rewarding team effort will communicate respect for everyone's efforts. Closure also implies letting go of things. There may be a need for grief work, the breaking up of a project team, letting go of the "old way," or releasing of an old mind-set. The need for grieving should not be underestimated during this phase. By dealing with these emotions, the individuals involved will be ready to move to the next project more quickly.

CONCLUSION

The challenges facing the health care industry in the next millennium are perhaps some of the toughest it has ever experienced. Meeting these challenges successfully will require every strength the organization and its people have to offer. Innovative, empowered employees will not be merely desirable but absolutely essential for survival of the organization.

Creating a climate and structure within an organization that empower clinical staff and managers alike takes a strong commitment and consistent effort on the part of the executive and leadership team. To make the leap from creative ideas to a new reality requires a process for managing innovation. It requires establishment of a supportive climate and individuals who have advanced skills in creativity, developing new ideas and plans, and the implementation of change. Transformation of the organization is the potential result.

REFERENCES

1. Manion J. *Change from Within: Nurse Intrapreneurs as Health Care Innovators.* Kansas City, MO: American Nurses' Association; 1990:1–11.
2. Post N. Managing human energy: An ancient tool of change experts. *OD Practitioner.* 1989; 21(4):14–16.
3. Post N. *Working Balance: Energy Management for Personal and Professional Well-Being.* Philadelphia: Post Enterprises; 1989.
4. Miller D. *Managing Change in Chaotic Times.* Minneapolis, MN: Kundschier-Manthey; June 1991. Satellite broadcast.
5. Manion J. Managing change: The leadership challenge of the 1990s. *Seminars for Nurse Managers,* 1994; 2(4):203–208.
6. Post N. Systems energetics. Presented at the Creative Nursing Management meeting; Minneapolis, MN; August 1991.

CHAPTER 6

Process Redesign: Beyond TQM and Reengineering

Bette Keeling, MSN, RN, CNAA
Sherry D. Baker, MSN, RN
Linda D. Thompson, BSN, RN
Cyndy B. Dunlap, MPA, RN
Kerry K. Seely, RN

Lower cost, higher quality, and improved access have been the mandates for survival in a managed care health care environment. A revolution intended to achieve these goals began in health care quality improvement with the introduction of total quality management (TQM) and reengineering. They have been recognized as acceptable methods for improving quality in organizations. Successes have been obtained with both methods, but anxiety about them still seems to be high. The focus of this chapter is to explore the TQM-reengineering relationships and to describe the organizational preparation needed to go beyond TQM and reengineering to process redesign.

WHAT IS TQM?

TQM is a group of quality improvement approaches that enable the improvement of existing structures and processes.[1] The central ideas of TQM are to add value for customers through continuous change and improvement instead of accepting the status quo. Value is added by including individuals who are closest to the work being examined, by applying analytical tools to measure improvements achieved, and by listening to the customer as the first step to achieving improvement.[2]

Key to the use of TQM as a method to improve quality is to assume that the basic structures and work processes that exist are sound. The tools of TQM (flowcharts, cause-and-effect diagrams, and histograms) assist teams of personnel to identify specific areas that are problematic. Through application of the tools to analyze problems, discrete tasks and structures are separated and isolated from the underlying work processes. Incremental improvements are achieved through the enhancements made in tasks and structures. Repeated measurements are made to evaluate the improvements that are achieved through TQM.

The focus of TQM is on specific, targeted tasks or functions. An example would be to use TQM techniques to consolidate several different preadmission forms into one document that is used consistently to gather information needed to preadmit patients. Since specific areas are isolated for improvement, bits and pieces of work may be improved, but the underlying problems are not altered.

Organizations had an incentive to adopt TQM, since it was embraced by the Joint Commission on Accreditation of Healthcare Organizations (Joint Commission) as the method to conduct root-cause analysis with identified problems.[3] For those health care organizations wanting to obtain or maintain accreditation, incorporating TQM was the way to proceed with quality improvement initiatives.

WHAT IS REENGINEERING?

Reengineering is the fundamental rethinking and radical redesign of business processes to achieve dramatic improvements in critical measures of performance, such as cost, quality, service, and speed.[4] Individuals who are closest to the work being changed are also included in reengineering. Other central ideas of adding value for customers through reengineering include the following:

- Organize work around outcomes instead of tasks.
- Incorporate information-processing work into the work of the individuals who produce the information.
- Capitalize on information technology to share data across geographically separate areas.
- Combine or link parallel processes as they occur.
- Build decision-making control into the point where the work is performed.
- Capture information only once, at the source.[4]

Fundamental to the use of reengineering to improve quality is to start with a clean slate. Reengineering requires the remaking of processes. This approach is what enables the "radical" part of redesign to occur. There is no assumption that parts of the current process need to be retained. The ultimate goal is to replace flawed existing processes with redesigned processes that run smoothly for all customers.

Reengineering's focus is on work processes, not individual tasks or activities. Processes are structured, measured sets of activities designed to produce a specified output for a particular customer or market.[5] Focusing on processes instead of individual tasks requires thoughtful consideration regarding how service is provided and not just consideration of the tasks that are grouped together to accomplish work.

In the example of the revision of the preadmission form, notice that in TQM, the structure of a form was changed. In reengineering, the approach would more likely be to revise the admission process, one subpart of which would be the preadmission process that would address the preadmission forms.

WHAT IS PROCESS REDESIGN?

Process redesign is the synergy achieved between combining approaches from TQM and reengineering, and goes beyond TQM and reengineering through the development of an organizational infrastructure to support the changes that are implemented. The focus of process redesign remains on adding value for customers. Implementation of process redesign seems to be more dramatic than implementation of TQM or reengineering alone because of the massive organizational efforts necessary to prepare all employees, especially management and leadership.[4]

How do TQM and reengineering work synergistically? Figure 6–1 demonstrates the cyclic relationship between TQM and reengineering that the authors envision. Reengineering is used to achieve the dramatic improvements needed to compete in today's world. In the implementation of the reengineered processes, organizations may encounter glitches along the way. TQM is used to identify the glitches and make the necessary improvements until the reengineered processes are fully in place. Once in place, the reengineered processes may be incrementally improved through TQM techniques, until the work processes are reengineered again. TQM techniques are then used to refine the redesigned processes and make small improvements.

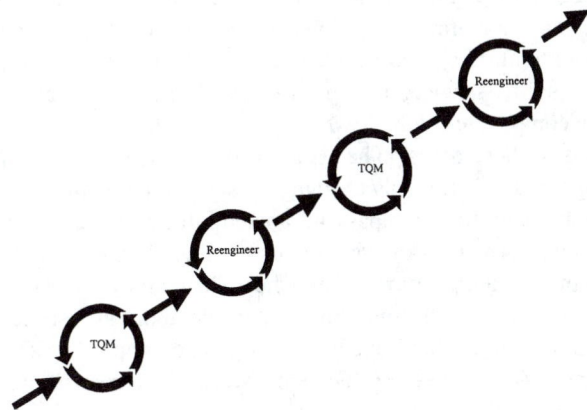

Figure 6–1 Cyclic Relationship between TQM and Reengineering To Achieve Process Redesign

WHAT IS ORGANIZATIONAL INFRASTRUCTURE?

Organizational infrastructure consists of the management behaviors and employee-employer relationships that act as barometers of "change readiness." Personnel often believe that managers are out of touch with the real work in the organization and may, therefore, distrust the intent of the change. In these instances, the managerial structure and the resulting employee-employer relationships are not change-ready. How does the organization become change-ready? A lot of preparation is necessary. While the list of preparations could go on ad nauseam, there are essential areas in which attention must be given to achieve success in implementing redesigned processes, which include communicating the scope of the changes, preparing management for the changes, and preparing the work force for the changes.

SCOPE OF THE CHANGES

TQM has been discussed as "playing with change" or as the "quick fix." Organizations are achieving incremental change with TQM but not the outcomes expected for the amount of time and effort expended to improve quality. Hammer[6] considers TQM as a mild, bottom-up approach to quality improvement. The scope of the changes implemented through TQM may change jobs slightly, but the changes do not typically cause job loss. Information gathering and analysis activities may remain separated. Automation of information gathering and use may not occur or, if it does occur, may not include existing positions within the organization. The number and types of positions may increase with TQM. For employees, the TQM scope may be less threatening than the reengineering scope.

Reengineering is a dramatic, top-down approach to quality improvement.[4] According to the literature,[1,4,6] radical changes must be made in work processes to achieve cost, quality, service, and speed goals. The incremental improvements that can be accomplished with TQM simply do not help organizations achieve dramatic gains in these areas.[4] The scope of the changes implemented through reengineering frequently not only change jobs significantly but may also result in job loss. As jobs begin to encompass automated information gathering processes and incorporate information analysis and use, the need for employees to conduct the activities in separate positions diminishes. The employees who remain in the reengineered organization become knowledgeable about all aspects of the process. Organizations have downsized, rightsized, and simply laid off employees, all in the name of reengineering. For employees, reengineering raises anxiety because of the fear of job loss.

Both TQM and reengineering can be affected by "scope creep." If the scope of the work is not clearly defined, the wrong task, function, structure, or work process will be improved. Close attention should be given to the problem definition statements. Exhibit 6–1 lists improvement opportunities, which have been identified in several different organizations, in which the authors have experience. Notice the difference in the titling and the scope. Most organizations that undertake TQM or reengineering efforts are truly trying to improve the accuracy of medication administration and not increase the medication error rate.

Managerial communication regarding the scope and nature of the anticipated changes at the beginning of the change is critical to gaining any level of trust with employees.[7] Process redesign requires new communication patterns. Because change is accelerated and the amount of information that needs to be shared is so large, traditional patterns of communicating may not work. The nature of the changes is personal in process redesign. Employees will have to change their work groups, working relationships, and mentors to survive.[8] As a result, communication needs to occur on a more personal level, with more frequent interactions with employees on a one-on-one basis.

PREPARING MANAGEMENT

Probably the biggest challenge facing any organization that plans to embark on a journey of process redesign is to prepare managers, especially senior management, to be enthusiastic role models for change and to let go of their turfs.[4] As the care delivery system is redesigned, collaboration among leaders from all areas will be essential.

The executive leader must be visionary in the approach to process redesign. Motivating employees to participate and be open to new ways of doing things will

---

Exhibit 6–1 Differences in Focus between TQM and Reengineering

TQM	*Reengineering*
Medication Errors	Medication Administration
Specimen Mislabeling	Specimen Identification
Operating Room Turnaround Time	The Surgical Process

require a positive enthusiasm for the changes, which must be reinforced by all managers in their communications to employees. Otherwise, actions will be taken to undermine or slow down the changes. Unrelenting efforts by the executive leader and senior management will increase the likelihood that the changes will be implemented and that resistance to change will be overcome.

Health care organizations have fairly rigid departmental and job boundaries that hinder the collaborative redesign of processes. The tendency of managers to "protect their turf" reinforces this rigidity. These barriers must be broken down to shift from a focus on tasks and structure to a focus on outcomes; otherwise, process redesign cannot succeed.[7] Senior managers have to move out of their comfort zones of managing budgets and people into managing communication and collaborative change efforts to achieve new outcomes across the continuum of patient care. Employees need to see that walls can come tumbling down at the administrative level. The role modeling that results enables employees to believe that it can also happen at their level.[7]

Change efforts often fail because of the lack of strong leadership at the highest level and a change agent to guide and support the redesign efforts.[7] A strong leadership coalition, linked with expertise in process redesign efforts, is necessary to achieve successful change. External consultants may be engaged as process redesign experts. However, the challenge for administrators is to retain control of the process redesign and not abdicate the responsibility to the external consultants. Successfully implementing redesign takes a team effort.

PREPARING THE WORK FORCE

Implementation of redesigned processes requires all employees to become learners. This is a massive undertaking for the following reasons:

- Jobs in the redesigned world are more complex, more highly technical, and require higher cognitive functioning to accomplish the information-processing requirements of data collection and analysis.
- There is not an unlimited pool of human resources waiting for jobs.
- Those who are available may be the least prepared to enter into jobs requiring employees to be highly technically competent, knowledgeable workers.[4]
- Previously confident and competent employees may not have all the necessary skills for the new work environment.

The only choice is to address the learning needs of the work force. The demographics of an area need to be considered when designing staff development programs for new hires and for existing employees. In addition to the role transition and technical skills that need to be taught for the redesigned processes, training will need to be conducted in the use of performance measurement data, interpersonal communication, and team dynamics.[7]

There is also a need to identify certain employees as "change support agents."[7] These employees are strategically placed in departments such as human resources, social services, or pastoral care. In addition to their work roles, they should be trained to listen, support, and assist employees through the rapid changes occurring in their work lives.[7] Change brings about anxiety. Support for employees becomes particularly important during times of high anxiety to enable them to continue to provide excellent customer service.

CONCLUSION

Process redesign requires increased communication, increased training and education, and highly visible executive involvement. Turf battles must be eliminated and change support agents must be in place for redesign to occur. The focus must be on total process redesign and the outcomes of those processes. With redesign, the work of employees becomes much more complex and, it is hoped, more empowering and stimulating.

The health care quality improvement revolution is fully under way. Further improvements can be achieved through the synergistic use of TQM and reengineering to achieve process redesign. However, organizational leaders should go into process redesign with their eyes open, knowing full well that change is costly, disruptive, and fraught with organizational and business risks.

To prepare for process redesign, massive management and employee retraining needs to occur to achieve the goals of lower costs, higher quality, and improved access across the continuum of care. The nature of the demands on the organization to achieve desired outcomes demands that organizational leaders understand that entering into process redesign is embarking on a long journey and not a quick trip.

REFERENCES

1. Lin B, Vassar JA. Implications of reengineering in health care. *Health Care Supervisor.* 1996; 15(2):63–68.
2. Health Care Advisory Board. *Total Quality Management.* Volume II. Washington, DC: The Advisory Board Co; 1992.
3. The Joint Commission on Accreditation of Healthcare Organizations. *Comprehensive Accreditation Manual for Healthcare.* Oakbrook Terrace, IL: Joint Commission; 1997.

4. Hammer M, Champy J. *Reengineering the Corporation: A Manifesto for Business Revolution.* New York: Harper Business; 1993.

5. Davenport T. *Process Innovation: Reengineering Work through Information Technology.* Boston, MA: Harvard Business School Press; 1993.

6. Hammer M. *Beyond Reengineering: How the Process-Centered Organization Is Changing Our Work and Our Lives.* New York: Harper Business; 1996.

7. Parsons ML, Murdaugh CL, O'Rourke RA. *Interdisciplinary Case Studies in Health Care Redesign.* Gaithersburg, MD: Aspen Publishers, Inc.; 1998.

8. Keeling EB, Linnen B. Managing communication in times of rapid change. *Sem Nurse Managers.* 1997; 5(1):18–24.

CHAPTER 7

Leading People through Organizational Transformation: The Human Side of Radical Change and Transformation

Edward L. Beard, Jr., MSN, RN, CNAA

Information on how to change an organization structurally is everywhere. It is in the literature, in seminars, and on the Internet. We are inundated with methodologies on how to restructure and how to improve the operations of the "body" (the processes of the whole organization). However, this information often lacks detail on how to deal with the behavioral ("mind") and cultural ("spirit") aspects of organizational change. Perhaps this is because leaders and managers lack basic skills in dealing with people on an emotional level. Or maybe it is because we as a society are uncomfortable with dealing with each other on an emotional or spiritual level. Another factor is that there is no overt reward system for dealing with the behavioral and cultural aspects of change. Our systems are designed to reward measurable outcomes—usually quality or financial outcomes. However, it is time for leaders to recognize that structural change without attention to the behavioral and cultural issues involved in change and transformation is unsuccessful. Ignoring these human needs will quickly derail any efforts at structural change.

Health care is undergoing massive change. An icon is being dismantled before our eyes—an icon built on systems development with a strong sense of value in the "goodness" of the system, self-centeredness, and power plays. As the fundamental driver of the industry—reimbursement—has changed, health care has been forced to go back to the beginning of process design and reengineer, to start over to build an improved, more efficient system, with the goal of delivering a higher quality, more cost-efficient product.[1]

This chapter examines the "human side" of radical change and transformation. Frequently referred to as the "soft" side of change, it is actually the most difficult piece in the overall transformation process. Issues to consider related to human needs in transformation are discussed, as well as strategies to ensure successful implementation.

THE PEOPLE SIDE

Health care is a product that cannot be delivered without people—professionals and technical human resources interacting intimately with consumers. These people have invested their time, effort, and energy into developing themselves and the systems in which they practice. This investment has led to a strong belief that the current state of the system is good and does not need to be changed. As such, it is common for resistance to develop when health care leaders attempt to introduce change.

People have their first experience with change within the family unit, where change abounds. They learn to live and work in a group as a family and become socialized to some degree around change initiatives. Often, how people learn to react to and cope with change in the family unit determines their future reactions to change. Leaders of a family unit are challenged to introduce change in a constructive way. They can succeed at this or introduce chaos. When people enter organizational life, they once again enter a family type of unit. Here, people tend to react to change in the way that they learned while growing up in a family. Past influences and learning directly affect the way people handle change in an organization.

The chaos of the health care environment over the past decade has stimulated leaders to introduce radical and far-reaching changes into the system. This change has been perceived and dealt with by organizations in varied ways. People have reacted to this change in many ways, often using the same coping mechanisms they learned in the family unit. Leaders have had to deal with these reactions and have often found it difficult, since there are so many varied responses to change.

People in organizations, just like children in a family, compose the core of the operation. Organizations would not exist if it were not for the asset of people. Leaders need to explore the needs of the people involved in organizational transformation and continual change as health care organizations continue to reengineer and move toward becoming fully process centered. Strategies to facilitate effective change must be developed and implemented. Outcomes to achieve regarding the human side or the "people" side of change need to be defined and evaluated.

EMPLOYEE NEEDS

It is no secret that change is often misguided and is introduced without attention to human needs. In the workplace today, employees are often performing at low levels of productivity and manifest many signs and symptoms of job frustration. Employees are frustrated; they are being asked to change but are not being provided with reasons to change.

Americans are socialized to make choices, to speak up, and to work together within a community to improve their personal and collective situation. The nation was founded on the principles of freedom of speech and freedom of choice. To many people, a mandate to change often feels like an inability to choose. Allen and Kraft[2] identified four key principles for ensuring effective change:

1. Involve the persons who are affected by the change initiative.
2. Establish clear goals, objectives, purposes, and tasks.
3. Transform from a sound base of information.
4. Demonstrate concern for people and reward for achievement.

It is essential that the human needs of trust, respect, and open communication become the basis from which leaders work through the change process.[3] When managers begin to introduce change, it is imperative that these guiding principles be kept in the forefront. Effective change is not possible without a buy-in from staff and employees. Employees will not accept change unless they understand it and it meets their needs.

What do those involved in a change want? Employees generally want the following from their organizations and managers: to be respected, to be heard, to be listened to, to be understood, to be appreciated, to be involved in the change, to be valued, to be informed, to be allowed to express fears of change, and to be given a chance to understand the change and actively participate in it. Paying attention to these needs will help ensure transformation that is effective and long lasting. Executives and managers need to include a needs analysis of the entire organization as it relates to change. This analysis can then be used to assist in developing a human needs plan for introducing radical change.

MANAGEMENT'S RESPONSIBILITY

When change is planned and initiated, management's responsibility is to be holistic. Managers not only must focus on the structural part of change, "the nuts and bolts" of process redesign, but also must plan for an effective mind and spirit change. This requires leaders who are knowledgeable about human behavior and have the ability to carefully manage the human response to change.[4]

Humans are basically capable of two emotions, happiness and fear. People often express emotions at the anger or sadness level without fully understanding the underlying emotion. Exploration of the feelings of anger and sadness will result in the realization that fear was the underlying emotion. Fear is expressed in the active form of anger and the passive form of sadness. Once anger and sadness are framed in this context, individuals can process the emotions and move forward. It is management's responsibility to ensure that a plan is developed that encompasses dealing with the human side of change. This includes strategies to deal with outward expressions and the signs and symptoms of change. Other expressions of change that management must be cognizant of include sabotage, increased absenteeism, increased tardiness, lower productivity, poor performance, attempts at unionization, burnout, insubordination, errors in care delivery, and voluntary termination of positions. Leaders must assess for and confront these possible reactions as radical change is introduced.

PLANNING FOR THE BEHAVIORAL AND CULTURAL SIDE OF CHANGE

In the past several years, many books have outlined strategies to increase personal effectiveness. The central theme of many of the outlined strategies is to "begin with the end in mind." In other words, decide what you want up front and then work toward it for achievement.

Strategies for Meeting Human Relations Needs

A plan for managing the human and cultural aspects of change ideally includes three elements:

1. definition of expected outcomes
2. education of all employees in the organization
3. development of effective communication and feedback mechanisms

When transforming organizations to become process centered, it is necessary to plan with specific goals in mind. Some likely goals of any plan for human relations in change include employee cooperation and participation, transformation of the organization, a "squashed" grapevine, lack of fear, retained job satisfaction, transformation of managers into change agents, enhanced professionalism, enhanced employee-management communication, transformation of human relations, and greater efficiency and effectiveness in process redesign. Goal establishment is critical to the overall plan development and also serves as an excellent indicator for evaluation of the plan. Exhibit 7–1 presents outcomes that can be used for plan evaluation.

A plan for meeting human relations needs should be developed by the entire management team. This type of group effort will provide greater assurance that managers develop a sense of "owning" the plan. Once the plan is perceived as being owned by the management team, the team will likely ensure the plan's success.

Exhibit 7–1 Outcomes To Evaluate the People Side of Change

1. *Understanding*—Staff fully understand the imperatives to change and embrace the reality of the need for transformation.
2. *Acceptance*—Staff accept the inevitability of the change and seek to communicate such in the work environment.
3. *Honesty*—Communication by the staff is honest and correct. The rumor mill does not exist.
4. *Belief*—Staff communicate belief in the new mission and vision of the organization as change is introduced.
5. *Cooperation*—Staff fully cooperate with the leadership and with each other as planned change is introduced.
6. *Fulfillment*—Staff's needs for information are fulfilled; they react appropriately to the planned change.
7. *Professionalism*—Staff practice in a professional manner and handle change initiatives professionally.
8. *Motivation*—Staff demonstrate real motivation in implementing the change. There is a sense of movement, excitement, and expectancy.
9. *Consistency*—There is consistency in the staff's response and actions related to the change process.
10. *Commitment*—Staff are committed to achieving the defined vision and the goals of the change. There is demonstrated belief in the new system.

A human relations plan should be written as an organizational document. It should be concise yet contain the critical elements needed to address employees' needs as change is introduced. The plan should be a written strategy that includes goals, interventions, and mechanisms for evaluation and redesign of the plan. Plan development should be led by the chief executive of the organization. The chief executive must believe in the plan and create high expectations for the management staff in implementing it properly. Lack of support by the chief executive is the most likely reason for plan failure.

The plan must be reviewed and presented in an inservice to the entire management team. Managers require a keen awareness of the purpose of the plan, the goals, and the proposed strategies that will be employed to meet human needs of the change process. Managers then need to communicate the plan to their staff. The staff need to understand the degree of commitment to the change by management and to feel that their needs and issues are being given priority consideration. The staff also need to be aware of how the plan will be implemented, along with specific time frames.

Defining Expected Outcomes

It is essential that the drivers of change, executive management, clearly define how the human aspect of change will be managed.[5] When change is approached with top managers unclear about their expectations, employees immediately sense the ambiguity and lack of clarity. This leads to development and sharing of misinformation and a lack of trust in the leadership of the organization.

As noted earlier, leaders are well educated in the structural aspects of change. However, carefully thinking through the aspects of how the change will occur allows leadership to "hash out" issues upfront and prevents "splitting" later in the process. The leadership group should consider the following questions:

1. How does the expected change relate to the vision of the organization?
2. What are the parameters of the change?
3. How will employees be involved in the change process?
4. What is expected of management and frontline staff in terms of communication?
5. How will employees be involved in the process?
6. In what time frame can employees expect change to occur?
7. What mechanisms will be available for communication and feedback regarding the change?
8. What can employees expect in terms of a timely response to their feedback?
9. What is the authority and responsibility of teams involved in the change process?
10. What rewards can be expected for effective change?

Defining expectations clearly from the top will lead to a greater sense of security as the change process unfolds.

Education of Employees in the Organization

Organizational leaders are charged with the task of analyzing the organization as a whole and working to improve its efficiency and effectiveness. In other words, when leaders introduce change, they have invested time in learning about issues so that they may clearly define the need for a change. Frontline professional and support staff have not had this same luxury. They are busy providing care and supportive functions for care, as this is what they are employed to do. Therefore, it is essential that all employees be given information within a framework that they can relate to their knowledge base.

To accomplish this task, the senior leadership group must develop the plan and content for the education of staff. Consideration must be given to the varying levels of education of the work force. It is unlikely that information given to managers would be easily understood by all other staff. Education must be tailored so that the employees can relate the need for change to their departmental functions and goals.

It is extremely helpful to begin the education with the broad changes occurring in health care. This provides the context within which the organizational changes are needed. Though such information often frustrates employees as they begin to understand the external forces driving the change in health care, it provides the needed perspective that change is required. It also provides the opportunity to reinforce what employees are doing well and how they can continue to improve to meet future challenges. Like senior leadership, they may not embrace the external forces, but they will understand that radical change is essential for the organization to thrive.

Once the contextual factors are outlined, the expected changes must be defined. It is essential that the changes be specific enough that employees can relate them to their everyday work. In addition, careful attention should be paid to avoid the use of esoteric terminology. Terms such as *reengineering* create the specter of job loss and result in mistrust. Employees cannot be expected to embrace the need for change when the description of the need is embedded in terminology that they cannot relate to or that they reject.

Development of Effective Communication and Feedback Mechanisms

Managing the human relations side of change involves careful attention to communication.[6] The new millennium is fast approaching. This new era will be focused on information and knowledge. When planning for change, there is often a misconception by managers that employees cannot handle information while it is in the formative stages. This is not true. When there is honesty, employees can handle much more than managers believe they can. When information is not shared with employees, they perceive the existence of a gap. The presence of this gap is the basis for the creation of what is commonly referred to as the "grapevine." A grapevine can be extremely damaging. It can be fraught with fantasies, misconceptions, harmful rumors, and other problems. It can grow exceedingly fast and squeeze the life out of an organization. Grapevines are nothing more than a community's attempt to have some information. It is not necessary that the information be factual. Rather, it is more essential that there be some information. Even distorted, untruthful information is better than no information at all. The premise to remember is that communication is the most needed and the most effective strategy for any human needs plan for change and transformation.

When ideas are in the formative stage it is perfectly acceptable to design a communication system that states this. Communications can be designed to include employees in the brainstorming phase of change. Instead of shying away from this traditional management function, managers should design a method for including employees in the idea-generation phase. Several methods should be considered:

1. *Brainstorming sessions.* These sessions should occur weekly with a group of representatives from departments involved in the change. They can be structured as short creative sessions in which employees brainstorm along with management. The leader must be adept at managing this process so that employees feel safe to share their input. Methods to facilitate group input (nominal group technique, round robin, etc.) should be employed. Building a reward system for those willing to participate in this process often improves interest and participation in the process.

2. *Regular written communication.* Let's face it—humans are creatures of habit! If employees know that clear, concise information will be communicated on a regular basis, a sense of security and a feeling of well-being ensues. However, information overload must be avoided. Today's health care environment is busy and complicated. Staff invest their energy where they see value. Most of the time staff work to implement their role in the organization. Communications about change should be concise, an "easy-read," and a value for the frontline employee's time investment.

3. *Electronic means.* In the new information age, electronic means of communication have become increasingly common in organizations. It is imperative that these communication methods be made available to all levels of employees as soon as is feasible. E-mail and electronic bulletin boards are excellent methods of communicating information within an organization. This method allows quick communication with many people. It also allows employees a "safe" way to communicate with leadership if they are uncomfortable and/or intimidated by the idea of having face-to-face communication.

4. *Rumor control.* Make rumor control a part of all team meetings. This is an effective strategy in drying up the grapevine. The author implemented this technique in the midst of massive organizational change. Leaders and frontline employees were discussing issues, using many "he said," "she said" quotes. Rumor control was adopted as an agenda item for every meeting. Typically, employees will not participate in this process unless they feel it is safe to do so. It is easy to create a safe zone by discussing rumors and asking if the group has heard any different twists on the rumor. Once rumors are laid on the table and individuals add the different variations on the

rumor that they have heard, the absurdity of most of the circulating rumors becomes self-evident. The leader then has the opportunity to clarify information.
5. *High visibility of leadership.* Leaders should maintain high visibility. Knox and Irving[6] identified that maintaining high visibility within the organization is key during radical change. Such action supports the principle of demonstrating concern for staff during a difficult time. It provides staff with an informal mechanism for asking questions and expressing their opinions. In addition, such access provides reassurance that communication goes directly to top leadership without being filtered through various layers of management or teams.

Leaders often approach communication from a framework of providing information. However, it is essential that communication be perceived from both a sender and a receiver perspective. Building feedback mechanisms into the communication process will promote a greater comfort level among staff.

CONCLUSION

Employees are the greatest commodity of an organization and must be viewed as such. Any change that is attempted without employee input and buy-in will be unsuccessful. Therefore, leaders must understand that when undertaking radical organizational transformation, effective planning and execution requires attention to not only structure and function but also to effective management of the mind and spirit of the individuals involved in the change. An investment in managing the human needs will result in a trusting and effective transformation process.

REFERENCES

1. Tonges M. The white water of change—A survivor's guide. *Nurs Manage.* 1997; 28(11):64–72.
2. Allen R, Kraft C. *The Organizational Unconscious. How To Create the Corporate Culture You Want and Need.* Morristown, NJ: Human Resources Institute; 1987.
3. Nagaike K. Understanding and managing change in health care organizations. *Nurs Adm Q.* 1997; 21(2):65–73.
4. Scott C, Diggins M. Managing the human side of change. *J Am Health Inf Manage Assoc.* 1994; 65(5):42, 44, 46–47.
5. Kerfoot K. The people side of transformations. *Nurs Economics.* 1997; 15(6):326–327.
6. Knox S, Irving J. Nurse manager perceptions of healthcare executive behaviors during organizational change. *J Nurs Adm.* 1997; 27(11):33–38.

CHAPTER 8

Teams: The Essential Work Unit

Patti Higginbotham, RN, CPHQ, FNAHQ

Teams have been the core of successful organizations from early experimentation with quality circles to the current fast-paced, continuously changing work environment. Teams come in a variety of packages: self-directed work teams, quality improvement teams, process teams, rapid action teams, and many others. The team of today focuses on a common objective; relies on measurement; maximizes human resources; and achieves increased productivity, lower costs, and improved quality. While some processes may be performed by individuals, most are performed by teams and cross departmental lines. This chapter will explore the concept of teams.

PROCESS TEAMS

Process teams are the essential work unit of a process-centered organization. The team has responsibility for performing, evaluating, and improving the tasks and processes that result in an activity or product that is of value to the customer.

Hammer states, "Process-centering takes the old functional department of the traditional organization and deconstructs it into two mechanisms: the process team, where work is done, and the center of excellence, where skills are enhanced and people are developed."[1(p.22)] The process teams appear equivalent to self-directed work teams or self-managing teams, where employees are involved in the daily management of their business. With self-directed work teams, the manager develops the skills of the work force and also functions as coach, team builder, champion, sponsor, and guidance counselor.[2] In both cases, the combination of work performance and human development composes the fundamental structure of the business.

Process teams are very similar to the patient-focused or patient-centered care models of the late 1980s and early 1990s. The tenet in those models was that designing the structure and processes involved in delivering care around the patient would improve efficiency and resource utilization. Patients were aggregated together in accordance with care requirements, that is, similar service demands as determined by protocols or pathways. Hospital nursing care units have traditionally been organized around groups of patients with similar diagnoses (e.g., orthopaedic, obstetrics, cardiac). What was different with patient-focused care was cross-training and multiskilling of team members, which were considered key factors in implementation of patient-focused care.[3] The unit secretary became a phlebotomist; a phlebotomist was trained to do routine vital signs; the pharmacist administered medications. The "new" model of patient-focused care came as a surprise and something of an insult to many health care professionals, who thought that was what they had been doing throughout their careers, as had health care workers before them.

Some hospitals began to reorganize and redefine work processes and to examine closely the level of staff needed to perform the functions. They asked, do we need to do this? If so, who will do it and how? Employees were asked to resubmit applications and qualifications for the reengineered jobs on patient areas where they had worked for several years. In some hospitals the new model was seen as the equivalent of "rightsizing"—matching qualifications with the job to be done and assigning jobs to the lowest level staff qualified and trained to perform the function. Those who shared successes with the patient-focused model, as reported in presentations at conferences or in discussions with peers from other settings, seemed to have been a part of the design team, were moving into new positions, or were part of a team designing a new unit or service. Patient-focused models were most successful when the environment was truly a fresh start—the clean slate espoused by reengineers. The culture and behavioral competencies of staff may not have been ready for such a radical approach in the reengineering of health care delivery systems. While patient-focused care may have been an early attempt at process centering, as described by Hammer, the model seems to have disappeared from the most recent journals.

What was important about this movement was that health care workers began to see their role as part of a process, rather than viewing only their task. The current health care environment with multidisciplinary clinical teams developing pathways and protocols, clear identification and understanding of key business processes (e.g., admissions, billing), and continuous performance improvement may be an indication that many health care organizations have in place the culture and infrastructure for process teams.

SUCCESS FACTORS FOR TEAMS

The success factors for process teams mentioned in Hammer's book[1] are consistent with success factors for improvement teams as well as process teams. Process-centered work is interpersonal work. Processes are not performed in isolation, and they cannot be successful unless there is mutual understanding among team members. Communication skills are essential. Team members provide feedback to each other on what is going well and what is not. Teams need to establish communication tools and methods not only for team members but also for others who perform the process or are customers of the process and can provide feedback.

Another essential element is measurement. The team, as well as the organization, needs to agree on what the key measures and desired performance levels are so it may measure and assess performance. Measurements of process and outcome need to be valid, reliable, and useful to the team. When given data about performance, teams and individuals react to improve and set the success bar higher.

Over the years, Deming's 14 Points[4] have been restated, renewed, redesigned, and reworked multiple times. These points were designed for business, and the applicability for process teams or health care may need to be demonstrated. Deming's principles continue to provide insight for creating a quality organization or a process-centered one.

TEAM ROLES

If an organization is to perform, it must be organized as a team. Within the team, each member must act as a responsible decision maker. Even so, an organization must be managed.[5(p.91)] This is seen in the process-centered organization and its team members. Many leading business thinkers compare business to football, and the positions on the team can be compared with the roles of an organization.[1(pp.109–115)]

All organizations have a senior executive, president, or chief executive officer. This is the organization's "head coach." The head coach creates the organizational culture, its vision and values, and its strategies and is responsible for motivating the team to achieve the overall business objectives.

The manager or coach has the responsibility of staffing the process with well-selected and well-trained people. It is his or her job to guide and mentor employees, to develop and maintain the supply of skilled individuals, to allocate resources, and to facilitate problem solving. In many health care organizations, the manager is also the offensive and defensive coordinator. He or she frequently designs the process and is responsible for deciding who does what and in what order. The manager may not be the most skilled worker, and in fact, the most skilled workers should be on the frontline. What the manager must have is a keen understanding of the company's business and of those processes for which he or she is responsible. The most important skill for the manager is developing other people's skills. Just as a great football player does not necessarily make a great coach, a great coach may not be a great football player.

Process design is not enough to ensure that the process will perform well. The team also needs team members (football players). The players are the workers who execute the process and have a common objective. In a process team the members must play *as* a team, not just on the team. Each member of the team becomes a skilled, knowledgeable professional, not just in his or her own discipline but in other tasks essential to the process. Just as Deming emphasized the need to train, educate, and retrain, the process-centered teams should be cross-trained.

Hammer believes that a process-centered worker is a "self-employed professional, a hybrid of a professional and an entrepeneur."[1(p.51)] The successful entrepreneur focuses on the customer and the customer's needs. He or she understands the process and does what it takes to get the job done. To be successful, the entrepreneur must see the bigger picture of the business universe and understand that success of the team and the process means success for the business and for the individual. The entrepreneurial approach may be difficult to visualize for those who have been employed by a hospital for the duration of their professional work life. An analogy can be drawn to outsourcing. Hospitals are more frequently outsourcing services, for example, dietary, housekeeping, transcription, and billing. Consider how an individual would behave if he or she owned the company that had been hired to provide transcription services. What performance expectations should be measured if the company is to continue to have the contract to provide the service? Who decides what is successful performance? Who are the customers? How does the company communicate and with whom?

THE NEXT CHALLENGES

The next challenges for teams in health care are how to make changes and improve processes more rapidly and, second, how to sustain improvements. The process team seems ideally placed to include process improvement and problem solving within its scope of authority and responsibility. However, rapid improvement seeks to eliminate waste and non–value-added activities. Can the process team be objective enough to make changes that may eliminate a team member's job? That question remains to be answered.

Several models for rapid change have appeared on the market from well-known consultants such as the Juran Institute and the Institute for Healthcare Improvement.[6,7] Some ideas for rapid change include the following:

- Clearly identify and state the problem.
- Understand the process and identify the root cause.

- Use subgroups to study and develop action plans for various parts of the process and use the full team meeting only to put it all together and to implement rapid whole-system changes.
- Collect and use minimal sample data.
- Take advantage of existing research and literature to model change.
- Spend time outside meetings for discussion, planning, and statistical analysis.
- Do the obvious—eliminate redundancy, wasteful steps, and duplicative procedures.
- Communicate frequently with those who will be affected by change.
- Implement change and have the process team monitor the progress.

CONCLUSION

Teams are tools, and each team has its own uses, characteristics, requirements, and limitations. Teamwork is neither good nor desirable—it is a fact. Whenever people work together, they do so as a team.[5(pp.101–102)] In the process-centered organization, the process team is the way people work. The process team members are not closely supervised drones. They are self-directed professionals focused on creating customer value. It is what they achieve that defines the capability of the process-centered organization.

REFERENCES

1. Hammer M. *Beyond Reengineering.* New York: Harper Business; 1996.
2. Williams R. Self-directed work teams: A competitive advantage. *Quality Digest.* 1995; (November):15(11).
3. Buchan J. Patient-focus pocus? *Nurs Manage (London).* 1995; 2(7):6–7.
4. Walton M. *The Deming Management Method.* New York: Dodd, Mead & Co; 1986:34–36.
5. Drucker P. *Managing in Times of Great Change.* New York: Truman Talley Books/Plume; 1995.
6. Alemi F, Moore S, Headrick L. Rapid improvement teams. *Joint Commission J Quality Improvement.* 1998; 24(3):119–129.
7. O'Malley S. Total quality now! Putting QI on the fast track. *Quality Letter.* 1997; (December): 2–10.

CHAPTER 9

Leading Upstream: Implementing Process-Centered Leadership Skills

Janice K. Bultema, MSN, RN, CNAA, NHA
Marcia A. Colone, PhD, LCSW

The essence of leadership is best understood by reflecting on parables told by Oriental masters.[1] One parable* tells the story of Emperor Liu Bang, in the third century B.C. To celebrate his achievement of consolidating China into a unified empire for the first time, the emperor held a celebratory banquet. In attendance were several important people, including Chen Cen, the master who provided enlightenment to Liu Bang throughout the campaign. During the course of the celebration, Chen Cen's disciples were baffled as they observed the emperor sitting at the head table among his expert heads of staff: a logistician, a tactician, and a strategist. Without noble birth or the knowledge possessed by his heads of staff, the disciples could not understand how it was that Liu Bang was the emperor.[1]

Chen Cen explained this phenomenon by telling stories of the spoked-wheel and sunlight. He explained that the strength of a spoked-wheel depends on the sturdiness of the spokes and the manner in which those spokes are spaced and connected. Therefore, when considering a wheel, one must consider not only the rim and the spokes but also the spaces in between. "The essence of wheelmaking lies in the craftsman's ability to conceive and create the space that holds and balances the spokes within the wheel."[1(p.128)]

When the disciples further queried how the craftsman secured the harmony between the spokes, Chen Cen reflected on how the sun nurtures plants and trees

Acknowledgments: The authors acknowledge Anne M. Bolger, Senior Vice President, Hospital Operations; Mary Kay Getzfrid, Manager, Transition Planning; and Jason Pinchot and Nicole Kemerer, all of Northwestern Memorial Hospital, Chicago, Illinois, for their support and assistance in the preparation of this manuscript.

by giving away its light, but in the end the plants and trees grow in the direction of the sun. He explained that by "placing individuals in positions that fully realize their potential he secures harmony among them by giving them all credit for their distinctive achievements."[1(p.128)] He further expounded that just "as the trees and flowers grow toward the giver, the sun, individuals grow toward Liu Bang with devotion."[1(p.128)]

In this ancient parable are many lessons of leadership that are particularly relevant for today's postindustrial-age organizations. During the industrial age, managers focused on building hierarchical organizations and managing rather than leading. These strategies were effective at the time, but they no longer facilitate the work to be done. Today's organizations are moving toward process-centered structures that require leaders.

Managers who were effective in the old structures must learn new skills to be effective. They will frequently feel like they are swimming against the currents of old behaviors and structures, and at times the currents will be so strong they will drift downstream to the familiar waters of hierarchy and management. But when leaders find that those old ways no longer work, they begin the swim upstream again, with the goal of surpassing the distance they swam before. To help tomorrow's leaders navigate in the strong currents and meet their goals, the authors describe the traits and behaviors required by leaders in process-centered organizations.

RESPONDING TO TODAY'S UPSTREAM ENVIRONMENT

New Roles

The leadership behaviors described in the Wheel and the Light* parable[1] are very similar to those Michael Hammer defined in *Beyond Reengineering: How the Process-Centered Organization Is Changing Our Work and Our Lives.*[2] Hammer would label the expert chiefs of staff as process owners, Chen Cen as the coach, and Liu Bang as the business leader. Hammer wrote that leaders in process-centered organizations are responsible for entire processes: the work itself and its outcome. However, he emphasized that process-centered leaders share the responsibility and accountability with all members of the process team.[2]

Liu Bang's tactician, for example, just like General Norman Schwarzkopf in the Gulf War, designed and shaped the offensive process of the battle but was not single-handedly responsible for the outcome of the battle. The soldiers on the

---

Source: Reprinted by permission of *Harvard Business Review*. An Excerpt From *Parables of Leadership* by W. Chan Kim and Renee A. Mauborgne, July–August 1992. Copyright © 1992 by the President and Fellows of Harvard College; all rights reserved.

frontlines were responsible and accountable for their roles in the battles and for responding to surprise attacks or maneuvers.[2] Like General Schwarzkopf, leaders in process-centered organizations must create processes; sustain the processes by developing the organization's resources, its employees; and renew and redesign the processes to remain responsive to the organizational changing environment (Figure 9–1). But leaders cannot achieve success independently. To be successful and responsive to the environment, leaders must enter into a partnership with the organization's customers and employees (Figure 9–2).

New Structures

Today's climate of rapid changes in society, markets, customers, competition, and technology[3] mandates that organizations restructure to be able to respond quickly and anticipate market demands. This requires moving beyond strategy, structure, and systems to a focus on processes and people.[4] Hammer suggested that "the kinds of work that people do, the jobs they hold, the skills they need, the ways in which their performance is measured and rewarded, the careers they follow, the roles managers play, the principles of strategy [they] follow"[2(p.xiii)] are all re-created in a process-centered world. No one recipe creates success in all organizations, but experts predict that a framework based on purpose, process, and

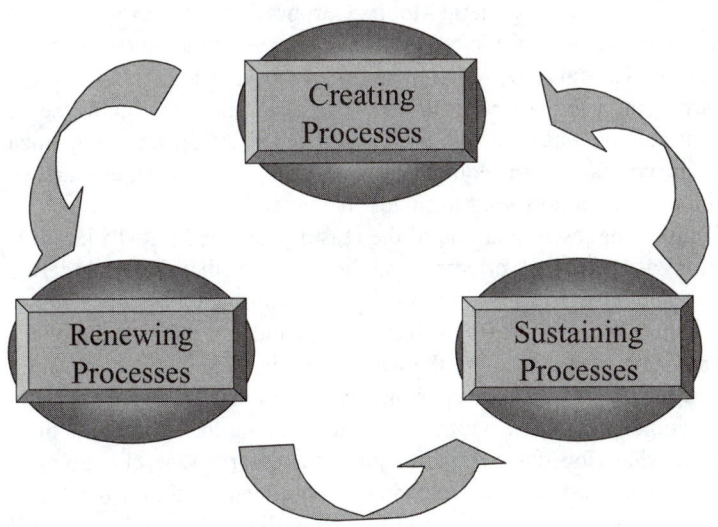

Figure 9–1 Process-Centered Leader's Core Functions

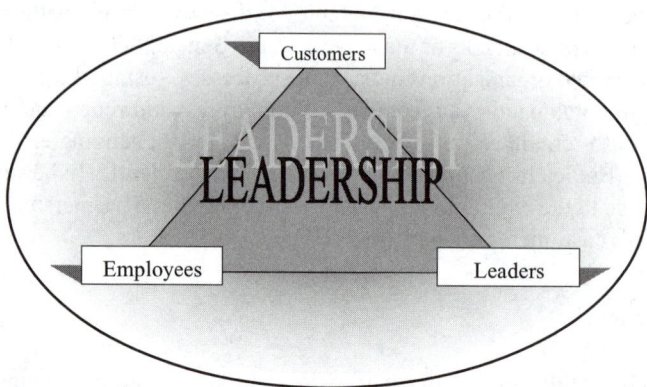

Figure 9–2 Process-Centered Organizational Partnership

---

people will best position organizations for fluid responses to the metamorphosing marketplace.[4]

Business literature is replete with models that organizations embraced to improve performance: developing learning organizations, initiating self-directed work teams, downsizing, rightsizing, empowering, and reengineering, to name a few.[4] These are all types of reorganization—a term that has become the organizational mantra of the century. General Motors Corporation is one example of a firm that has reorganized 30 times in the last 30 years, and at the time of this writing it is about to undergo its 31st reorganization.[5] According to Peter Drucker, the world is rearranging itself so drastically that two generations from now we will not be able to imagine what life was like in this decade.[6] Constant reorganization and restructuring have been required because most of the change models have not resulted in measurable long-term positive outcomes.

Hammer suggested that one of the reasons for this limited success is that the solutions are often task oriented, and the problems that afflict modern organizations are not task problems but rather process problems.[2] Task solutions are akin to examining one part of the problem versus understanding and solving a related group of tasks that constitute the whole. Another reason various change models have met with limited success is that organizations often apply the new models with a cookbook approach rather than customizing the structure to the organization and changing basic organizational behaviors.[7] One change agent wrote, "People, like rivers, may try to change their course, and they may even succeed for a while, but eventually they return to familiar habits and paths."[8(p.90)] Indeed this will be the outcome of many process changes and reorganizations because the new structures and systems are not properly supplemented by leadership and culture changes.

Each organization must build on its history and culture to define its own path toward process-centered operations. Some organizations will transform to a total process-centered structure, while others will superimpose processes on the existing hierarchical organization. Both alternatives have their challenges, and skilled leaders are essential for the transformation. Whatever the organizational structure, key leadership traits and behaviors are indicated to maximize organizational performance in a process-centered environment.

This chapter is not intended to be an exhaustive discussion of all leadership characteristics but instead a synopsis of fundamental skills required for success in process-centered organizations. These essential leadership skills are described using the framework of process-centered leaders' core functions: creating processes, sustaining processes by developing resources, and renewing and redesigning processes (Figure 9–3).

CREATING PROCESSES

Leaders in process-centered organizations do not create new processes; instead, they redefine the work of the organization in relation to its customers. This requires recognizing individual tasks and activities that historically were performed in separate departments, and linking them together. Since one individual does not possess the entire body of detailed knowledge, the process leader relies on the

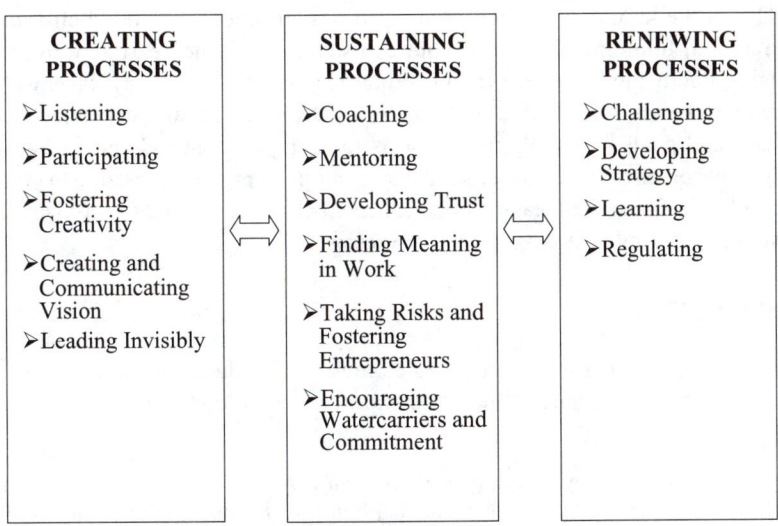

Figure 9–3 Process-Centered Leadership Skills

expertise of the team members to design a comprehensive process. However, the leader maintains a critical role, ensuring that the process meets the needs of the customers and the organization.[2] Following is a discussion of the essential skills required for creating processes.

Listening

Since processes need to be built around customer needs in a responsive organization, the process designer needs to be able to hear what the customer verbalizes and does not verbalize. The required listening skills are best explained by another parable.* In the third century A.D., King Ts'ao sent his son, Prince T'ai to study under a great master.[1] The master sent Prince T'ai to the forest for one year with the assignment that upon return, he was to describe the forest sounds. Prince T'ai returned in one year and described the sounds of the wildlife and wind to the master. The master responded by sending Prince T'ai back to the forest to listen again. After listening for days and nights on this second journey to the forest, Prince T'ai started to hear new sounds and was convinced these were the sounds the master wished him to hear. He returned to the master and reported that he could hear the flowers opening, the grass drinking the dew, and the sun warming the earth. The master was pleased with his student and said, "Only when a ruler has learned to listen closely to the people's hearts, hearing their feelings uncommunicated, pains unexpressed, and complaints not spoken of, can he hope to inspire confidence in his people, understand when something is wrong, and meet the true needs of his citizens."[1(p.124)]

This is the kind of listening required to design processes around customer's current and future needs, and it requires listening with the heart as well as the mind.[9] Effective leaders need to know their customers and employees as well as they know themselves. This includes knowing their beliefs, cultures, perceptions, values, and goals.[10] Equally important is listening without judgment,[9] because judgment serves as an unconscious filter to our perceptions. To be able to engage in this level of listening, leaders must constantly be out among the employees and customers. Listening is not a one-time exercise.

Participating

Successful process design requires teamwork. Phil Jackson, former coach of the Chicago Bulls, stated, "Good teams become great ones when the members

---

Source: Reprinted by permission of *Harvard Business Review.* An Excerpt From *Parables of Leadership* by W. Chan Kim and Renee A. Mauborgne, July–August 1992. Copyright © 1992 by the President and Fellows of Harvard College; all rights reserved.

trust each other enough to surrender the 'me' for the 'we.'"[9(p.21)] This takes equal participation of team members with diverse talents and abilities. Just as Jackson needed to teach Michael Jordan, whom he referred to as the Michelangelo of basketball, that "the true measure of a star was his ability to make the people around him look good,"[9(p.172)] leaders need to empower their stars while connecting them with the team.

The reason participatory process design is so important is explained in The Wisdom of the Mountain* parable.[1] Lao-li, a disciple of a great master who lived on a mountain, studied for more than 20 years but had not reached enlightenment. He finally decided that he should give up hope, and told the master that he was going to leave the mountain. The master offered to walk down the mountain with Lao-li. Before they started their descent, the master asked Lao-li to describe what he saw. Lao-li described the sunrise, the village below, and the mountains in the horizon. They then started their descent. Part way down the mountain, the master again asked Lao-li to describe what he could see. This time Lao-li described the livestock and children he could see in the valley. The master smiled and they continued to climb down from the mountain. When they finally reached the town, the master asked Lao-li what he had learned, but Lao-li had no response. After a prolonged silence, the master explained that what could be seen from the top of the mountain was different than what one could see from the bottom. He then added, "Alone one sees only so much—which in truth is not much at all."[1(p.127)]

As explained by this parable, one person alone, regardless of skill, has a limited view and limited insight. As Max De Pree, chairman of the board of Herman Miller wrote: "Leaders need an ability to look through a variety of lenses. We need to look through the lens of a follower."[11(p.7)] Organizations can only design a comprehensive process by engaging others from various levels in the organization and with diverse perspectives and abilities. The leader plays an important role in facilitating this participation. Sometimes employees on the frontlines and customers are limited in their vocabulary, are uncomfortable speaking, or intervene at inappropriate times; but that does not make their perspective or opinion less valuable.[3] The leader must help others listen with an open mind.

Leaders must encourage team members to express their views and encourage others to challenge those views and present their own. This will result in tension because some members feel strongly about their viewpoints. The leader must be able to defuse the defensiveness without squelching the exchange and help the team build consensus.[8] When consensus is reached, each team member feels own-

---

*Source: Reprinted by permission of *Harvard Business Review.* An Excerpt From *Parables of Leadership* by W. Chan Kim and Renee A. Mauborgne, July–August 1992. Copyright © 1992 by the President and Fellows of Harvard College; all rights reserved.

ership of the process. This does not happen quickly. However, in today's environment, time is critical and the leader may need to help the group agree that the process defined is the best for that time and that the team needs to initiate action. The risk of not acting is to get locked in process-definition paralysis while the organization's competition moves forward and captures market share.

Fostering Creativity

Overlaying or transplanting a process that has worked in another organization is tempting, but it is doomed to failure. Process transplants face the same potential for rejection as organ transplants if they are not matched to the organization and its customers.[8] To redesign a process around the customers' and organizations' needs, process leaders and team members need to think outside of normal boundaries. This requires creativity. Innovative strategies need to be enlisted to generate this kind of thinking.

Phil Jackson often used movie clips as a teaching device. For postgame review sessions, he spliced clips from games with movies such as *The Wizard of Oz* and *An Officer and a Gentleman.* The players, while laughing at themselves, learned valuable lessons about their performance.[9] Likewise, one of the authors recently used the movie, *Babe,* for a team session on leadership. The resulting list of leadership traits matched most textbook lists, but by using a creative learning strategy, the team members engaged in the session and internalized the content more quickly. It also helped them to discover fresh and original leadership characteristics.[9(p.164)]

Using metaphors rather than logic is another way of fostering creativity. Employees of a car company who were working to improve their customers' satisfaction with the shopping experience compared their operations to chocolate. The employees described chocolate as one of their favorite foods and then described the characteristics of chocolate that they found most pleasing. Once that was defined, they set about creating a customer shopping experience that, like chocolate, would be smooth, sweet, and comforting. By mixing up the concepts, they were able to creatively redefine their operations without being biased by existing paradigms.[12]

Hand and hand with creativity comes risk taking. Encouraging autonomy and creativity will certainly result in successes and failures. As a leader in health care stated: "I know that 80 percent of every plan will work smoothly, but consistently 20 percent will cause problems and the need for revisions. . . . I expect 'stumbling blocks,' and I know that some things aren't going to go as planned. As a leader, I am there to support people and help them figure out how to get around the problems."[8(p.94)] Leaders must be able to allow people to learn from mistakes and must deflect requests for instructions by asking employees their own opinions on the preferred course of action. This action develops employees' potential.

Creating and Communicating Vision

Participation is as important in creating a vision as it is in defining a process. Phil Jackson wrote: "Visions are never the sole property of one man or one woman. Before a vision can become reality, it must be owned by every single member of the group."[9(p.100)] He added, "When your vision is based on a clear-sighted, realistic assessment of your resources, alchemy often mysteriously occurs and a team transforms into a force greater than the sum of its individual parts."[9(p.100)] Jackson's six National Basketball Association championships were a testament to his ability to create this chemistry with independent and diverse superstars like Michael Jordan, Scottie Pippin, and Dennis Rodman.

Creating a vision for a process starts with looking at the positive aspects of the current process rather than focusing on what is wrong with the process.[8] Once the team is clear about what the process should look like, the team can begin to develop strategies to accomplish that purpose. The process and desired outcome need to be worded to catch the employees' interest and passion.[4,13]

To stay alive, a vision must be communicated. Clear communication relies on using a variety of communication vehicles[8]: Say it, write it, and visualize it. Several years ago, Frank Dale, who was hired as the new chief executive officer (CEO) of the Los Angeles Herald-Examiner after a violent 10-year strike, provided an excellent example of communicating a vision. The building had been barricaded and empty for eight years, so the new CEO had to enter the building through the back door on his initial day of work. The first thing he did was suggest to the employees that they open the front door. Letting the sunshine in was a symbolic step toward a new future. Dale also developed a missile metaphor to communicate the challenge of catching up to their main competitor newspaper. He displayed missile posters throughout the facility, and he equipped his office chair with an airplane seatbelt that he fastened each day as he took his post. Every employee was clear about the new mission of the Herald-Examiner.[14]

Jan Carlzon, CEO of Swedish Air, is another good example of an effective communicator. In his first two years at Swedish Air, he realigned the company's mission to be customer driven and spent half of his time out in the field communicating to employees. This communication included Carlzon explaining the mission, giving examples of the new empowered employee role, and listening to the employees. He wrote that listening to the employees helped him shape his strategic thinking, win the employees' support, and accomplish their goals. Carlzon believed in clear and simple messages. The company wrote a booklet to present the mission and expected employee role. Each page contained only a few words in big print and animated cartoons of an airplane smiling, frowning, and so forth. Carlzon related that this booklet was widely criticized for being too simplistic but that it was successful internally because it used simple messages and symbols.[13]

Leading Invisibly

In successful process design, the leader is behind the scenes. Phil Jackson's goal as a coach was to be invisible. He believed that a coach's best method of building a team was working with the players and "shaping their role."[9(p.161)] This is the message the master taught in the Wheel and the Light* parable when he said that an essential part of the wheel was the space between the spokes.[1] Phil Jackson strove to be an effective leader by being the space between the spokes.[9]

Another metaphor that explains this concept is that of a bowl.* In describing a bowl, one must consider the material the bowl is made from as well as the hollow—the space that creates the bowl's shape and size.[1] Without the hollow, it would not be a bowl. Leading by invisibility may seem to be contrary to the charismatic leadership style advocated by many leadership experts. But in a team-oriented, process-centered environment, it is essential. Leaders must think of the good of the organization and their team rather than their own recognition and reward.[15]

The parable of Fire and Water* further explains this concept.[1] In the fourth century B.C., Duke Chuang, who governed a small district, realized that the district was deteriorating under his rule. He set out to visit the great master Mu-sun to seek his guidance. Mu-sun silently walked him to a river where they sat and meditated for a time. Then, still without speaking, Mu-sun built a fire. After meditating on the fire for hours, Mu-sun turned to Chuang to ask if he now understood how the district prospered under the former leader but declined under Chuang's rule. Since Chuang had not grasped the answer, Mu-sun proceeded to reflect how the strong fire had burned intensely, savagely, and loudly for several hours, and that it would have overcome whatever had come in its path. The fire, in the end, had been consumed by its own fierceness and turned into a handful of ashes. Mu-sun contrasted the fire to the water that had started as a stream in the mountains. The river continually flowed downward, sometimes rapidly and loudly and sometimes so slowly that it could not be heard. Unlike the fire, the river did not come to an end but became deeper and more powerful as it traveled toward the ocean, nurturing all that came in its path. Mu-sun counseled, "For as it is not fire but water that envelops all and is the well of life, so it is not mighty and authoritative

---

*Source: Reprinted by permission of *Harvard Business Review*. An Excerpt From *Parables of Leadership* by W. Chan Kim and Renee A. Mauborgne, July–August 1992. Copyright © 1992 by the President and Fellows of Harvard College; all rights reserved.

rulers but rulers with humbleness and deep-reaching inner strength who capture the people's hearts and are springs of prosperity to their states."[1(p.125)]

The best leaders, as this parable* teaches, are those who humble themselves to their followers. It is their job to be behind the scene, supporting and empowering the followers. The leader invisibly nourishes the followers just as the water in the soil that seeps from the riverbed provides sustenance to the trees and flowers that grow above the soil.

SUSTAINING PROCESSES

Regardless of how well the process is designed, the right employees are necessary to implement it. Leaders in process-centered organizations must develop the team and its members, who are expected to perform as professionals—able to direct, problem solve, and make decisions autonomously.[2] However, many employees in organizations do not currently fit that description. Leaders have a responsibility to develop those team members. They also have a responsibility to hire employees who exemplify the requirements needed by the organization and the process.[2]

Organizations must begin the work of sustaining processes by rethinking their strategies for developing the employees. They must challenge their thinking by asking key questions: How do we select, develop, and improve our best resources—our employees? How do we prepare our culture, including leaders and staff, for a shift to process-centered operations? What leadership attributes and skills are necessary to ensure the organization is truly shifting its perspective to a process-oriented organization concerned with results, not with what it takes to produce them?

Traditionally, organizations have not given substantive attention to employee training and continued personal development in a manner that enables them to perform their new roles in an effective manner. To be effective, process-centered organizations must behave in a radically different manner toward their employees and the processes that make them viable organizations. Employees must not only understand and redesign the processes necessary to achieve outcomes; they must participate at key levels and receive the coaching and mentoring that is often only available in small doses in organizations. The challenge for leaders is to go beyond determining what needs to be done differently and to execute actions that have the greatest possibility for success.[16]

---

*Source: Reprinted by permission of *Harvard Business Review.* An Excerpt From *Parables of Leadership* by W. Chan Kim and Renee A. Mauborgne, July–August 1992. Copyright © 1992 by the President and Fellows of Harvard College; all rights reserved.

Coaching

Coaching represents a critical attribute of leadership. It is the key to how well the organization succeeds in developing employees and sustaining its processes. Similar to their counterparts in sports, organizational coaches must take the raw resources, the employees/players, and turn them into the most valuable resource for a winning team.[2] Coaches must nurture, facilitate, teach, and provide enough growing room for employees to take calculated risks and learn from each other and from the processes. The coach is responsible for developing "team think" and the requisite skills needed to ensure successful organizational outcomes.

In a process-centered organization, the leader as coach has ultimate responsibility to develop the supply of skilled individuals, allocate resources, guide and mentor employees, and resolve performance problems.[2] The skills inherent in coaching include those associated with "developing other people's skills: teaching, listening, evaluating, [and] advising."[2(p.121)] Without the multifaceted role of the coach, employees are back at square one, devoid of the opportunity to truly participate and develop in the organization.

A key responsibility of the coaching leader is to ensure the supply of skilled employees. If processes are to work effectively, the availability of well-trained employees is essential. The leader must formulate an overall recruitment strategy to ensure the supply of workers is sufficient to meet the demand. Hiring strategy, orientation programs, and continuing education are critical components of this role.

The allocation of resources is another key component of the coach role. Employees are assessed as to their skills, knowledge, and abilities and are matched with the appropriate job. A balance must be struck between the immediate needs of the process-centered leader who is trying to fill a job and the long-term, developmental needs of the employee. The coaching leader is the person who must ultimately decide whether this person is right for this job at this point in time.

A coach also attends to performance problems and intervenes to find a solution in a manner that ensures that the employee is treated fairly and with respect. Regardless of how well an organization functions, there will always be human relations, performance, and other issues that require a balanced and objective point of view. Such issues need immediate attention and clarification to assess the source of the problem and the best method for its resolution.

Mentoring

The leader must also guide and mentor employees. Mentoring of employees, if available at all in traditional organizations, is often cursory and not available in a systematic manner that helps employees grow and develop as professionals over time. In the process-centered environment, however, mentoring is a responsibility of all leaders.

A mentor is available to the employee who needs advice, career counseling, or personal attention. Mentoring requires spending the requisite time with the employee to ensure that issues are properly identified and to guide the employee toward resolution. Because the employee is truly a vital human resource for the organization, time spent on mentoring is an expected part of the leadership role and critical for the organization.

Mentors must guide the professional development of employees. In process-centered organizations, employees must be self-motivated, self-reliant, and disciplined. They also must recognize the importance of their work, be enthusiastic and sincere about it, and be committed to doing whatever is ethically necessary to achieve the desired outcome.[2] Employees need to cultivate their creativity, imagination, and intuition.[15] These are not attributes that individuals are taught in educational programs but must be continually nurtured in a work environment.

Developing Trust

Creating an atmosphere of mutual trust and respect in the work environment is the goal of most organizations. One leadership expert suggested that goals are achieved proportionately "to the extent that the organization can achieve a climate where members can level with one another in open and trusting interpersonal relationships."[17(p.174)] Total quality management is an example of how horizontal processes foster team building and the development of employee-leader trust. This approach cuts across the boundaries separating organizational units to create dynamic processes involving the special expertise of both employees and leaders.[18] The effectiveness of this approach lies in the leaders' ability to listen, facilitate, and coach their team into inventing new and more dynamic processes. But the employee must also be an astute listener and an active participant in the process. Moreover, both leaders and employees must commit to the value of "the greater good," which is at the very root of mutual trust and commitment.

"Good teams become great ones when the members trust each other enough to surrender the *me* for the *we*."[9(p.21)] As Bill Cartwright, former center for the Chicago Bulls stated, "What it takes is to give yourself over to the team and play your part."[9(p.6)] That takes a level of trust in your teammates. This level of trust is just as important in process-centered teams as it is on the basketball court. Often, team members must rely on each other's judgments and commitments, and they have responsibilities for activities over which they have little control. To establish this environment of trust, leaders need to develop practices of fairness and openness.[18]

An environment of mutual trust occurs over time, issue by issue, problem by problem. It is not something that can be talked about, published in organizational policies and publications, and given only face value. As with any changing environment, "The leader creates the conditions for diverse groups to talk to one another about the challenges facing them, to frame and debate issues, and to clarify the assumptions behind competing perspectives and values."[3(p.127)] Each time a leader creates a situation where dialogue can occur between and among employees and leaders, trust begins to take root and bud.

Finding Meaning in Work

Finding meaning in one's work life is an age-old issue that has new meaning in today's environment. Institutions such as families, churches, and communities are changing in nature and form, so employees are turning more to organizations to find their identity, meaning, and affiliative support.[4] On the other hand, there is no such thing anymore as an employment contract.[19] Today, the average employee is expected to work for multiple organizations, and many will pursue diverse career paths during their work years.

Employees ask, "How do I find meaning in my work, and who is ultimately responsible for ensuring that there is meaning in my work life?" Organizations ask, "How can we develop a psychological contract with our employees, and how do we garner their loyalty?" Simple answers to these questions are not readily available. Each question is intensely personal and depends on diverse personal and organizational characteristics.

Setting aside personal characteristics, the organization that creates a work environment focused on human relationships, employee development, and participation in all aspects of the work process will more likely have satisfied employees who find meaning in their work. Further, the environment must be a place where fairness, coupled with high organizational expectations, is standard operating procedure.

The employee, by virtue of being a professional, also has a responsibility for bringing values, attitudes, and purpose to an organization. Being a professional means that one has an inherent interest in finding meaning in work and making a contribution to the organization. If professionals can expect to enter into dialogue, be coached to develop new skills, and supported as they take new risks, they will feel genuinely respected and capable of creating new processes. Finding meaning in one's work is an expected outcome of an environment where respect for the individual is an article of faith and a commitment from both leaders and employees.

Taking Risks and Fostering Entrepreneurs

Most traditional organizations are conservative in nature and adhere to a hierarchical structure specifically designed to control behavior and minimize risk.[18]

Risk taking among leaders and employees is not often encouraged or supported. This cautiousness, however, is not necessary or desirable. If an initiative does not initially work or turn a profit, there generally are multiple opportunities to redesign the process or product. In the last 20 years, entrepreneurship as a business strategy in organizations has grown steadily.

The role of entrepreneurial initiatives is critical for both employees and leaders because it fosters a culture that places genuine faith in the abilities of individuals. Such a culture breeds mutual respect, ongoing dialogue, and breakthrough initiatives. William L. McKnight, 3M's leader from 1929 to 1966, believed that "the company was best served when management trusted those with direct knowledge of the market, the operations, or the technology."[18(p.89)] He stated, "Mistakes will be made, but if a person is essentially right, the mistakes he or she makes are not nearly as serious in the long run as the mistakes management will make if it is dictatorial and undertakes to tell those under its authority how they must do their jobs."[18(p.89)]

Entrepreneurship is not a process that can be developed spontaneously and left to its own accord. To create a culture where entrepreneurship can flourish, leaders bear a significant responsibility to instill discipline, establish organizationwide leadership practices and expectations, and create a supportive and nurturing atmosphere. Employees, too, must enter into the entrepreneurial process by abiding by required practices and delivering on their promises and commitments. At 3M, leaders allow employees to spend 15 percent of their time on processes and projects that are not established business lines. Many of these projects fail, but some have become major business initiatives. These success stories and the "15 percent rule" ensure continued experimentation and creativity.[4]

Encouraging Watercarriers and Commitment

To sustain the processes, the leader also must shape the culture and values. This is often more difficult than developing and sharing the vision because it relies on informal communication and implicit beliefs.[4] Max De Pree fostered the development of culture carriers at Herman Miller, referring to them as watercarriers. In American Indian tribes, the person who carried water was highly respected because water was as vital to their survival as food and air. De Pree described the watercarriers in his organization as the people who "transfer the essence of the institution to new people who arrive to help us and, eventually, to replace us."[11(p.69)] He further described them as the people who perpetuate quality, foster unity, and exemplify commitment. To express his appreciation of the watercarriers, and to encourage emulation of their behavior, De Pree commissioned a watercarrier sculpture to be erected at the company's headquarters.

Likewise, Ingvar Kamprad, founder of Ikea, the Swedish home-furnishing stores located in 20 countries, positioned culture bearers throughout the organization.

He conducted extensive training on the organization's history, culture, and values with individuals identified as future leaders. He then assigned these company ambassadors to key positions worldwide. This strategy facilitated propagation of the culture, effective communication, and ongoing commitment to the company's mission.[19]

The commitment that is required to sustain processes is also described in the parable* of the Babbling Brook.[1] In the fourth century B.C., a messenger brought a report on the preparations for an upcoming battle to the grand general of the Chin state. The messenger reported that the Chin regiment was favored to win the battle because their troops far outnumbered the competition and the troops were well fed and prepared for battle. However, after the report, the grand general was convinced that the battle would be lost. When a soon-to-be-appointed general, Meung, asked him why he was so discouraged in light of this positive report, the grand general brought him to a large lake. Once at the lake, he threw a small piece of paper into the lake. The paper floated but barely moved. After watching the paper for an hour, Meung asked what it meant. Rather than replying, the grand general took Meung to a narrow, babbling brook, and again threw a piece of paper into the water. This time the paper moved quickly downstream and disappeared. The grand general then explained that their regiment was like the piece of paper in the lake—large and well equipped with weapons. The competitors, on the other hand, were so inferior in number and weapons that the general placed himself at the front of the battle, with the rear of the regiment against the river— a position of win or die. "His commitment to die in order to win," the grand general predicted, "will beget the troop's commitment in turn. Just as the babbling brook, which rushes in one direction, carries the paper easily while the large lake cannot, so it is that a regiment small in size but unified in commitment will win."[1(p.126)]

RENEWING AND REDESIGNING PROCESSES

Designing a process is not a static process. The most effective leaders continually clarify, refine, renew, and redesign their processes and goals to meet changing customer needs and technological changes.[4] As stated by Yoshio Maruta, former chairman of the Kao Corporation: "Past wisdom must not be a constraint but something to be challenged. Yesterday's success formula is often today's obsolete dogma. My challenge is to have the organization continually question the past so we can renew ourselves every day."[18(p.94)] It was exactly this kind of renewal that helped Kao, a former soap manufacturer, translate its expertise in fat and emulsification into a new business line and become Japan's second largest cosmetic company. They also used their expertise in powders and coating to become a leading manufacturer of floppy disks.[18]

Some organizations need radical redesign as Kao demonstrated, while others need to be tweaked to stay in tune with their markets. For example, Canon also created new business lines through the renewal process, from cameras to calculators to photocopiers. These products seem to share more similarity than soap, cosmetics, and floppy disks, but their development was still a renewal of Canon's core business. According to researchers Ghoshal and Bartlett, "People at Canon believe in creative destruction and the idea that the company should make its products obsolete by coming out with the next generation before the competition does."[18(p.95)]

Challenging

The ability to renew or reengineer relies on the leaders' ability to challenge the status quo. When the cofounders of Intel were exploring their business strategies, they asked, "What would a new top-management team do?"[18(p.96)] This direct question helped them to discern the obvious answer. They challenged themselves to figuratively leave the organization, reenter, and redesign their business initiatives.[18]

Similar questions of challenge include: What is best for our customers? What do our customers want? What services would the community like us to provide? All of these questions frame the work of organizations around the customer. But before leaders and followers can openly entertain these questions, they must ask themselves how open they are to new ideas. Can they step back and look at the organization from the balcony?[3] They must question their receptiveness to perceptions and opinions that are contrary to their own and contrary to the way the organization has always conducted its business.[11]

Developing Strategy

Process improvements must be connected to the organization's strategy to be successful.[20] Strategic planning takes on a new focus in customer-driven process-centered organizations. Rather than engaging in developing a plan over several months, the process-centered organization needs to be able to shift gears rapidly and repeatedly. Leaders can promote this activity by incorporating it into daily activities.

Beginning with the naming of a new vice-chairman in 1993, PepsiCo started a series of retreats to foster strategic thinking. The vice-chairman invited the company's next generation leaders to a retreat and instructed each to bring a cutting-edge business proposal. After discussing and fine-tuning the plans, the leaders instituted them. They came back 90 days later to report their progress and plan further action. This repeated activity stimulated strategic thinking throughout the organization and proved to be a dynamic method for shaping the organization's direction.[19]

Developing strategy to keep ahead of the competition in today's market requires faster decision making than in years past. Prewitt encourages the concept of fast-cycle decision making, which, he wrote, "is accomplished not by simply 'pedaling faster,' but by systematically changing the way your team processes information."[21(p.8)] He suggested that organizations must adopt the philosophy of Asea Brown Boveri's (ABB) CEO, Percy Barnevik, who advocated a "7-3 formula" in which "it's better to make a decision quickly and be right seven times out of ten than to delay while searching for the perfect solution."[21(p.8)] To ensure that 70 percent of decisions are the right ones, Prewitt suggested that a few tools leaders can rely on are intuition, interconnection, and market testing. He pointed out that intuition is not a soft skill, as some suggest, but is based on leveraging the leader's knowledge.[21] By using themselves—their perspectives, hunches, unconscious thoughts, and feelings—leaders transform years of education and training into the art of leadership. This is the true integration or synthesis of all other leadership skills.

Another tool to aid fast-cycle decision making is electronic interconnecting. With access to e-mail and the Internet, leaders can benchmark best practices and collaborate with thousands of experts in real time. Not only does this help leaders make decisions more quickly, but also the decisions are bound to be better. As discussed previously in the parable* of the Wisdom of the Mountain,[1] the holistic perspective of an issue is gained by incorporating the thoughts and opinions of employees from all levels of the organization. Likewise, as ideas and concepts are bantered about worldwide by diverse thinkers, decisions emerge.[21]

Market testing finds new meaning among rapidly competing organizations. Rather than relying on extensive market research and analysis, there is a place in today's organizations for beta testing. Software manufacturers put a product on the market to test consumer response and enlist consumer help in identifying and correcting defects, and other organizations could use the same strategy.[21] This may involve piloting a product or service or virtually testing it on the Internet.

---

*Source: Reprinted by permission of *Harvard Business Review.* An Excerpt From *Parables of Leadership* by W. Chan Kim and Renee A. Mauborgne, July–August 1992. Copyright © 1992 by the President and Fellows of Harvard College; all rights reserved.

Learning

Leaders can foster renewal by creating learning organizations. Senge emphasized the need for employees to continually stretch and grow.[22] This includes acquiring and assimilating new knowledge as well as changing behaviors to integrate that new knowledge.[8] Leaders must role model continual learning and support employees in the organization in their individual pursuits.[15]

Senge and colleagues in their book, *The Fifth Discipline Fieldbook*, wrote that most leaders want to know how to fix things quickly.[23] However, leaders cannot permanently fix things just by applying a bandage. Instead, leaders must apply theories, methods, and tools to increase their own skills and those of the employees. Only when leaders experiment with redesigning the organization's infrastructure will a new type of organization emerge. It will be a learning organization that will be able to deal with the problems and opportunities of today because its members are continually focused on enhancing and expanding their collective awareness and capabilities. The focus is on building collective capabilities and understanding processes at the level needed to bring about lasting change.

"Learning in organizations means the continuous testing of experience, and the transformation of that experience into knowledge—accessible to the whole organization, and relevant to its core purpose."[23(p.49)] For an organization to focus on processes and continual learning, members of the organization at every level must change the way they interact. This means becoming aware of the nearly invisible patterns of interaction between people and processes. Organizational barriers are viewed as employee-leader made and hence amenable to change. Organizational renewal requires collective awareness of interactions and processes and the capacity to choose differently.

Regulating

As organizations shift processes and engage in continual learning, employees can begin to feel that they are in a pressure cooker. Heifetz and Laurie suggested fundamental leadership tasks that help control this pressure and ensure continued employee motivation.[3] Using the pressure cooker analogy, they emphasized that some heat is required to keep things cooking, but the steam needs to escape periodically or the pot will explode. Thus, the leader has to pace the changes and challenges to avoid a state of organizational frenzy.

The leader must provide the ongoing direction of the organization, clarifying the environmental realities and the organizational vision.[3] Continually, the leader serves as a checkpoint for the organization and the employees.[15] Without this regulation, the organization could easily drift downstream, away from its strategic vision.

The leader must be able to surface and manage the expected tension and conflict that arise in a participatory environment.[2,3] Properly exposed and channeled, conflict fosters creativity and provides the heat needed for productive processes. Unchanneled, conflict will stall process work and divert it from the organizational vision.

Finally, leaders must be able to regulate themselves, maintaining presence and poise.[3] Heifetz and Laurie wrote: "A leader has to have the emotional capacity to tolerate uncertainty, frustration, and pain. He has to be able to raise tough questions without getting too anxious himself."[3(p.128)] One is reminded here of the lesson of the parable of Fire and Water* that was previously described.[1]

A leader's poise is fragile.[11] We have all experienced the difficulty of following a leader who becomes anxious and scattered, and therefore we know the importance of self-regulation on the part of leaders. Effective leaders are a positive force[10] in process-centered organizations, not a hindrance. To prepare for this, leaders must develop themselves in all facets, professionally and personally. De Pree wrote, "Polishing one's gifts requires the tumbling of experience and the grit of great discipline."[11(p.42)] This requires more than reading books or taking part in formal education programs. "Real preparation consists of hard work and wandering in the desert, of much feedback, much forgiveness, and the yeast of failure."[11(pp.42–43)]

CONCLUSION

The challenges for the process-centered leader are diverse, and the path outlined is not an easy one to follow. Leaders will often feel that they are swimming upstream—against the currents of the organization and the status quo and against their own learned management behaviors. Just as we started this chapter with the wisdom of an ancient Chinese parable, we turn to the sagacious writings of Niccolo Machiavelli's, *The Prince,* written in 1515, to sustain process-centered leaders as they lead upstream: "And it ought to be remembered that there is nothing more difficult to take in hand, more perilous to conduct, or more uncertain in its success, than to take the lead in the introduction of a new order of things. Because the innovator has for enemies all those who have done well under the old conditions, and lukewarm defenders in those who may do well under the new."[24(p.9)]

Source: Reprinted by permission of *Harvard Business Review.* An Excerpt From *Parables of Leadership* by W. Chan Kim and Renee A. Mauborgne, July–August 1992. Copyright © 1992 by the President and Fellows of Harvard College; all rights reserved.

REFERENCES

1. Kim WC, Mauborgne RA. Parables of leadership. *Harvard Business Rev.* 1992; 70(4):123–128.
2. Hammer M. *Beyond Reengineering: How the Process-Centered Organization Is Changing Our Work and Our Lives.* New York: Harper Business; 1996.
3. Heifetz RA, Laurie DL. The work of leadership. *Harvard Business Rev.* 1997; 75(1):124–134.
4. Bartlett CA, Ghoshal S. Changing the role of top management: Beyond strategy to purpose. *Harvard Business Rev.* 1994; 72(6):79–88.
5. Mateja J. GM to make 31st attempt at general reorganization. *Chicago Tribune.* 1998 (July 31); 3:1.
6. Drucker P. New society of organizations. *Harvard Business Rev.* 1992; 70(5):95–104.
7. Kotter JP. *Leading Change.* Boston: Harvard Business School Press; 1996.
8. Hanson RB, Sayers B. *Work and Role Redesign: Tools and Techniques for the Health Care Setting.* Chicago: American Hospital; 1995.
9. Jackson P, Delehanty H. *Sacred Hoops: Spiritual Lessons of a Hardwood Warrior.* New York: Hyperion; 1995.
10. Kouzes JM, Posner BZ. *The Leadership Challenge: How To Get Extraordinary Things Done in Organizations.* San Francisco: Jossey-Bass; 1995.
11. De Pree M. *Leadership Jazz.* New York: Dell; 1992.
12. Sweetman KJ. Cultivating creativity: Unleash the genie. *Harvard Business Rev.* 1997; 75(2): 11–12.
13. Carlzon J. *Moments of Truth.* Cambridge, MA: Ballinger; 1987.
14. Bennis W, Nanus B. *Leaders: The Strategies for Taking Charge.* New York: Harper & Row; 1985.
15. Kohles MK, Baker WG, Donaho, BA. *Transformational Leadership: Renewing Fundamental Values and Achieving New Relationships in Health Care.* Chicago: American Hospital; 1995.
16. Conner D. *Managing at the Speed of Change.* New York: Villard Books; 1992.
17. Bennis W. *An Invented Life: Reflections on Leadership and Change.* Reading, MA: Addison-Wesley; 1993.
18. Ghoshal S, Bartlett CA. Changing the role of top management: Beyond structure to processes. *Harvard Business Rev.* 1995; 73(1):86–96.
19. Bartlett CA, Ghoshal S. Changing the role of top management: Beyond systems to people. *Harvard Business Rev.* 1995; 73(3):132-142.
20. Hout TM, Carter, JC. Getting it done: New roles for senior executives. *Harvard Business Rev.* 1995; 73(6):133–141.
21. Prewitt E. Fast-cycle decision making. *Harvard Management Update.* 1998; 3(8):8–9.
22. Senge PM. *The Fifth Discipline: The Art and Practice of the Learning Organization.* New York: Doubleday/Currency; 1990.
23. Senge P, Kleiner A, Roberts C, Ross R, Smith B. *The Fifth Discipline Fieldbook.* New York: Doubleday/Currency; 1994.
24. Machiavelli N. *The Prince.* In: Hutchins RM, ed., Marriott WK, trans. *Great Books of the Western World.* Vol. 23. Chicago: Encyclopedia Britannica; 1952. (Original work published in 1515.)

CHAPTER 10

Management and Organizational Restructuring: Reforming the Corporate System

Dominick L. Flarey, PhD, MBA, RN,CS, CNAA, FACHE
Suzanne P. Smith, EdD, RN, FAAN

Inherent in the concept of reengineering is radical change. When a change occurs through process reengineering, change ensues throughout the organization. To successfully reengineer, organizations must redesign their management roles and restructure traditional hierarchal, bureaucratic, and line-reporting relationships. A new organizational structure that will support ongoing reengineering needs to be created.

When creating a new organizational structure, it is important to keep in mind that, as processes and systems are reengineered, major components of restructuring and role redesign will evolve. Thus, restructuring and role redesign will change as the organization is re-created. This chapter details the planned and evolving changes occurring in organizational structures and management roles as an imperative and as outcomes for reengineering processes and systems. Leadership imperatives and matrix structures are also discussed.

RE-CREATING MANAGEMENT ROLES

To support an environment for organizationwide reengineering, management roles need to be re-created. Although changes in various responsibilities will evolve

Acknowledgment: The authors thank Jack Kenneson, BSME, mechanical engineer, for typesetting the figures in this chapter.

Source: Reprinted from D. Flarey, and S. Smith Blancett, Management and Organizational Restructuring: Reforming the Corporate System, in *Reengineering Nursing and Health Care: The Handbook for Organizational Transformation*, S. Smith Blancett and D. Flarey, eds., pp. 75–86, © 1995, Aspen Publishers, Inc.

as an outcome of reengineering, the imperative for strong leadership remains constant. The most important leadership skill for driving reengineering is communication. Since reengineering is a change initiative, communication must be ongoing and sensitive to the information needs of various stakeholders in the reengineering process. Open communication will increase confidence and trust in the staff, which can lead to increased risk-taking behavior and creativity. This communication allays employee fears and ensures that everyone in the organization understands how change will occur.

Two additional characteristics must also be designed into the leadership role if reengineering is to be successful. Leaders must become visionaries and motivators for the change initiative.[1] These characteristics require leaders to maintain accountability for the overall rethinking of the organization and to constantly provide the staff with the motivation necessary to bring the vision to reality.

In terms of role structure, reengineering initiatives require a different approach than other, more recent projects for initiating change, such as total quality management, continuous quality improvement, and quality circles. In those approaches, change is generally initiated from the bottom of the organization, with staff driving the project while receiving support from top management. In reengineering, the initiative must be led by one person or a group at the top level of management; if it is led from the bottom up, it will be blocked by organizational barriers.[2] This phenomenon is due in large part to the radical change inherent in the reengineering project.

"'Who fills the leader's role?' The role requires someone who has enough authority over all stakeholders in the process(es) that will undergo reengineering to ensure that reengineering can happen."[1(p.104)] This requirement is essential because the reengineering process crosses many organizational boundaries. As a consequence, issues of turf protection need to be successfully confronted and resolved. Thus, the leader must possess the inherent authority to make reengineering happen. The top leadership is accountable for the judicious allocation of resources and must make them available if reengineering is to succeed. When organizations re-create themselves through major reengineering initiatives, many new roles emerge. Hammer and Champy[1] define five major new roles that are created through and developed by reengineering initiatives:

1. *Leader*—A leader must emerge who can oversee the entire project[2] and ensure that it happens. This reengineering leader, in most instances, should be the chief executive officer or the chief operating officer so that top management will continue to be engaged and committed to the project. This top-level leadership will also solidify the perception by the entire organization that top executive management is truly living out their responsibility to lead the organization through its re-creation.

2. ***Process owner***—Process owners are generally the managers who are responsible for specific processes. The major imperative for their role is to facilitate process reengineering and to ensure the integration of departments that is necessary to recreate the organization. They must think differently and support the facilitation of an organizationwide change initiative. It is their responsibility to remove the traditional barriers and boundaries that have slowed the organization down in its past attempts to respond swiftly to the changing external environment.

3. ***Reengineering team***—The reengineering team is the group that actually reengineers processes and systems. Its membership generally consists of multidisciplinary representatives throughout the organization. As reengineering team members, they take on a true leadership role. One of their primary responsibilities is to sell the change concept to everyone in the organization and to be role models for change. These members lead by doing and, as a direct consequence, motivate others to cooperate with the actual reengineering process.

4. ***Steering committee***—The steering committee is generally made up of senior and middle managers who assume accountability for developing policy and standards related to reengineering efforts. They also serve as the primary body responsible for the ongoing evolution of the project. Their other major responsibility is to evaluate the need for additional resources for reengineering and to ensure that such resources are available to the reengineering team.

5. ***Reengineering czar***—Every organization that reengineers needs a full-time leader who is an expert in process reengineering and serves as a teacher and mentor to the reengineering team. This new leader must also be well versed in the use of specific tools for process reengineering, as well as in the tools and statistical analyses used to evaluate reengineering projects. In this role, the reengineering czar serves as an internal consultant to the organization for its reengineering initiatives.

As previously discussed, one of the major roles of management in any reengineering effort is to help others work through change.[3] Creating an environment for change is the single most important task for driving success in reengineering. Based on this change imperative for change movement, it is essential that the organization's leaders undergo major shifts in the transformation of their roles.

Flarey identified 15 paradigm shifts in the role transformation of the nurse manager.[4(p.42)] Such transformations are applicable for all leaders involved in reengineering projects. These shifts demand that leaders change roles from:

1. manager to leader
2. director to coach
3. boss to mentor
4. quality assurance to continuous quality improvement
5. department perspective to organizational perspective
6. clinical audits to research
7. coordinator to project manager
8. participatory management to self-governance
9. turf protection to collaboration
10. control to partnership
11. planning to strategic vision
12. vertical management to horizontal management
13. budgeting to fiscal accountability
14. status quo to innovation
15. department focus to product-line focus

The authors believe that shifts to these new roles will support the overall reengineering initiatives by the organization and also assist in re-creating the organizational culture and climate for ongoing reengineering and change processes. We believe reengineering cannot happen unless this transformation occurs. Such a transformation must be led by top executive management through intense management education and development, as well as role modeling.

THE NEW NURSE MANAGER

The one role that has undergone change and will continue to transform itself in the future is that of the nurse manager.[5] In the context of reengineering, this transformation becomes more critical. The business of health care organizations is the delivery of patient care. This primary product is delivered at the bedside. Consequently, many of the reengineering initiatives in health care are focused on the delivery system of care. Care is delivered by nurses. Thus, the nurse manager role is pivotal to the successful re-creation of care delivery and of the organization.

Nurse managers must be included in all phases of the reengineering initiatives and should be assigned a leadership role on the reengineering team. For reengineering to successfully drive change in the delivery of patient care at the bedside, the nurse manager role must be redesigned.

Flarey[5] has identified 10 visionary outcomes for the transformation of the nurse manager role. Exhibit 10–1 presents these defined outcomes. These outcomes drive the redesign of the nurse manager role, which must be led by the nurse executive and supported by the chief executive officer and the chief operating

Exhibit 10–1 Ten Role Outcomes for Nurse Managers

1. ***Postentrepreneurial style:*** the ability to relinquish bureaucratic styles of leadership; more employee-person centered, with core characteristics of innovation, efficiency, and reward of outcomes; authority derived from expertise and experimentation.[1]

2. ***Empowerment:*** ability to empower self and staff for quality patient outcomes; ability to influence organizational policy development as related to patient care.

3. ***Vision:*** ability to foresee the growth and development of nursing and management practice and strategically to plan to assist processes.

4. ***Enhancement of image:*** ability to identify self as a professional nurse and manager, perceiving self as a leader and enhancing the profession of nursing within the profession, community, and organization.

5. ***Flexibility:*** ability to adapt to turbulence in the institution and the practice environment; ability to assess outcomes and design new and better processes in patient care and management to achieve quality and superior service.

6. ***Clinical expertise:*** ability to identify with those who are managed; staying close to the client and the practice environment to manage the delivery of health care effectively.

7. ***Analytic thinking:*** ability to problem solve effectively using logic and decision support systems and models; ability to conduct research in nursing and management.

8. ***Leadership role identity:*** ability to see self as a leader, mentor, and nurse/patient advocate; ability to assist in meeting institutional goals and objectives through effective performance; ability to "get things done."

9. ***Autonomy:*** ability to practice nursing and management in a highly decentralized environment without alienation of executive leadership.

10. ***"Change Master":*** ability to identify, cope with, introduce, and assimilate change successfully in the practice environment.[2]

(1) Moss-Kanter R. *When Giants Learn To Dance: Mastering the Challenge of Strategy, Management, and Careers in the 1990s.* New York: Simon & Schuster, Inc; 1989.

(2) Moss-Kanter R. *The Change Masters: Innovation and Entrepreneurship in the American Corporation.* New York: Simon & Schuster, Inc; 1983.

Source: Reprinted with permission from D Flarey. Redesigning Management Roles: The Executive Challenge, *Journal of Nursing Administration,* Vol. 21, No. 2, pp. 40–45, © 1991, J.B. Lippincott Company.

officer. Based on these visionary outcomes, coupled with the support and direction of executive management, nurse managers can actually redesign their roles to facilitate the change necessary in the practice environment to support ongoing reengineering of the delivery system. Redesign of the nurse manager role is not an option; it is a must if health care organizations are to successfully re-create themselves to deal with the new environment.

THE MATRIX STRUCTURE

The hospital, ostensibly a part of the free-market economy, yet resembling it only to the extent of capital needs and profitability, must operate differently from general businesses, requiring new ideas, management approaches, and information systems that allow managers to find their way effectively in a hybrid, quasi-free enterprise environment.[6(p.23)]

This phenomenon is certainly true for health care organizations that are undertaking radical changes through reengineering. The successful recreation of the organization through reengineering requires a hybrid structure. This concept is supported by the gurus of reengineering, Hammer and Champy.[1] A hybrid organization structure is one that combines the characteristics of both a product structure and a functional structure. In this structure, functions important to each product or market are decentralized, whereas other functions are centralized.[7]

Because health care organizations are so complex, it is advisable to go beyond a traditional hybrid structure to a matrix structure to support reengineering. For reengineering, health care organizations need an organizational chart that assigns priority to functional activities and product lines simultaneously. "The unique characteristic of the matrix organization is that both product and functional structures are implemented simultaneously in each department."[7(p.242)]

Figure 10–1 details our version of a matrix structure for reengineering in health care organizations. In this structure, the organization retains a semblance of some traditional vertical line reporting around major functions such as (1) patient care services, (2) ancillary and plant services, (3) finance, (4) medical affairs, (5) human resources, and (6) managed care.

Horizontally, a team-based structure that crosses the traditional, functional boundaries is developed. This team-based structure focuses on ongoing, major imperatives for re-creating the organization through reengineering. For health care organizations to re-create themselves and to develop and support an environment for reengineering, we propose that the hospital component of the matrix structure be developed around the following self-directed teams:

1. *Reengineering team*—This team is the top-level team and is the pivotal point of the horizontal structure. There is an open relationship between the reengineering team and all of the other established teams. Thus, the process between teams is interactive, and the teams support each other in goal attainment. The reengineering team is led by a reengineering executive who reports to the chief executive officer (CEO) or the chief operating officer.

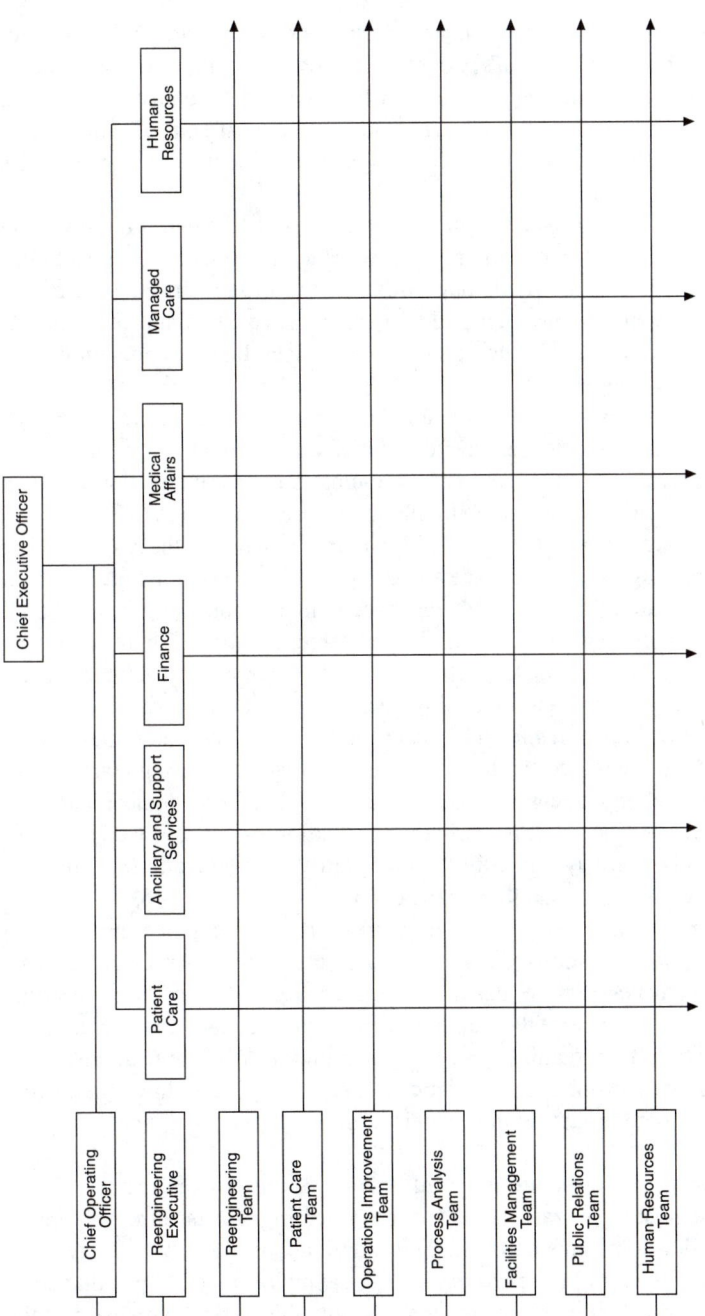

Figure 10–1 Matrix Structure for Reengineering in Health Care Organizations

2. *Patient care team*—This team exists to oversee the integration and re-creation of the organization's patient care delivery system. It constantly seeks to reengineer the delivery system on the basis of imperatives of quality, speed and efficiency, customer satisfaction, and cost control. The team is instrumental in assessing the delivery system and identifying opportunities for reengineering.

3. *Operations improvement team*—This team is challenged with assessing the internal environment and seeking ways to reengineer processes to improve specific and overall operations in the organization. It is multi-disciplinary and focuses on patient care improvements and other operations improvements, such as maintenance services, business operations, and utilization management.

4. *Process analysis team*—This team is made up of members who, through education and experience, have developed an expertise in the analysis of existing processes, as well as process re-creation. Their interaction will help all other teams to create value in the overall reengineering efforts.

5. *Facilities management team*—This team is charged with the responsibility for overseeing the maintenance and design of the physical plant. The team conducts plant inspections and makes recommendations for redesign based on government regulations as well as customer feedback. This team works with other reengineering teams to add value to the initiative where the physical plant is a component of a reengineering project.

6. *Employee relations team*—This team focuses on the critical issues around "people" in reengineering initiatives. It assists reengineering teams in developing and implementing a communications plan for the project. The team also works to reengineer performance evaluation systems, as well as recognition and reward systems, for the newly created organization. Labor relations issues are also handled by the team.

7. *Public relations team*—This team works with all reengineering teams to develop public relations plans for the projects. It also focuses on the marketing of any new services that may have been created through reengineering. Another major focus of the team is to involve physicians, vendors, and other customers in the organization's reengineering efforts. The team also edits and produces an internal newsletter to keep everyone in the organization updated on the progress with reengineering.

Although this team structure is not all-inclusive, these seven teams will adequately serve most organizations in their reengineering efforts. However, organizations must develop teams based on their individual needs.

Regardless of the types of teams developed, the major imperative is that all of the teams are interactive with each other and within the vertical dimension of the matrix structure. This interaction will give maximum value to all reengineering efforts and will drive a fundamental change in the way health care organizations manage their business.

Our matrix model will assist health care organizations to dissolve boundaries and become more integrated. The need to integrate health care organizations more fully, both internally and externally, is a major imperative today in health care reform. "At the strategic level, boundaries are being redrawn as the outlines of integrated health care systems begin to emerge. Physicians, hospitals, payers, and insurers are reconfiguring their boundaries in ways that reflect changing conceptions of what business they are in."[8(p.68)] The future challenge of health care organizations will be to create a boundaryless system; one that is fully integrated and provides for a full continuum of health care services. A matrix organizational structure will facilitate that goal.

RETHINKING THE ORGANIZATION

Through reengineering, newer organizational structures will evolve. These newer structures will be focused on simplicity so that organizations can respond more quickly to rapid changes in both the internal and external environments. We envision the evolution of a new structure that depicts the newly created organization. Figure 10–2 is a representation of that vision.

To enhance the inherent simplicity and focus on the future imperative for health care organizations, this new structure is called the interactive model. This model depicts three core, structured elements of the new organization: (1) human resources, (2) finance and operations, and (3) clinical services. A circular structure is used for each element to depict its high degree of interactiveness. Each of the core elements further interacts with each of the others. This integrated structure also demonstrates the further need to flatten the hierarchical structure of organizations.

Peter Drucker asserts, "The typical large organization, such as large businesses or a government agency, twenty years hence will have no more than half the levels of management of its counterpart today, and no more than a third the number of 'managers.'"[9(p.207)] This reality is evolving for health care organizations and will be realized in the near future. As Figure 10–2 demonstrates, only three executive positions besides the CEO will be needed in the newly integrated health care organization. All activities within the core elements of the new structure will be team based. Remaining managers will not function as they have traditionally. In the coming era, managers within the core elements will function as teachers, team coaches, and mentors. Traditional management duties and responsibilities will be incorporated into the established self-directed teams and will be accomplished by the teams.

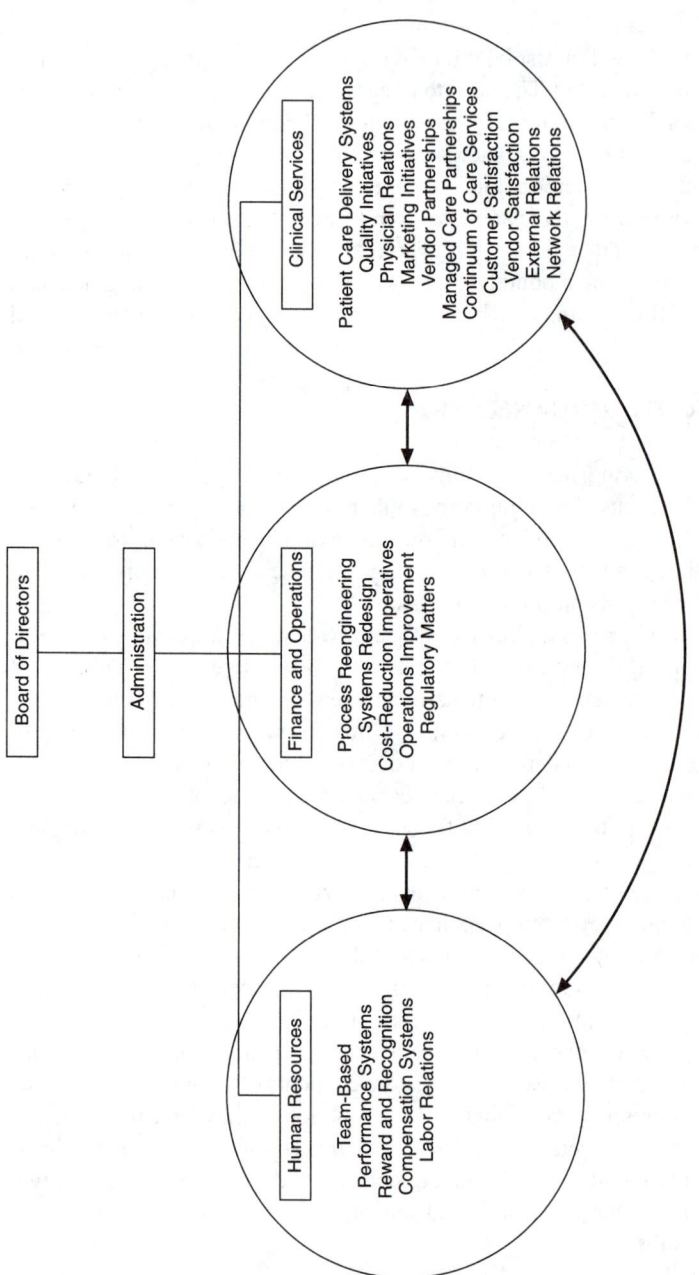

Figure 10–2 The Interactive Organization

This new structure will also drive changes in the redesign of senior management roles. "We must rethink what we want our senior managers to be accountable for. At the same time, we need to align authority and responsibility with that new notion of accountability."[10(p.103)] In the newly created organization, the core competencies of senior managers will be to:

- provide visionary leadership
- remove barriers of organizational transformation
- constantly drive the re-creation of the organization
- support organizational integration
- develop the continuum of care services
- establish partnerships with the organization's internal and external customers
- ensure that managers are accountable for moving the organization forward
- empower everyone in the organization
- create a knowledge-intense, learning organization
- constantly communicate with the members of the organization
- ensure decision making at the staff level

In creating the new integrated organization for the support of ongoing reengineering, Hammer and Champy[1] describe eight major shifts that need to occur throughout the entire organization:

1. a change from functional departments to teams
2. job change through redesign—from simple tasks to multidimensional tasks
3. a move from control to empowerment
4. a shift from training to ongoing education
5. a change from focus on the evaluation of activities to measurement of results
6. a change in management roles from that of supervisor to that of coach
7. organizational structure changes from hierarchical to flat
8. a transformation of executives into leaders

A health care organization that truly re-creates itself through reengineering will experience these shifts, and these shifts will further support the environment necessary for ongoing reengineering. As the organization is re-created and a new structure emerges, some radical changes in reporting relationships will occur. "Executives must challenge the prevailing attitude that people in a particular occupation must report to individuals of a like occupation (accountant to an accountant, nurses to a nurse, pharmacist to a pharmacist)."[11(p.79)]

In a newly created organization, one founded on integration and a team-based structure, reporting relationships will need to change. Even with this inevitable change, the core element of patients' services in the new integrated structure (see Figure 10–2) should be under the leadership of a nurse executive—the one executive on the management team whose primary educational preparation was in patient care delivery. The nurse executive role will emerge as the pivotal role in the newly integrated system. It will be the nurse executive who will undoubtedly lead the reengineering of overall care delivery and who will sustain the organization and continue to move it forward in its overall transformation. Thus, it is imperative that nurse executives acquire new skill sets of transformational leadership because they will be leading not only the nursing practice environment but, in partnership with the CEO and a few other senior executives, an entire integrated system of care delivery.

CONCLUSION

To successfully reengineer and create an organizational culture that continually seeks ways to do things better through reengineering, organizations must be re-created. Essential to this transformation are (1) leaders who think and act in ways dramatically different from the past and (2) organizational structures that are simple, flexible, and adaptable to change. These two factors are critical if organizations are to be successful in the future.

REFERENCES

1. Hammer M, Champy J. *Reengineering the Corporation: A Manifesto for Business Revolution.* New York: Harper Business; 1993.
2. Stewart TA. Reengineering: The hot new management tool. *Fortune.* 1993; 128(4):41–48.
3. Wachel W. Reengineering: Beyond incremental change. *Healthcare Executive.* 1994; 9(July/August):18–21.
4. Flarey D. The changing role of the nurse manager: Redesign for the 1990s and beyond. *Semin Nurse Managers.* 1993; 1(1):41–48.
5. Flarey D. Redesigning management roles: The executive challenge. *J Nurs Adm.* 1991; 21(2): 40–45.
6. Helppie RD. A time for reengineering. *Comput Healthcare.* 1992; 13(1):22–24.
7. Daft R. *Organizational Theory and Design.* 2nd ed. St. Paul, MN: West Publishing Co; 1986.
8. Gilmore T, Hirschhorn L, O'Connor M. The boundaryless organization. *Healthcare Forum J.* 1994; 37(4):68–72.
9. Drucker P. *The New Realities.* New York: Harper & Row; 1989.
10. Lathrop J. *Restructuring Health Care: The Patient-Focused Paradigm.* San Francisco: Jossey-Bass, Inc, Publishers; 1993.
11. Shelley S, Jones L. The turnaround process: Management, board, and cultural changes. In: Baehr R, ed. *Engineering a Hospital Turnaround.* Chicago: American Hospital Publishing, Inc; 1993.

CHAPTER 11

Management in the Process-Centered Environment

Anita Gottlieb, MA, RNP, CPHQ

Changing practices and processes with the goal of containing cost and improving quality has become common practice within health care institutions. However, even with continued efforts to control costs, the United States spends 12 percent of its gross national product on health care.[1] Technological advances have been credited with having the greatest impact on cost and contribute to the United States spending more than any other industrialized nation. Accelerated alignment of clinical and management processes, systems integration, and health care redesign are required to achieve the goal of lowered cost, improved quality, and better access.[2] In his book, *Beyond Engineering,* Hammer writes that superior process performance is achieved by having a superior practice design, the right people, and the right environment for them to work in.[3] It has become imperative to identify the organization's mission and vision and to ensure that it is appropriately supported by the key processes.

While providing high-quality patient services and practicing cost containment are major health care goals, the process and supporting structures are not always aligned to support patient care in the most cost-effective and efficient manner. When waiting in an admissions area of a hospital or emergency department, have you ever thought that you have received better service at a fast-food establishment? Needless to say, the provision of health care services is more intense and specialized than the preparation of a taco or a hamburger, but in each case there are certain processes that are necessary to achieve appropriate outcomes. In the health care environment, it is necessary to identify key processes for patient care

Acknowledgment: The author thanks Kaye Earney for technical assistance in manuscript preparation.

and make changes within the structure of the institutions to be competitive. This chapter addresses key processes in a variety of health care settings and the evolvement of management roles to support them.

MANAGEMENT ROLES IN THE PROCESS-CENTERED ORGANIZATION

As hospitals and other health care settings review their practices and take steps to make changes to meet the demands of patients and payers, the roles and responsibilities of employees at all levels of the institution are affected. To support the process-centered environment, management roles will be realigned to support the key processes. The need for strong leadership and open communication throughout the institution is imperative. As in reengineering, leaders in the process-centered workplace must continue to be visionary and encourage continued improvement. The key processes must be clearly defined, simple, direct, low cost, and flexible. Workers must be capable of performing process-focused jobs that require autonomy and responsibility for decision making. The traditional boss and employee roles are drastically affected when institutions focus on processes and become less fragmented and task orientated. In *Beyond Reengineering*,[3] the role of the traditional department manager has been described as giving way to the new role of process owner, and employees are process performers. Hammer defines these role changes as follows:

- *Process Performer.* The process performer is the individual performing the functions necessary to support his or her assigned key process. In the process-centered organization, employees are provided with the necessary and appropriate tools, as well as information on customer expectations, and are treated with respect and guided by clearly defined expectations.
- *Process Owner.* The process owner is the individual concerned with ensuring the successful realization and completion of a process from beginning to end. Thus, the process owner has responsibility for the design of the process, implementation, documentation, evaluation, and training for process performers. The process owner must be the expert in the process as a whole and responsible for supporting those performing the process. In the process-centered organization, quality improvement is not a peripheral activity but the essence of managing. Figure 11–1 illustrates the ongoing cycle of quality improvement and its adaptation in process-centered health care. In some settings, the process owner role may replace the traditional manager role. In others, it may replace the department head or vice president role. In other words, modifications are made, as appropriate, for support of the organiza-

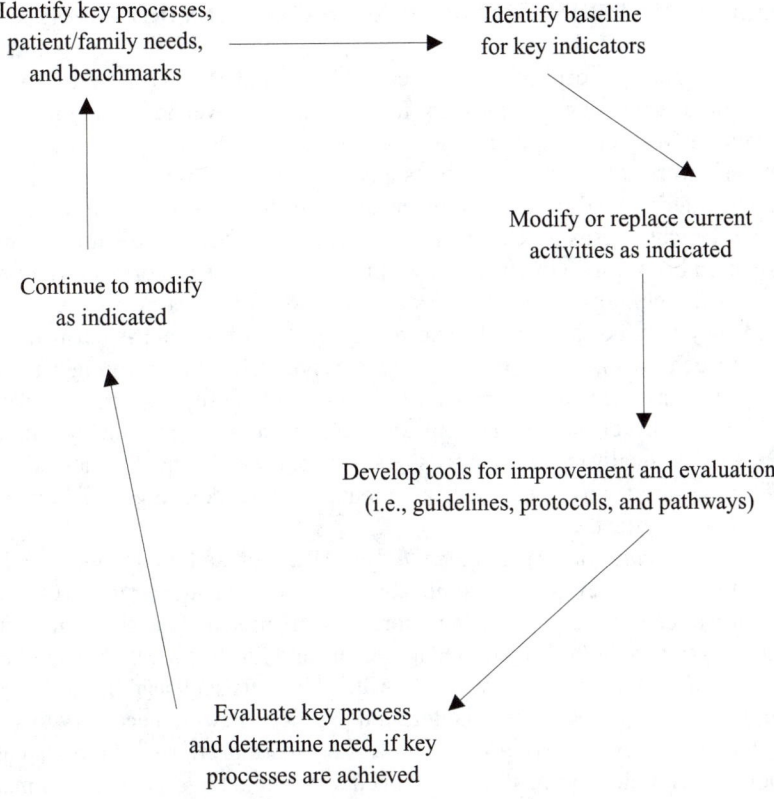

Figure 11–1 Continuous Quality Improvement for Key Processes

tion's key processes and will vary from institution to institution. According to Hammer,[3] in the process-centered world, the following are functions of the process owner:

- responsibility for ensuring there is a high-level performance process for the specified key process or processes
- coaching and support of the process performers
- leadership and responsibility for shaping and designing the overall environment
- continuous evaluation and support of improvement processes

PROCESS CENTERING IN THE HEALTH CARE ENVIRONMENT

Embracing the concept of process-centered care and support from the leadership of the organization is necessary for successful conversion to the process-centered environment. Although the health care industry was not the focus of Hammer's work, the customer focus supports patient-focused care nicely, and process centering readily adapts to the health care arena.[3] It specifies a customer or patient focus versus a department or organization focus, and patient/family satisfaction becomes the focus of the employee or process performers. Hammer describes the employees in a process-centered workplace as professionals, although they may not have an advanced degree. A professional is defined as a cross between a worker and a manager and is responsible for performing the work and ensuring its successful completion. This definition and expectation adapts well to the health care setting. The impact of all employees in a health care setting feeling professionally responsible for supporting or providing quality patient care, whether they are a part of the medical, nursing, or housekeeping staff, can only have a positive effect.

In *Reengineering Nursing and Health Care*,[4] Blancett and Flarey present a list of paradigm shifts they consider applicable for the nurse manager involved in an institution undergoing reengineering efforts. A comparison of the similarities and differences in paradigm shifts for reengineering and for the process-centered environment is presented in Exhibit 11–1. Although shifts such as those described represent major changes in both beliefs and practice, they are necessary to support the overall reengineering and/or process-centering efforts. These changes cannot happen unless a transformation occurs that is led by top executive management and is supported by education and role modeling. The application of the paradigm shifts should include traditional management roles, as well as employees at all levels.

Application of process centering in a hospital or ambulatory health care setting involves many of the same role changes Hammer describes as necessary for other industries. Some workers will adapt well and thrive, while others will not. Shifting to new roles within the same jobs or positions will be necessary to support improvement and process change. Recently, some health care institutions developed and implemented product line services and/or centers of excellence. Such changes reflect the move toward a process-centered environment. Roles in the specialized health care setting, such as nurse manager, have already incorporated some of the characteristics of the process owner. For example, the nursing manager for a hematology unit may have responsibility for the design of the process, training of the process performers, evaluation, and continuous quality improvement efforts. He or she is the expert in the process as a whole and responsible for coaching the unit staff. However, in most settings, for true process centering to

Exhibit 11–1 Comparison of Paradigm Shifts for Reengineering and Process Centering

Reengineering	*Process Centering*
Manager to leader	Manager to process owner
Director to coach	Similar
Boss to mentor	Mentor and advocate
Quality assurance to quality improvement	Continuous quality improvement focus
Department perspective to organizational perspective	Similar
Clinical audits to research	Continued evaluation and monitoring
Coordinator to project manager	Process owner and team leader
Participatory management to self-governance	From direct supervision to monitoring outcomes
Turf protection to collaboration	Collaboration and interaction between services
Control to partnership	Decreased department and increased interdepartment focus related to processes
Planning to strategic vision	Vision related to identified key processes
Vertical management to horizontal management	Similar
Budgeting to fiscal accountability	Similar
Status quo to innovation	Innovation and initiative
Department focus to product line	Product line and centers of excellence

Source: Data from S. Smith Blancett and D.L. Flarey, *Reengineering Nursing and Health Care,* © 1995, pp. 77–78, Aspen Publishers, Inc.

occur, there must be a paradigm shift in the organization that is readily apparent to all employees. Responsibility for the budget, patient/family satisfaction, and evaluation of the employees, or process performers, as well as patient outcomes, would be included in the role of the process owner.

STRUCTURES SUPPORTING THE KEY PROCESSES

Many of the tools and support structures used in quality improvement and reengineering efforts are applicable and necessary for identification and support of key processes. Quality improvement or reengineering teams can be a key element in developing a process-centered environment. The team leader for a clinical pathway or quality improvement team may essentially be the process owner. Just as a team-based structure is appropriate for organizations undergoing reengineering, it is equally applicable in developing a process-centered environment. The focus of teams used in reengineering efforts include patient care, operations improvement, process analysis, facilities management, employee relations, and public relations.[4] Although not all-inclusive, the list includes areas that would benefit those developing a process-centered institution. Regardless of the types of teams developed and whether they are temporary or permanent, they must interface well with the mission and vision of the institution and positively support patient care areas. The team approach also supports a system that has no boundaries and helps decrease departmentalization and improve multidisciplinary relationships.

Use of clinical pathways and protocols is also helpful in supporting the key process of a specific diagnosis or treatment area.[5] A team approach is usually used for pathway development, and the team leader should be the process owner in most instances. Pathways are designed to outline the crucial steps in caring for a patient with a specific diagnosis, using a multidisciplinary approach. The usual goal is to provide high-quality care while lowering cost and decreasing length of hospitalization. Clinical pathways should be part of the foundation developed to support process-centered health care.

CONCLUSION

The ever-changing health care environment is best described by Charles Dickens in *A Tale of Two Cities:* "It was the best of times, it was the worst of times." To survive in today's managed care environment, it is necessary to continually develop methods for keeping up with the changing technology while maintaining cost. Organizational leaders need to provide the vision, mission, and key processes, and communicate these to all employees. Process ownership and identification of all employees as professionals will be the "keys to the kingdom" in a process-centered environment. Managers in health care have different roles and responsibilities than they did a few years ago, and their jobs and responsibilities will continue to change. Adaptation to these changes is imperative. Medical technology has lengthened the average life span and improved the overall quality of life. However, to continue to serve patients and families and survive in the era of medical cost containment, institutions must look for ways, such as process centering, to support their survival efforts.

REFERENCES

1. Banta HD. Future health care technology and the hospital. *Health Policy.* 1990; 14(1):61–71.
2. Lin B, Vassar JA. Implications of reengineering in health care. *Health Care Supervisor.* 1996; 15(2):63–68.
3. Hammer M. *Beyond Reengineering.* New York: Harper Business; 1996.
4. Blancett SS, Flarey DL. Management and organizational restructuring: Reform in the corporate system. In: Blancett SS, Flarey DL, eds. *Reengineering Nursing and Health Care.* Gaithersburg, MD: Aspen Publishers, Inc.; 1995:75–86.
5. Blancett SS, Flarey DL. The future of collaborative path-based practice. In: *Health Care Outcomes Collaborative, Path Based Approaches.* Gaithersburg, MD: Aspen Publishers, Inc.; 1998: 18–31.

CHAPTER 12

Reengineering Patient Care in a Multi-Institutional System

Marjorie Beyers, PhD, RN, FAAN

Reengineering patient care delivery takes many forms and may settle in either broadly at the organizational level or narrowly at the task level. It may focus on a whole new way of delivering care. This chapter provides (1) an overview of ways in which multi-institutional systems can approach the redesign of patient care, (2) a perspective on the potential for redesigning health care, and (3) considerations and approaches to reengineering patient care delivery.

In today's practice, the broadest approach to reengineering patient care is found in the development of networks and new types of systems. This formation of health care networks and community care systems emphasizes patient care services from wellness to death. Nursing's knowledge base is being tapped in this reengineering. Nursing care knowledge and competence, which are demonstrated in patient assessment, care planning, and continuity of care, are highly valued. Other health professions and the public are picking up and using nursing's language. The language once formerly heard in nursing circles now appears in the *Wall Street Journal*. Nursing has a good opportunity to reposition patient care in the broader arena by claiming its own work and building on it.

Health care networks of different types are being formed as part of health care reform. These emerging types of health care networks are reflected in new types of corporate structures—arrangements and alignments between and among hospitals, long-term care facilities, and other health care institutions. Emphasis on physician-hospital bonding prevails. The general environment offers untapped possibilities for nursing that can be nurtured.[1] Nursing's capability to provide

Source: Adapted from M. Beyers, Reengineering Patient Care in a Multi-Institutional System in *Reengineering Nursing and Health Care: The Handbook for Organizational Transformation*, S. Smith Blancett and D. Flarey, eds., pp. 223–237, © 1995, Aspen Publishers, Inc.

care along the entire spectrum of care for communities is an asset that nurses must claim and use, or else others will adapt and adopt it. Nurses now have an opportunity to shape and define clinical nursing roles that contribute significantly to health care in ways that realize the potential to serve and contribute to the nation's health.

REENGINEERING: THE IMPORTANCE OF LANGUAGE

Cycles of change are very short in today's world, and the words used to describe the phenomena are being developed quickly and used loosely. Today's language lacks precision sufficient to describe reengineering, multi-institutional systems, and other key concepts. Although reengineering, restructuring, redesigning, and reform have been differentiated, they are more alike than different in that they mean change. It is quite possible to have a lengthy discussion of reengineering among experts without a significant meeting of the minds. The importance of a common language to describe the emerging patient care systems and networks cannot be overemphasized as an imperative in reengineering initiatives. A multi-institutional system has an advantage because it can create its own glossary of terms for systemwide communication, which is a powerful tool in creating both vision and common understanding in redesign initiatives. Electronic mail and agile minds are both needed to keep up with the short change cycles in the evolution of health care.

REENGINEERING IN A CORPORATE STRUCTURE

Multi-Institutional Systems As Corporate Structures

For simplicity, multi-institutional systems are referred to as corporations in this chapter. A multi-institutional system is a corporate body with health care services provided in multiple settings. The term corporate in health care has been associated with multi-institutional systems, even though free-standing hospitals may be corporations. The multi-institutional systems may comprise different types of services. For example, a multihospital system is defined as two or more hospitals or a horizontally organized system. A multi-institutional system may include hospitals, long-term care facilities, home care, and ambulatory care. These systems are referred to as vertically integrated systems, meaning that they have comprehensive service capability for the continuum of care. For purposes of this chapter, the loosely applied term *corporation* is used to refer to the multi-institutional system.

Focus on Nursing Services

Although this article focuses on nursing services, it is unlikely that reengineering initiatives will concentrate solely on nursing services. Because nursing care is so integrated in the total care the patient receives, reengineering nursing services naturally implies a more broadly based approach: patient care. It also naturally implies involvement of physicians, pharmacists, and other health care professionals in the reengineering process.[2] Nurses in a multi-institutional system have a distinct advantage by working together to define and position clinical nursing care in the broad arena of health care systems. Another advantage to nurses who participate in reengineering nursing services in a multi-institutional system is the energy and growth for nurses, physicians, administrators, and others involved.

The Design of Reengineering

Reengineering is simply changing what is to what could be. In a corporation, the initiative may involve reengineering the corporation.[3] Examples are formation of a system or network of care—a specific type of service or job category within the corporation. Health care corporations have been influenced just as other businesses, by futurists. Visions of the future conjure up images of a world in which electronic communication prevails and one in which data and information are available to anyone who has access to a computer and software.[4] This world is very different from the one we have known. An outcome of this information age is that the traditional power structures of organization give way to more fluid forms of decision making and participation. Health care is as influenced by these changes as other businesses. The economic constraints in health care, however, tend to mask the widespread societal and technological changes. Even so, hospitals, like businesses, are being reshaped, refinanced, realigned, and reformed.[5]

One can conclude that radical change in all types of organizations is inevitable and that one of health care's general precepts is that the changes must effectively address economic constraints. Health care is subject to societal changes influencing business in general. Power in the future lies not in traditional structures but in designing the reengineered organization. Being in control is of the essence.

After Accepting the Need To Change

The inevitability of change is an underlying assumption that significantly influences decisions about redesigning. What to reengineer, which methodology for redesign to use, and how to implement the change process are the important questions. How to evaluate the outcomes of change is the greatest challenge. In a sense, formation of the multi-institutional system—a different type of corporate structure for most health care entities—is a "redesign." It is also an example of how change that focuses on one aspect of the organization eventually influences all other parts. Only recently has nursing service in a corporation been significantly influenced by reengineered corporate structures. The emergence of clinical services as the reason for being, which has been made clear in health care reform debates, has opened up avenues for increasing the visibility of clinical services.[6] Needless to say, nursing is a major clinical service, recognized by many as one of the significant, fundamental services for which health care corporations exist.

Clinical services are rising to the front lines now because more care is being delivered in ambulatory, home, and nontraditional settings. These services delivered in multiple sites are seen without the mantle of the hospital or the service infrastructure the hospital conveys. The captive hospitalized patient with a captive staff is giving way to an informed participative client who expects excellent, competent, quality care. This imposing list of adjectives is used to indicate that clinical services may be provided in a variety of settings with equally good results if the caregivers are competent and have the appropriate resources. The increasing mobility of clinical health professionals supported by mobile technology allows many new approaches to care delivery.

Another indication that clinical services have been discovered by the public and by payers is the attention being given to methodologies in care delivery. Care planning, for example, in the form of clinical pathways, is now used as a way to define clinical services, control the cost, promote understanding of health care in the business world, and ensure a measure for utilization of health care resources and productivity. The public is hungry for something tangible to use in managing health care. The expert judgment and clinical knowledge that have been the health professionals' commodities continue to be poorly understood because the outcomes of decision making are more measurable and visible than the decision-making process. Defining health care outcomes continues to be an area of discovery that has yet to fulfill the public expectation of a tangible, visible expression of professional clinical care.[7] This matter remains fundamental in any redesign initiative.

The Scope of Reengineering

Reengineering has to start somewhere. Choices have to be made about the best way to introduce reengineering in a corporation or any of its organizations. Consider the range of possibilities for where to start redesigning:

- the organizational structure
- leadership
- access to care
- the system for care delivery in a region or community
- the way clinical care is delivered within a system
- the work of the organization: patient care delivery
- the way clinical care is delivered in any given entity (e.g., in a long-term care facility or on a patient care unit)
- the way nurses work with other health care professionals
- the way patients access and use the health care system
- ways patients and families participate in the care of patients
- an information system that supports patient care delivery
- admitting and discharge processes for care episodes
- staffing to include a qualified team
- services to provide comprehensive care
- care planning to provide continuity of care

This list of possibilities provides a brief view of the complexity of decision making regarding reengineering. It is neither inclusive nor proven. Reengineering initiatives in health care as well as in business have not been tested or verified through research.[8] The culture of reengineering is emerging from the lore of anecdotal information, expert observations, and the natural order of adaptation to a changing world. Storytelling has become an important way of transmitting information about reengineering, the methods and processes used, and the barriers to change. The question of where to start with redesigning initiatives is thus open to debate and influenced by business imperatives, patient or community priorities, and the talents and predilections of the grass roots and leaders who are redesigning organizations.

INITIATING REENGINEERING EFFORTS

Reengineering is initiated as soon as the decision is made to think about and plan for the change. Reengineering is all about change. The literature offers contrasting viewpoints about the optimum way to initiate change. Terms such as reengineering, restructuring, redesigning, and reform are used. Definition of the meaning of each of these terms is a moot point when people are experiencing change. Some argue for a top-down approach, whereas others believe in a grass roots approach.[9] The fact is that reengineering, redesigning, restructuring, or reforming initiatives will not be effective unless the whole organization is engaged in meaningful ways. The approach to restructuring in a corporation is more complex than in a single organization. If the change is to be corporatewide, should the change be designed at the corporate office level and then implemented in each organization?

Another view of how to initiate and implement change within a corporation is to introduce the change in one or more of the corporation's organizations and then spread to the remainder, over time. This approach allows testing of the reengineering initiative and an opportunity to learn from the pioneer implementers. The possible pitfall is that the redesign initiative will be tailored to a given organization. The question of replicability must be addressed in this approach. Resistance from other corporate sites can stem from the question of whether the same reengineering design will work in every organization in the corporation. One organization within the corporation can reengineer effectively without significantly changing the corporation as a whole.

BUILDING ON STRENGTHS

Multi-institutional systems have an advantage of systemwide sponsorship, mission, values, and, usually, a vision of the current state as well as the future. Consistency in these important elements provides a unifying thread that expands the perspective of restructuring. One can depersonalize change in a corporation by transcending any one organization's response to change. When all organizations within the corporation are experiencing similar change effects, the perspective of organizational change as a global phenomenon can override the tendency to be paranoid about local power and motivational issues. The perspective of change rather than interpersonal or departmental conflict changes the playing field. A corporation also has the advantage of networking and sharing among peers in a noncompetitive environment to promote understanding of change and acceptance. When managed well, the strength of shared experiences can become stimulating and supportive. One can share in a group in which all are members of the same corporation more easily than with those eyeing one's market share. Competition to perform does exist in corporations, which can facilitate good performance.

THE CRITICAL ELEMENT IN REENGINEERING: THE WORKER

In either multi-institutional corporations or single organizations, successful reengineering is dependent on recognizing that the worker is critical to the organization's success. Consequently, change has to involve the workers to gain commitment and participation. Change processes grounded in enhancing, improving, or strengthening the relationships between and among people at all levels in the organization are more likely to be successful. Early restructuring initiatives tended to follow more traditional change processes that began with creating readiness to change before implementing great change. In today's world, this approach is referred to as incremental change, which may not be bold enough or fast enough to keep up with the times. Any initiative or process that provides a pathway to restructure by making people more comfortable with their own decisions, with change, and with team approaches to problem solving and decision making is useful.[10]

Truly radical change engages people in fundamental ways. Radical change implies a new reality. The world as we know it no longer exists, and new ways must be found. Such change involves not only the workers but also their workplace, the materials and technology they use to perform work, and their communication. Technology is the operative word in radical change.[11] The point is that change is inevitable; there are different avenues for initiating change, and the approach to change must be as carefully designed as the desired change.

A CORPORATE APPROACH TO CHANGE

Entry points to reengineering by corporations may range from a broad approach, such as changing the corporate organizational structure, to a very specific approach, such as a task analysis and work reengineering initiative. Some highlights of change particular to corporations deserve consideration:

- reengineering organizational structures
- centralization versus decentralization
- the centralized, decentralized, and combined reengineering models
- common themes in reengineering processes

Reengineerng Organizational Structures

In the broadest sense, multi-institutional systems are the result of a form of organizational reengineering. Establishment of a health corporation with multiple entities unites them in a corporate body that may achieve both economy of scale and economy of scope.[12] Shared financing, purchasing, and policies and procedures improve efficiency if applied appropriately. Corporations, because of the variety of entities that make up the whole, may also develop a broader perspective of health care. Formation of health care networks to provide care throughout the life span—the continuum of care—is an example of a broader perspective, allowing not only shared resources but also more comprehensive services.

The corporate structure reengineering focuses on the function of the corporate office in relation to the entities. Commonly centralized functions are finance, purchasing contracts, human resource policies, and quality management.

Should executive management and operational aspects of the services be centralized? If the answer to this question is yes, then the corporate structure reflects centralized policy and decision making, with model management structures put in place in each of the corporate entities. For example, chief executive officers are generally employed by the corporation. In centralized corporations, finance officers and human resource executives are also corporate employees. A reporting-line authority is typical of centralization.

If the answer to the question is no, corporate office functions may focus on administrative matters involving the corporation as a whole, with each entity managing its own business. In this case, it is typical to establish management goals and objectives that local managers must meet.

Centralization versus Decentralization

Reengineering the corporation may involve changing from a centralized to a decentralized structure or vice versa. Centralized structures allow more control and a sense of "systemness," whereas decentralized structures provide for shared governance models with local decision making. Health care services by nature tend to be local, owing to the unique relationship between the services and persons who use them. A community hospital, home care agency, or ambulatory service is locally based in relation to the persons served. Corporations, to be successful, attend to the local nature of health care when designing the structure. Even academic health science centers, which serve a wider range of persons from geographically distant locations, are community and culturally based.

The two key questions are:

1. Which health care services and/or management structures should be centralized to achieve an advantage in the marketplace and which should be decentralized?
2. Which functions are best provided centrally and which are best provided locally?

Corporations with organizations in different geographic locations must be sensitive to local culture. A health care organization, to be effective, must provide services commensurate with local expectations. The strength of local influence on the organization may override corporate influence on some matters. Meeting local expectations is important. Corporations may have designed image, approach, and service structures sufficiently unique and replicable to be implemented in different settings. Psychiatric services of the 1980s were organized and implemented in such a way. General medical-surgical services generally have not been designed for such generalized application.

Three Models

Three models of corporate reengineering can be applied to nursing services.

1. *Centralized model*—In a centralized model, which is compatible with a centralized system, change is planned for systemwide implementation.
2. *Decentralized model*—In a decentralized model, corporate entities may be unified by mission, values, and financing, but the management and operations of health care delivery are locally defined and controlled.
3. *Combined model*—In combined models, functions that affect all entities equally, such as human resources, purchasing, or quality management, are centralized; the other functions are not centralized.

Health care corporations that include a number of hospitals and perhaps a long-term care facility and home care services may be centralized, decentralized, or a combination of both.

Centralized Reengineering Model

Reengineering in a centralized model is accomplished by deciding what the redesigned structure should look like, planning the process to accomplish the redesigned structure, and implementing the change. The decision-making process can be approached in several ways. Consultants may be engaged to design the model. The consultants usually work with selected corporate staff in this design and may also implement the model. In some cases, the corporate staff, working with representatives of each entity, may implement the redesigning. A centralized approach is advantageous because it allows for one plan, one design team, a common implementation strategy, and objectives. Disadvantages include the local nature of health care, with variety in culture, patient population, and staff expertise in each of the corporate entities. All of these factors must be considered when planning the most appropriate redesign initiatives.

In general, either very specific or very general approaches to reengineering work best with the centralized model.

Assessing readiness for change in each setting is basic to implementation. When the restructuring has to do with work redesign or changing staff tasks, the temptation to implement the "boilerplate" can be very strong. Centralized reengineering works best if staff employees are included in planning and implementation and if the initiatives are kept in perspective to the whole.

Decentralized Reengineering Model

In an effort led by corporate staff with or without consultants, decentralized reengineering models are planned and implemented in the local organization. In the decentralized approach, the corporate entities may share educational programs and visioning sessions to determine what the future should look like, and they may agree on major themes and concepts integral to redesign. Each entity then takes its learning and works out the redesign plan and implementation locally. The advantage of this approach is that people in each location are empowered to think through the reengineering process and to structure the plan and implementation in ways that suit the local institution, while also meeting the corporate objectives for redesign.

The result is an approach compatible with local culture and resources. Disadvantages include costly repeated discovery of what works and what does not, uneven change due to different resources and leadership, and less consistent results. Decentralized reengineering requires development of clear performance outcomes that serve as guidelines or outcomes to be achieved. Otherwise each organization may define its own level of performance.

Combination Reengineering Model

Both centralized and decentralized aspects of reengineering are included in the combination reengineering model. The centralized model features include visioning of the future, consideration of possibilities, and agreement on priorities by all participating entities in the corporation. Commonly shared materials and resources may then be developed to save time and money in the development process. Local autonomy is respected in that each entity selects its own plan to implement the changes but with commonly held corporate objectives for change. Some aspects of change, such as a task analysis, a job or work redesign process, or a service line plan may be implemented in all settings. The way in which more specific change is implemented and related to the whole is designed locally.

Advantages of this model include savings from selected planned interventions or changes, while local needs and control issues are accommodated. Disadvantages of this combined model relate to the difficulty in selecting change initiatives and plans that can be used with equal results by each entity and that fit into each different structure. More process is required to retain the focus on objectives for redesigning. Local events may distract from the reengineering, yielding uneven results and intervening factors that may be interpreted as negative to the desired change.

The models for reengineering fit different types of corporations. In all three, the decision must be made about what to reengineer. Consider the possibilities: the list of where to begin reengineering offers a brief glance at the complexity of reengineering.

In addition, corporations may consider reengineering to be a way to form alliances with physician groups or to acquire new entities to expand markets. The range of possibilities is usually translated into "opportunities" to improve, enhance, or streamline the organization.

Common Themes in Reengineering Processes

Corporations have an advantage in reengineering afforded by the networking and sharing that go beyond one setting. Within a corporation, peers may work together and share ideas without the constraints of competition. In today's health care environment, changes are inevitable. The emphasis on health care reform has accelerated redesign initiatives. Now, leaders of these initiatives must decide whether to redesign from the inside out to create integrated networks for care. This inside-out approach fundamentally changes the relationship among entities providing patient care such as home care, long-term care, and acute care. Another option is to focus on the arrangements between and among the various settings where health care is delivered, without significantly changing each setting. In light of today's challenges, some of the redesigning initiatives that seemed bold now fade in comparison with the new care networks being formed.

Reengineering patient care delivery in the corporate structure allows a broad view of the delivery system. If the corporation includes primary care, acute care, long-term care, and home care entities, the broad view leads to reengineering to provide the continuum of care in ways that change each entity.

All entities must have representation in planning and development to foster successful reengineering attributes, which are as follows:

1. Commitment
2. Common vision
   - organization of services around patients
   - premise of optimized resources: higher quality and lower costs
   - optimal use of resources

- increased flexibility, increased responsiveness to patients
- continuity of care
  - in-hospital component
  - for episode of care (time limited and across settings) and managed care (continuum from wellness to illness care, over time, and across settings)
- qualified staff
- expanded roles and functions
- integrated teams
- a key role of registered nurse as patient care coordinator

SPECIAL CONSIDERATIONS FOR REENGINEERING CLINICAL SERVICES

Some reengineering initiatives focus directly on clinical services. These initiatives must be sensitive to the fact that clinical services are embedded in both professional disciplines and organizational habit. In many reengineering efforts, formation of clinical care teams causes much soul searching, and in some cases, an identity crisis.[13] In some reengineering initiatives, issues to be addressed must be considered throughout the redesign process.

Most clinicians will be concerned about the following three issues:

1. Who is accountable for care outcomes?
   - physician
   - nurse
   - team
2. How can staff be motivated to accept accountability?
3. Which clinical services and management structures should be consolidated? What criteria should be used for consolidation?

MANAGING THE ISSUES

Assessment

Reengineering is facilitated by assessment of patient care and nursing services in the corporation. This assessment provides insights about initiation, implementation, and evaluation from the outset. The assessment includes eight key aspects as follows:

1. determination of what should be the same (standardized) and what should be differentiated

2. framework for patient care delivery
3. principles for application to patient care
4. guidelines for patient services delivery in the continuum
5. clarification of roles and functions of nurses and other clinicians
6. definition of relationships and decision-making process
7. community involvement
8. proposal for system of care delivery

Participation

Leaders from the many organizations within a corporation gain by sharing and learning to work with each other's cultures.[14] For example, some may sense that their hospital is very open and people oriented. Others may perceive that differences in employee satisfaction and involvement are significant and may serve as barriers. They feel that "mixing cultures" will result in some lost identity.

Risk Taking

Formal and informal leaders emerge in reengineering efforts. These persons are risk takers who take the lead in supporting and shaping a different model for patient care delivery. In the early stages of reengineering, understanding and awareness may be provided for key staff by having them read and research reengineering and by having them talk to others who have experienced similar changes. These methods help prepare people for change. Risk takers usually emerge in this awareness-heightening stage of the process.

Consultants

Whether to use and how to use consultants in the redesign process are important considerations. Are consultants needed to help prepare a design team? To design the change? To provide for cultural team building? Often, consultants are engaged to lead key staff in the thinking and visioning phases, to ensure consistency in expectations and goals for the change process. This shared visioning also begins the processes of building implementation teams, to draw people into doing the work of reengineering. Inclusion of appropriate groups—care providers, ancillary staff, and support workers on the team in training—is necessary for effective change.

Assessment of readiness for change may be helpful to put the process on a fast track. One common approach is to deal with attitudes about patient care and services provided for clinical and nonclinical aspects of care. How does a patient perceive the care provided? If the readiness for change must be developed and if the staff is not prepared for empowerment and leadership, the reengineering may be initiated in discrete ways. An example is work reengineering analysis in which work processes are examined, tasks are sequenced for efficiency, and staff implement the new task sequence. One pitfall in this approach is that almost anyone can perform one or two tasks. Unless decision making is provided for, and unless oversight is provided to ensure that tasks are performed correctly and appropriately, the discrete task analysis approach can reduce the success of the outcome in the long term and the credibility of the change process in the short term.

Incentives for Reengineering

One of the challenges of reengineering is gaining the support of employees and retaining it through the change process. Initiatives such as gain-sharing programs, which develop responsible teams whose performance is measured against organizationwide targets for financial and clinical outcomes, serve to help team members perceive the team as a part of the organization as a whole. To be effective, team goals must be quantifiable, attainable, and relate to the whole institution. Evaluation of outcomes is used as a performance measure for salary increases, gain sharing, or other financial rewards. The best incentive is involving staff in the study of what and how to reengineer.

Retaining the Commitment

The downside of reengineering is that, if it is not managed appropriately, staff may suffer loss of identity, alienation, loss of pride, nonconstructive competition, and loss of commitment.

Reengineering that starts with or that involves nursing services is best fostered when the following features are attended to:

- common philosophy to determine the model
- model to try out what works best
- common decision regarding framework and attributes of change
- linkages with centralized functions, such as accounting
- patient-centered value system
- team skill—a specialized task or skill efficiency
- sense of oneness
- commitment to patient
- commitment to improvement

CONCLUSION

It is easier to put a model on paper than to figure out how it works. Often, the desired impact on patient care is different from what is expected. Questions of accountability are inevitable. Can several people on a team be accountable for coordinated effort or does there need to be a standard-bearer for key aspects?

The code words for reengineering, restructuring, redesign, and reforming are similar: work "smarter," consolidate, avoid duplication, eliminate unnecessary processes or steps, and look for ways to improve outcomes without using more resources. For nurses responsible for patient care delivery, these code words continue to be compelling. Nurses, perhaps because of gender characteristics, education, or sheer practicality, are by nature resource conservationists. In fact, this tendency of nurses may be the greatest barrier to nursing's capability to effectively reposition itself in the future.

The approaches to reengineering may be global or very specific. Reengineering activities become increasingly more defined as the process flows from conceptualization to application. Initial design is more abstract and allows room for brainstorming and creativity. Implementation plans become more specific and less open to discussion and debate. Application to practice becomes even more defined and specific. It is easy to flow with the reengineering movement and to become focused on "the project" or the redesign activities. It is important to view these focused activities as means to an end. The opportunity to enhance nursing's future capability to serve communities, patients, and families lies in keeping the global view alive. Most reengineering initiatives decrease layers in organizations, disperse decision making, and expand the scope of employees. Nursing must retain a perspective of global redesign, in which nursing care is a major component of health care in the continuum. Real change lies in this global perspective.

REFERENCES

1. Sovie M. Exceptional executive leadership shapes nursing's future. *Nurs Econ.* 1987; 5(1): 13–20.
2. Keeney R. Creativity in decision making with value-focused thinking. *Sloan Manage Rev.* 1994; 35(4):33–44.
3. Hammer M, Champy J. *Reengineering the Corporation: Manifesto for Business Revolution.* New York: HarperBusiness; 1993.
4. Tonges MC, Lawrenz E. Reengineering, the work redesign-technology link. *J Nsg Admin.* 1993; 23(10):15–22.
5. Krepinevich A. Keeping pace with military-technological revolution. *Issues Sci Technol.* 1994; 10(4):23–29.
6. Madden MJ, Ponte P. Advanced practice roles in the managed care environment. *J Nsg Admin.* 1994; 24(1):56–62.

7. Bandeian SH, Lewin L. What we don't know about health care reform. *Issues Sci Technol.* 1994; 10(3):52–59.

8. Caldwell B. Special report: Missteps, miscues. *Information Week.* June 20, 1994:50–60.

9. Jansen E, Eccles D, Changler G. Innovation and restrictive conformity among hospital employees: Individual outcomes and organizational considerations. *Hosp Health Services Adm.* 1994; 39(1):63–80.

10. Wilson B, Laschinger S. Staff nurse perception of job empowerment and organizational commitment: A test of Kanter's theory of structural power in organizations. *J Nsg Admin.* 1994; 24(45)(suppl):39–47.

11. Sewer A. Lessons from America's fastest-growing companies. *Fortune.* August 8, 1994: 42–60.

12. Stuckey J, White D. When and when not to vertically integrate. *Sloan Manage Rev.* 1993; 34(3):71–83.

13. Velianoff G, Neely C, Hall S. Developmental levels of interdisciplinary collaborative practice committees. *J Nsg Admin.* 1993; 23(7,8):26–29.

14. Sandrick KM. Prepare for change. *Trustee.* 1994; 47(7):6–9.

CHAPTER 13

Managing Diversity

Magdalena A. Mateo, PhD, RN, FAAN

Culture comprises the patterns of thoughts, feelings, behaviors, and symbols that recur throughout the organization.[1(p.34)] Each organization has cultures that guide decision-making processes. In a health care system, each unit has a subculture unique to the staff's professional values about how things are done. In reengineering, units or services may be combined, resulting in a new configuration of staff who have differing values, expectations, and subcultures. Differences in processes used when making decisions related to practice changes or conflict management could lead to culture clashes. The goal is to encourage diversity yet find a common ground to achieve cultural cohesion. When cultural cohesion is achieved, the group works toward common goals instead of against competing goals, thereby capitalizing on individual staff strengths and assisting others to grow. This chapter describes methods to manage diversity through involvement of all staff.

PROMOTING CULTURAL COHESION

Cultural diversity is defined as differences in perspective that stem from cultural backgrounds, and professional and life experiences. Although there are advantages and disadvantages to achieving diversity (Exhibit 13–1), the advantages outweigh the disadvantages.[2]

There is a great need to achieve multiculturalism at all levels of the work force in order to serve the diverse community. The long process required for achieving this goal has to be carefully planned and evaluated by monitoring milestones that are identified in the initial phases of the efforts. Interface between leadership and staff and harmony between an organization's values, norms, and policies with diversity are essential.[3,4] Organizational processes that enrich, recruit, and retain

Exhibit 13–1 Examples of Advantages and Disadvantages of Diversity in Organizations

---

Advantages

- Work force is more representative of consumers.
- Having multiple perspectives enhances problem solving and innovations in practice.
- Knowledge and understanding of other customs and cultures increase.
- Recruitment and retention of talented persons with various backgrounds are promoted.

Disadvantages

- Subgroups may exist, thus hindering unity.
- Addressing the concerns or issues of numerous groups is time consuming.
- Efforts to achieve diversity may be seen as mandated versus desired by an organization.
- Openness in resolving conflicts may be challenging.

---

a diverse work force are crucial in making diversity management come alive following reengineering efforts when there may be fear of losing jobs and stress that is triggered by coping with change. To maintain a fully functioning staff amidst diversity, processes must be established to promote cultural cohesion.

Nash and Everett[5] reported on the practical application of the Model for Cultural Cohesion by Cartwright and Cooper.[6] Effective cultural integration includes

- an understanding of existing cultures
- unfreezing of existing cultures and recognition that a degree of cultural integration or change is vital within a realistic time
- presentation of a positive and realistic view of the future
- full cooperation of members
- a process for monitoring the progress of cultural integration or change

ELEMENTS OF DIVERSITY MANAGEMENT

Managing diversity means that each person will be valued and will be assisted to perform to his or her potential. Leaders assume an important role in promoting a work environment that supports diversity. Bhimani and Acorn reported on closely related issues in managing a culturally diverse environment[7]: (1) the importance for staff to understand cultural norms of patients whose cultural background differs from their background and (2) the need for managers to understand cultural norms of staff whose cultural background differs from their background. They suggested the following approaches for managers in promoting a culturally diverse work environment:

- Subscribe to the belief that diversity is an organizational strength.
- Facilitate staff awareness of cultural blind spots that get in the way of understanding others.
- Promote a broad definition of diversity that includes race, religion, nationality, language, sex, age, education, work experiences, marital status, gender, and sexual orientation.
- Structure informal staff meetings to identify and discuss culturally based work problems.
- Be sensitive to the effect of speaking a language that patients do not understand.
- Plan to celebrate holidays specific to a culture.
- Make cultural assessment part of practice.

To manage diversity it is essential to gain knowledge of the overall organizational culture as well as work unit subcultures. Assessing staff attitudes and perceptions toward diversity is a necessary process to identify biases and ways to overcome problems that may be hindering participation in the organization's diversity efforts. Individuals could be encouraged to assist each other in sharing observations that may uncover biases. For example, staff can ask colleagues to observe them during interactions with people who have different professional or cultural backgrounds so that they may identify whether these interactions differ from their interactions with people who are similar to them. Exhibit 13-2 presents 10 guidelines that can be used to manage diversity.[8]

A culture audit is a tool used by organizations to assist leaders to assess current culture in relation to diversity.[1] There are five phases in a culture audit.

Phase One—Needs Awareness. When there are major organizational changes such as reengineering, administrators and clinical leaders recognize the need to make changes in policies, procedures, and staff roles.

Phase Two—Cultural Diagnosis. Outside consultants, in collaboration with the organizational advisory groups, gather data from staff through observations, structured focus groups, individual interviews, or surveys. Examples of questions include the way practice changes are made, how staff react to role changes, or the presence of systems that contribute to the success of staff in fulfilling their roles. Pertinent organizational data such as reporting structures and committees are also collected. Although organizations differ, similar indicators that contribute to suc-

Exhibit 13–2 Guidelines for Learning Diversity Management

1. Clarify the motivation for desiring diversity.
2. Clarify the vision of the meaning of diversity in an environment where each person's potential contributes to the mission.
3. Expand a focus of diversity to encompass a work force that is reflective of society.
4. Conduct a culture audit.
5. Modify assumptions that respect multiculturalism versus traditional group culture definitions (e.g., adhering only to the traditional definition of a family—father, mother, and children living together).
6. Modify systems such as promotions, mentorship, and sponsorship to advance in the organization.
7. Modify models of leadership, manager, and staff behaviors.
8. Help staff be pioneers of change.
9. Apply the special consideration test. For example, "Will a program contribute to everyone's success, or will it only be an advantage to one group?"
10. Continue affirmative action to achieve work force diversity at every level.

Source: Adapted and reprinted by permission of *Harvard Business Review,* "From Affirmative Action to Affirming Diversity," by R. Roosevelt Thomas, Jr., March/April 1990. Copyright © 1990 by the President and Fellows of Harvard College; all rights reserved.

cess are shared.[9] There are four signs that indicate an organization's overall health, adaptability, strength, and vigor of functional systems:

1. Power: Do employees believe they can make things happen?
2. Identity: Do employees narrowly identify with subgroups or with the organization as a whole?
3. Conflict: How do staff members handle conflict? Is conflict confronted and resolved?
4. Learning: How does the organization learn? How does it deal with new ideas?

Phase Three—The Plan for Change. The organization determines whether the result of the culture audit presents a culture that will enhance or deter the changes required. Processes included in this phase are

- comparing the culture with organizational characteristics such as the structure and systems for decision making and the responsibilities of leaders and staff
- determining the characteristics that hinder a change, for example, determining whether committee structures have adequate staff representation from

varied cultural backgrounds or what process the organization will use to obtain input from staff whose role is affected by a change in a policy or procedure

- identifying the desired goal of achieving cultural cohesion

Phase Four—Action. The organization moves toward cultural cohesion by establishing systems to be used for promoting and monitoring decision-making processes and implementing changes that facilitate the inclusion of all staff and outcomes of initiatives.

Phase Five—Evaluation. The organization assesses the progress of change as reflected by performance, for example, employee productivity and involvement in activities, including diversity initiatives.

STRATEGIES FOR PROMOTING DIVERSITY EFFORTS

Managing the diversity that results from changing systems and structures is critical. For example, memberships of teams, communication patterns, conflict resolution methods, and operations that relate to goals all require change following reengineering. Successful organizations have the ability to revitalize systems and structures by eliciting participation from all staff. Involvement of all staff and working toward common goals empower staff to participate in diversity efforts. It is essential to foster skill development, determine a process for integration of cultures, monitor the plan, and evaluate outcomes. The following strategies are useful in promoting diversity.

Foster Staff Commitment to Diversity

Common strategies to gain commitment from all levels of staff are educational programs and inclusion of diversity in competencies and performance evaluation. Essential to success are organizational and leadership support and an emphasis on strategies to overcome barriers.[10] Prejudices and attitudes that get in the way of diversity must be identified. For example, a barrier that might hinder diversity efforts is assuming that staff members communicate or deal with change in similar ways. To avoid such assumptions, staff can be encouraged to validate their perceptions of a situation before judging.

Recruit Staff Champions

To spearhead efforts, identify and provide ongoing support for staff who have a great interest in diversity. The staff champions could take the lead in identifying realistic plans, implementing the organizational plan, and evaluating outcomes.

Stress Group Similarities

Stress group similarities while highlighting how differences enrich the organization. Patient care goals are accomplished more easily when differences are valued and shared by all staff. These goals could be stressed as the similarities that everyone shares. Differences may emerge in the role and perceptions of others' roles. Identifying the way these differences add value to excellent patient care highlights the importance of promoting diversity. For example, the staff role in assisting patients with discharge planning includes patient education and ensuring that there is a caregiver if the patient is not able to be independent with activities of daily living after leaving the hospital. The primary nurse or case manager may feel primarily responsible for assisting the patient with discharge planning, while social workers may feel that it is their responsibility. While there is a need to delineate responsibilities, the differences in the perspectives of the primary nurse (e.g., immediate care needs following discharge), case manager (e.g., seamless transition to home or placement), and social worker (e.g., long-term plans for placement, if required) benefit the patient. Clarifying roles decreases duplication and stresses the value of each health care team member.

Foster Skill Development

Empower staff by fostering skill development. An essential aspect of skill development is an ongoing assessment of strengths and areas of growth of the staff in relation to the missions and goals of the organization, including diversity. Developing a feasible process is helpful, such as a skill development grid for staff nurses (Table 13–1). Staff could use the grid to monitor their progress in meeting goals and share the information with their managers so that they may get appropriate support. The demands of health care organizations require the continuous and simultaneous development of staff skills in the areas of practice, education, research, and administration. For example, with regard to diversity initiatives, it is vital to have the ability to provide excellent care to patients from other ethnic groups. The approach to education of patients who are unable to communicate in English requires resourcefulness from the caregiver in communicating the essential aspects of a health condition in an understandable manner.

Table 13–1 Skill Development Grid Example

Focus of Skill Development	Strengths	Areas for Growth	Key Points for Development & Target Dates	Indicators of Success
Practice • Care of diverse patient population • Collaboration Intradisciplinary Interdisciplinary Multidisciplinary	Experience providing care to a patient with an Asian cultural background, which differs from my cultural background	Obtain knowledge of cultural background of a patient since it may not be obvious from physical attributes	Suggest to colleagues the inclusion in admission assessment, inquiry about patient's cultural backgrounds by 1/99	Ongoing inclusion in admission assessment form questions on the cultural background of a patient
Education • Orientation of staff • Preceptor experience • Preparation and presentation of classes to diverse groups	Knowledge of various teaching strategies	Frequently assumes that everyone learns the same way that I learn	Use tools to evaluate learning styles of participants if possible before a presentation. Develop a method for matching personal styles of a preceptor and the orientee by 6/99	Considers learner's styles and adapts teaching strategies to enhance learning
Research • Use of various types of literature for seeking solutions to clinical problems • Evaluation of outcomes from multiple perspectives • Evidence-based practice • Participation in development of data collection tools • Responding to initiatives of the organization, e.g., surveys • Presentation of data	Ability to understand and read research reports	Acceptance that not all staff have the capability to read and understand research articles	Interpret research language and communicate relevant information to practitioners in a way that information applies to practice by 12/98	Use of research results in practice protocols, development of critical path

continues

Table 13–1 continued

Focus of Skill Development	Strengths	Areas for Growth	Key Points for Development & Target Dates	Indicators of Success

Administration
• Management
• Leadership
• Facilitation and conduct of meetings
• Communication
  • Written
  • Verbal
• Performance evaluation
• Giving & receiving critical feedback
• Self-evaluation
	Provide critical feedback to colleagues who have the same cultural background	Give critical feedback to colleagues whose cultural backgrounds differ from mine	Acquire knowledge of communication patterns of one of my colleagues whose cultural background is different from mine by 12/98	Able to give critical feedback in a respectful manner and is accepted well by the recipient

Other • Support for diversity • Use of technology	Knowledge that I have prejudices about people from some cultures, for example, colleagues who do not respond instantly to requests but prefer to think things over before responding	Confront and do something about my prejudices so that my interactions with these people are not influenced in a negative manner and assume that the person is incapable of fulfilling responsibilities	Seek help from colleagues in evaluating biases that may be identified during my interactions with a staff by 1/99	Gain objectivity and not judge a staff's actions based on my prejudices

Evaluate

Evaluate the organization's progress in the stages toward achieving multi-culturalism. Integrating cultures and subcultures occurs in stages, as described by Bruhn.[2]

- *Stage 1.* Awareness, education, and modeling are achieved through education programs, diverse work teams, and the visible commitment and modeling of managers. During this stage, commitment to diversity efforts is conveyed by sponsoring organizationwide activities during work time, assisting staff to develop goals with identified target dates, and getting input from staff regarding the support required for them to successfully meet their goals.
- *Stage 2.* A change in attitudes, behaviors, and values of the organization is reflected in all employees. Indicators are a change in management style, career development for all employees, the recruitment and retention program, and diverse staff members teaching diversity programs. Managers conduct follow-up meetings with staff to identify progress toward individual goals. Meetings with new employees include an assessment of their perception of the organizational culture, for example, whether they feel welcomed or included in activities. Providing critical feedback to new employees, which includes strengths and areas of growth, is important during the first two years so that adjustment issues are identified and addressed in a timely manner.
- *Stage 3.* Diversity is fully integrated in organizational structure and operations. The indicators for achieving this stage include valuing and managing diversity, existence of and adherence to a unified policy on diversity, high employee morale, and diversity of the work force at all staff levels. The organization's annual plan reflects progress with regard to numbers of staff recruited and retention rates. Staff at all levels evaluate diversity initiatives and their effect on the work environment.

CONCLUSION

Successful organizations with high productivity, a strong bottom line, and a high quality of work life possess similar cultural characteristics related to leaders, organization, and staff involvement.[1] Leaders have a vision and the structures for providing high-quality products and services, as defined by their customers. They have a full commitment to employee empowerment, authority, responsibility, decision making, and participation in continuous learning and improvement. Effective leaders facilitate the formation of internal communication mechanisms that value unique employee contributions to an organization. They believe that diversity works and provides positive rewards to staff who help to make it work. Organizations that support diversity reflect it in their policies and procedures. Diversity of the work force is manifested in a multicultural way in leadership, direct caregivers, and support staff. Recruitment and retention efforts reflect the commitment to a diverse work force. Staff involvement in planning, implementing, and evaluating diversity efforts is conveyed through their active participation in all facets of the organization's activities such as attendance and presentation of seminars focusing on diversity.

REFERENCES

1. Wilkof R, Ziegenfuss JT. Culture audits: A tool for change. *Health Progress.* 1995; 76(4): 34–38.

2. Bruhn JG. Creating an organizational climate for multiculturalism. *Health Care Superv.* 1996; 14(4):11–18.

3. Gardenswartz L, Rowe A. Diversity management: Practical application in a health care organization. *Frontiers of Health Serv Manage.* 1994; 11(2):36–40.

4. Gardenswartz L, Rowe A. *Managing Diversity in Health Care.* San Francisco, CA: Jossey-Bass; 1998.

5. Nash MG, Everett LN. Cultural cohesion versus collision. *J Nurs Adm.* 1996; 26(7/8):11–18.

6. Cartwright S, Cooper CL. *Mergers and Acquisitions.* Oxford, England: Butterworth-Heinemann; 1992.

7. Bhimani R, Acorn S. Managing within a culturally diverse environment. *Canadian Nurse.* 1998; 94(8):32–36.

8. Thomas RR Jr. From affirmative action to affirming diversity. *Harvard Business Rev.* 1990; 68(2):107–117.

9. Pascale R, Millemann M, Gioja L. Changing the way we change. *Harvard Business Rev.* 1997; 75(6):126–139.

10. Taylor R. Check your cultural competence. *J Nurs Manage.* 1998; 29(8):30–32.

CHAPTER 14

The Learning Team

Hussein A. Tahan, MS, RN, CNA

Through our learning, we create ourselves.

—Peter Senge

It is crucial that health care organizations engaged in reengineering, restructuring, or redesign efforts share Peter Senge's limitless regard for the power and importance of ongoing and conscious learning. Effective learning can prepare health care providers, teams, and organizations for unending success and prosperity. It also prevents failure and sustains survival. Today's health care organizations are seeking learning not only to achieve excellence in care provision but also to maintain or improve it. Billions of dollars are spent on reengineering as the concerns of administrators and executives regarding the pressures of the health care environment (e.g., cost reduction, quality improvement, competition, and consumer and employee satisfaction) continue to intensify. A considerable amount of money is also spent on training and education of staff. This chapter examines the issues surrounding learning in the reengineered/process-centered organization and provides health care administrators with an alternative view to teaching and education.

TEACHING, EDUCATING, OR LEARNING

Reengineered health care organizations cannot continue to rely on their traditional educational capabilities. They need to establish new ways of learning; otherwise their reengineering efforts are sentenced to fail. The revolution of reengineering in the health care industry has led to the re-creation of work teams, particularly because of a shift in interest to improving the processes of care delivery. The productivity of the team is based on its characteristics (i.e., teamwork, unity, cohesiveness, comfort, knowledge, and ability to learn) and the balance between the goals of each individual member, the team goals, and the goals of the health care organization. Learning is an important characteristic of the work team. The ability of the team members to acquire new skills and gain new knowledge improves the care delivery processes, enhances team performance and productivity, and increases the chances for success.

Restructured operations require redesigned learning/educational services. The demand for learning changes as the organizational operations and systems move toward a philosophy of teamwork, reliance on work teams, team goals, team productivity and performance, peer coaching and mentoring, and team-based process ownership. In the reengineered/process-centered organization, individual learning activities are tied to team-based thinking and a process-based learning. Focusing on team-based learning is an important philosophy because learning together leads to working together, provides a variety of opportunities for continued learning, enhances better understanding of problems and solutions, and results in creativity and innovation. Working and learning together in work teams enhances the process of developing mutual trust and respect. In addition, team members become better able to recognize each others' contribution to team performance, productivity, and learning. Thus, a person's worth is more appreciated.

During the life after reengineering, the use of the terms *teaching* or *educating* in a health care organization is replaced with use of the word *learning*. It is important to differentiate between these terms since their meanings have significant effects on the operations of the reengineered environment, especially in the areas of developing new skills and knowledge, and thus competent performance. Teaching and educating denote instructing, whereas learning implies gaining knowledge. While the use of the terms *educating* and *teaching* means providing staff with information or facts needed for job performance, it is unclear whether the tasks of teaching and educating result in the staff developing the skills necessary for satisfactory performance and productivity. Educating and/or teaching imply that one person is sharing information with another. However, these tasks do not establish whether the person receiving the information is able to understand it, use it, or apply it in performing the job for which he or she is accountable.

Using an alternate term such as *learning* eliminates this dilemma. Learning denotes the act of gaining knowledge, understanding, and/or skill. Learning deals with building knowledge beyond the task of sharing information. Switching to the use of the term *learning* during or after the reengineering process is important because it entails the process of teaching as well as the outcome of teaching (i.e., learning/building knowledge), whereas the terms *teaching* and *educating* are limited to the process of instructing only.

Learning may occur in different forms. One may learn from other team members, the team leader, members of other teams, or from one's experiences. Thus, learning is not limited to one person learning from another (i.e., educator) as is the situation in the traditional teaching and educational practices employed prior to reengineering. A health care professional may learn while performing the care processes for which he or she is accountable through experimentation, discovery, and realization. Thus, a health care professional may gain knowledge through work functions and experiences or through working and interacting with others; that is, members of the work team. In the rest of this chapter, the term *learning* is used instead of *teaching* or *educating*.

HEALTH CARE REENGINEERING AND LEARNING

Reengineering has been viewed as an essential survival tool that provides organizations with incredible promise and hope to meet the demands of the health care system, counteracts the pressures of the environment, improves performance/productivity, and sustains marketability and survival. Reengineering is defined as "the fundamental rethinking and radical redesign of business processes to achieve dramatic improvements in critical, contemporary measures of performance, such as cost, quality, service, and speed."[1(p.32)] The key elements of this definition are fundamental, radical, dramatic, and processes. The impact of these elements on health care organizations undergoing (or already having undergone) reengineering is discussed in other chapters of this book. This chapter, however, addresses the relationship between these elements and organizational and team learning.

Reengineering in regard to learning is the fundamental and radical change in the health care organization's learning processes to achieve higher standards of care as evidenced by staff's knowledge, skills, and competence in performing their patient care activities and processes. These learning efforts must then lead to dramatic patient care outcomes (e.g., high quality and improved consumer satisfaction) as well as organizational outcomes (e.g., lower cost and better marketability). This results in a paradigm shift from a traditional focus on teaching and education to an innovative focus on learning. The critical components of reengineering are the care provider's attitude toward patients and families, skills and knowledge of care activities, competence in care delivery, willingness to work in teams, and especially openness to continuous learning. The new environment of learning allows the staff to acquire these qualities during and after the process of reengineering to meet the needs and demands of patients, families, and fellow staff. Such qualities will then result in the provision of cost-effective care, superior quality, and superb consumer satisfaction.

RELATING THE FOUR KEY ELEMENTS OF REENGINEERING TO LEARNING

The real challenge to fundamentally, radically, and drastically changing the processes of care delivery and learning lies in the hands of the health care organization's work force, including executives, management, and workers. The staff's ability to change the way they work, how they think, and how they gain new knowledge and skills is an important determining factor of success in the reengineering effort. Performance and productivity in the process-centered environment of care should be built on new ideas and innovative approaches to care delivery and learning rather than focusing on past processes and what seemed to have worked. The environment of care must enhance the staff's ability to identify and pursue new learning opportunities that result in competitive care that meets the needs and demands of their consumers. Learning in the reengineered health care organization is dramatically different than traditional learning practices. Exhibit 14–1 presents a summary of the shifts associated with learning that take place after successful reengineering.

Exhibit 14–1 Learning Shifts as a Result of Successful Reengineering

From	*To*
• Teaching and educating	• Learning
• Instructing and information sharing	• Knowledge and skills building
• Task-based thinking	• Process-based thinking
• Task-based learning	• Process-based learning
• Classroom setting	• On-the-job setting
• Educator-based teaching	• Peer-based coaching
• Retrospective teaching	• Concurrent learning
• Centralized support	• Work team–based support
• Planned teaching	• Opportunistic/situational learning
• Mandatory/imposed teaching sessions	• Voluntary approach/self-identified needs
• Individual specialization	• Multiskilled staff
• Teaching at once	• Layered/incremental learning
• Teaching within disciplines	• Learning across disciplines
• Sporadic teaching	• Continuous/ongoing learning
• Past and present focus	• Future focus
• Time and space boundaries	• No boundaries
• Classroom teaching strategies	• Adult learning strategies

Learning opportunities in the reengineered organization can be fundamentally changed through a critical examination of the organization's educational practices (training and development and continuing education practices). Questions such as why employee education is important, why educational sessions are held that way, whether there are any alternative or better ways of educating staff, and what educational practices fit the new and reengineered processes of care delivery must be answered so that innovative practices can be developed. The process-centered organization is then able to focus its educational practices on the processes of care delivery; that is, learning opportunities become process based, untied to time or space, and unbound to a specific person. Hence, a futuristic vision of learning is born, wherein staff members are constantly learning as they provide patient care instead of learning in the classroom setting. In fact, classroom-based education is reduced and perhaps completely eliminated in the completely reengineered, process-centered health care organization.

This shift in educational practices is affected by a shift in thinking as well. The focus of the reengineered organization becomes learning rather than teaching and educating. Thereby, an emphasis on outcomes of the teaching and educational practices arises. Productivity and performance in relation to teaching are then measured by what staff learned and were able to apply to the patient care (work) processes rather than by the number of teaching sessions or encounters. This shift is of great benefit because of the new focus on the applicability of the subject matter learned and the skills acquired to the work environment and processes of care, and thus on its effects on patient and organizational outcomes.

Focusing on learning rather than teaching results in a radical change in the teaching and educational practices of the reengineered health care organization. Radically redesigning education means that its roots are completely thrown away and the process of learning is completely reinvented rather than modified or enhanced.[1] The traditional educational practices (i.e., classroom-based education) are given up and replaced with creative and ongoing work processes–based learning (i.e., on-the-job peer learning). The size of the training and education department shrinks dramatically after reengineering because the responsibility of staff's learning is shifted to the work team level. The work teams created during reengineering become the basis for learning. Team members educate and train each other as they perform their work responsibilities. This way of learning is feasible since the skills and knowledge bases of the team members are often complementary.

Each team member becomes both an educator/trainer and an active learner. Learning in the reengineered environment is the individual's responsibility rather than that of the training and education department. Each member is empowered to identify his or her learning needs and to pursue them through the guidance and coaching of other team members, and in some instances the team leader. The training and education department is brought along only as a support service when the team is unable to provide the learning needed. In most cases, the team leader is the one responsible for coordinating the learning activities. The team leader is also responsible for mentoring and coaching the team members and ensuring that they develop the skills and gain the knowledge required for satisfactory job performance. This learning environment, as it is void of bureaucracy, increases the capabilities of the health care organization, individual staff member, and work team to flex and adapt quickly to new demands and to find answers easily when questions, ambiguities, or uncertainties arise.

Because the approach to learning in the reengineered organization bears no resemblance to past educational practices, organizational opportunities for learning are dramatically changed. Learning then takes place as the need arises rather than on a planned basis. Concurrent learning becomes the norm of the learning team instead of retrospective learning. For example, if a nursing assistant is unable to withdraw a blood specimen from a patient due to a deficit in the skills needed for successful completion of the task, a registered professional nurse or a competent phlebotomy technician may guide the nursing assistant through the phlebotomy process at the time that a blood specimen is needed. The technician may demonstrate to the nursing assistant the techniques of blood withdrawal and explain each step in the process. The nursing assistant, through this on-the-job learning opportunity and after multiple demonstrations, develops the needed skill and eventually becomes able to perform this function independently. In this example, a fellow team member acted as a mentor for the nursing assistant. Learning occurred in a real work situation and at the same time that the need for a blood specimen existed. Prior to reengineering, the nursing assistant would have been scheduled for a phlebotomy class to be held at a later date and time, conducted by an educator who is not a fellow team member, and the skill demonstrated using a dummy. Thus, performance of the individual member, the team as a unit, and the organization as a global entity in the new learning environment witnesses "quantum leaps" in outcomes. Integral to the success are the decentralized approach to learning with the responsibility based in the individual staff member and the work team; the environment of openness, trust, and respect for each member's rights and duties toward learning and coaching; and the support provided by the management staff, especially the team leader.

The environment of care after reengineering shifts its focus from tasks to processes. The same is true for learning. The process of learning gains greater importance in the process-centered health care organization. Adult learning strategies such as peer coaching and on-the-job training become more popular. Work teams are empowered to apply a process-based thinking approach to learning instead of task-based thinking. Such a paradigm shift is conducive to team learning, in which team members seek opportunities for learning voluntarily rather than wait for someone to impose education or teaching on them. Mandatory educational practices disappear, and learning becomes an act of choice and a need for survival in the organization. Team members view learning as an essential process for improving individual performance and team productivity and for sustaining organizational survival and marketability.

THE LEARNING WORK TEAM

It is not enough to reengineer the work processes and environment of care alone. It is just as important to reengineer the work force, especially the managerial staff who will be functioning as leaders of the work teams. Neglecting to redesign the role of each staff member to fit the new and reengineered environment results in organizational failure. As the environment and work processes change, the roles of those who will perform or oversee the processes must be changed as well. A health care organization is not considered a process-centered organization unless the roles assumed by the staff match those required by the redesigned work processes. Reengineering the health care organization results in a diminished role for hierarchy and bureaucracy, a state that allows for a dramatic shift in power to the work teams directly involved in patient care provision. Hammer calls this environment "the end of the organizational chart."[2(p.116)] Therefore, the role of the team leader gains increased importance and power. The team leader becomes the coach and mentor for members of the work team.

Work Team Leader/Process Owner

The role of the traditional manager no longer fits in the reengineered/process-centered organization. The traditional manager's role is to make sure that staff do the right things. In the process-centered organization, members of work teams are capable of performing process-focused jobs that demand understanding, independence, responsibility, and autonomous decision making. The responsibilities of members of the work teams in the new organization become larger, broader, and more complex. The intensity and complexity of the new roles demand highly qualified workers. Therefore, work teams do not require supervision. As a result, the need for the traditional manager disappears and a new role emerges—the role of the process owner.[2] Process owners replace traditional managers. Their role is neither to supervise the work team nor to ensure that members are "doing the right thing." It is rather to enable the work team to perform competently, to facilitate its work and simplify work processes, and to coach those who need to acquire new skills.

In the process-centered organization, the team leader is the process owner who is responsible for ensuring that work processes are organized in an efficient and effective manner and that team members responsible for performing the work are well selected and well trained and possess an open mind and heart for lifelong learning. A successful process owner is able to redirect the thinking and change the behaviors of his or her team members to meet the demands of the work processes the team is responsible for and the outcomes of the processes and the value of the product consumers are interested in. An effective process owner must be able to instill enthusiasm for learning in the team members. He or she has an obligation to make sure, through learning and coaching, that members of the team develop the knowledge and skills necessary for worthy performance and increased productivity.

Work processes in a process-centered organization are usually simplified. As hierarchy is eliminated, non–value-adding work processes are dissolved. Non–value-adding work processes are ones that can be eliminated and not change the outcome/product or its quality. Examples are administrative hassles, obtaining permission from superiors, or awaiting direction before performing a certain task. The process owner then is given more power and authority to act autonomously to ensure that processes that are considered to be waste—those that neither add nor enable value in the product—are eliminated or replaced with value-adding work processes. Value-adding processes are those that are absolutely necessary for producing a product and if eliminated would result in a poor quality product. An example is asking a hospitalized patient to identify the kind of food he or she prefers before serving the meal. The successful process owner facilitates the creation of an environment that is conducive to learning wherein members of the work team learn together how to differentiate value-adding from non–value-adding processes. He or she also provides team members with the authority to either get rid of processes considered waste or replace them with ones that improve the team performance and increase the value of the product, thus improving consumers' perception of the quality of the product they receive.

In regard to health care delivery, an effective process owner in oncology services, for example, is one who demonstrates the ability to involve his or her team members in redesigning the care delivery processes to a seamless approach to care. As a result, consumers are cared for in a patient-centered environment in which services such as diagnostic testing (e.g., X-rays, phlebotomy), radiation therapy, and chemotherapy are brought to the consumer, thus simplifying the processes of accessing health care services and care delivery. Such changes may improve the quality of care delivered, increase consumer satisfaction with care, and enhance the work environment.

A major role of the process owner is helping the work team through difficult and challenging situations. When uncommon or unfamiliar issues surface, the process owner becomes the mentor or the coach of the team. When members of the team face such issues and are unable to resolve the situation, a perfect opportunity is created for team learning. The process owner capitalizes on these opportunities to enhance the skills of his or her team members, expand their knowledge and understanding of the work processes, and improve their competence in job performance. With his or her understanding, expertise, and competence regarding the whole work processes, the process owner is able to assist the work team in its learning at the appropriate time. He or she facilitates the team learning process through explaining and demonstrating the solution to the challenging situation and answering any question members of the team may ask. The process owner ensures that members of the work team are free to exercise their skills in making the process work by helping them handle unusual situations and by providing them with the knowledge, skills, and tools necessary for better job performance.[2] Thereby, through coaching and mentoring, learning takes place, and team performance and productivity in future situations are potentially improved. Exhibit 14–2 shows the responsibilities of the process owner regarding work team learning.

Hendricks identified 10 values necessary for effective coaching.[3] These values are essential for a successful process owner. They facilitate his or her ability to develop a learning work team. These values are

- *Clarity*—clear communication and strong sense of direction and purpose
- *Supportiveness*—standing behind members of the work team and providing them with the help they need whether that help means advise, support, counseling, understanding, encouragement, or information sharing
- *Confidence building*—believing in members of the work teams and in what they do and rewarding them on their successes and accomplishments
- *Mutuality*—sharing a vision of common goals and a true partnership orientation
- *Perspective*—understanding work teams from the inside out and focusing on the performance and productivity of the entire work team as well as the individual member
- *Risk*—letting work team members know it is acceptable to take risks and understanding that not all risks taken are going to be successful but that risk taking encourages learning
- *Patience*—balancing learning and performance (business demands/productivity) and viewing time as necessary for avoiding hasty reactions/responses to problems
- *Involvement*—caring for work team members enough, attempting to understand their experiences, and allowing them to control their work processes
- *Confidentiality*—protecting the work team members' right to privacy

Exhibit 14–2 Process Owner Responsibilities toward Learning

1. Enhance the capabilities of work team members that are necessary for completing their job responsibilities, thus improving their skills, knowledge, and competencies.
2. Assess the present and future demands of the market and ensure that the work team is able to attend to these demands. Make the necessary training and learning experiences available to the work team.
3. Facilitate the work team's process of learning, and ensure that members of the team are consumer focused and produce products of great value to the customer.
4. Create a learning environment conducive to producing superior process performance, the right work teams to perform these processes, and the right environment for them to work in.[2]
5. Guide and mentor members of the work team.
6. Intervene when a team member experiences difficulty in a particular work process by facilitating learning while resolving the situation.
7. Develop plans for learning; that is, hold ongoing learning sessions, whether on the job or in the classroom.
8. Create opportunities for mentoring among team members to enhance learning from member to member, exchange of knowledge, and sharing of skills and expertise.
9. Enable work teams to exercise their skills and capabilities to the fullest extent possible. This enhances creativity and promotes innovation. Enabling and learning go hand in hand. So, during this process, learning opportunities may arise that allow the team members to share experiences, knowledge, and skills and therefore enhance their learning.
10. View mistakes as part of the learning process. Empowered teams will learn as they are given the chance to exercise their knowledge.
11. Mobilize individual creativity by listening to team members' ideas and acting upon them.
12. Set expectations for team learning and member mentoring.
13. Transfer authority for initiating learning down to members of the work team.

A process owner must possess certain skills to be able to perform his or her duties effectively.

- *Respect*—valuing work team members and seeing the treasures they possess

It is necessary for the process owner to use these values when examining alternative ways in which to affect the work team's performance and productivity. As the process owner assesses the performance of each member, he or she is able to identify, in collaboration with team members, where the individual team member is in terms of mastering the work processes and contributing to the team's performance. Next, the process owner determines the team member's growth potential based on the current performance level. Together, the process owner and team members establish the improvement goals and design the action plan for learning. The learning plan may require the process owner to function as a coach if the member's performance is above standard, as a mentor if performance is average, or as a counselor if performance is below standard. The process owner also ensures that the team member, regardless of performance level, is integrated into the work team in a positive and productive way. Therefore, each member's respect, integrity, self-confidence, and self-esteem are protected. The emphasis on healthy and positive integration of each member into the work team is essential for a continuous and uninterrupted learning process.

The Work Team Member and Learning

Any work team is able to achieve new and higher levels of performance, given that the process owner provides members of the team with the right vision, guidance, and learning opportunities and that the team is able to agree on mutual goals, is committed to team work, and understands the importance of each team member in meeting the goals. In the reengineered/process-centered health care organization, members of each work team share the same vision and goals. They are able to work together as one unit, maintain their mutual respect and appreciation of each member's contribution toward team performance, and assist each other in learning and developing. The process-centered organization results in changing the boundaries of traditional jobs, expanding their scope and breadth so that waste and non–value-adding processes are eliminated. This is achieved by creating jobs that encompass a larger number of value-adding processes.[2] As work processes become more complex and bigger, the people needed to perform these processes are required to possess more complex skills, wider knowledge, and more varied experiences. They are also required to be able to live up to the demands of the work environment and its culture and values. Learning is essential for such teams to be successful. Exhibit 14–3 illustrates the elements necessary for work team learning to occur.

As members of work teams in a process-centered health care organization seek excellence in their performance, they also emphasize the importance of learning to stay afloat, flexible, open-minded, intelligent, autonomous, accountable, responsive, ready, knowledgeable, and successful. Each member feels responsible for facilitating the learning activities of the work team and its members. Learning

Exhibit 14–3 Key Elements in Effective Work Team Learning

For learning to occur, members of the work team must be able to do the following:

- Communicate clearly with each other and be interpersonally savvy.
- Mentor and teach other members.
- Trust and respect people.
- Deal with the unexpected.
- Function autonomously.
- Feel accountable for the work processes.
- Ask for help and help others when needed.
- Take initiative.
- Tolerate change and participate in the process of change.
- Listen to others.
- Adapt to the work environment as it constantly changes and is at times uncertain and unpredictable.
- Learn constantly.
- Be people oriented.
- Be open to new experiences and ideas.
- Cherish risk taking.
- Recognize the need for team learning and its benefit.
- Pursue the assistance of the process owner as the need arises.

in such an environment takes place through questioning, experimentation, risk taking, role modeling, mutual support and respect, and constant feedback. These strategies enhance the development and advancement of the work team and its individual members so that performance and productivity are improved.

Process-centered health care organizations allow work team members to "concentrate on substantive work that capitalizes on their [team members] imagination and resourcefulness. People are too important, too valuable, and too capable of doing important work."[2(p.40)] They are independent human beings and are capable of meeting the demands of their jobs successfully once they are provided with the requisite knowledge and a clear understanding of their goals. Members of work teams in the process-centered organization are usually multiskilled professionals. They share certain responsibilities such as answering the telephone, responding to patients requesting help, transportation, and so forth. However, each member is also a specialist in certain patient care activities/processes. For example, registered nurses are accountable for managing and coordinating the patient care activities, whereas patient care associates (support staff) are accountable for environmental services. Together, all members constitute an autonomous and independent work team that is capable of responding to the various needs of patients. Over time, members assist each other in learning the activities/processes they lack skills in until eventually the team becomes a solid and integrated whole. Members share their knowledge and expertise with others until everyone learns the necessary skills required for responding to patients' needs appropriately. In some situations, work team members may not be able to facilitate learning because of a lack of expertise in certain aspects of the work processes. Thus, the process owner is called upon for assistance. He or she is usually someone who understands the whole work process, is able to design an appropriate team learning plan, and is able to successfully coordinate the required learning activities so that the learning needs of the team are met. The process owner may personally function as the coach or mentor or may call on the help of others.

The work team usually experiences a process of learning whereby the opportunities for learning vary in relation to the five different phases of the process (Figure 14–1): chaos, clarity, comfort, cohesion, and confirmation. As the team attains its individual identity and becomes cohesive, and members are able and willing to share mutual and common goals, learning is at its best and becomes a daily activity every member is involved in. Learning becomes the work team's "second nature." Opportunities for work team learning depend on the team's developmental stage. The degree of learning increases as the team progresses in its development from forming to transforming. Exhibit 14–4 summarizes the

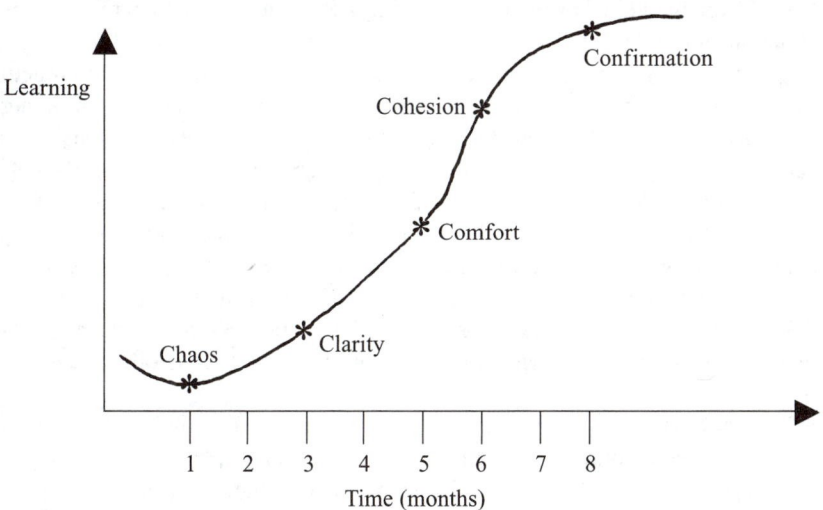

Figure 14–1 The Process of Work Team Learning

Exhibit 14–4 Opportunities for Work Team Learning

Developmental Stage[4]	Learning Stage	Opportunity for Learning
Forming and Storming	Chaos	Rare to nonexistent
Norming	Clarity	Minimal
Performing	Comfort and cohesion	Moderate
Transforming	Confirmation	Extensive

opportunities for work team learning as they relate to the team's developmental stages.

When the team is still forming, every member is preoccupied with transitioning into a process-centered work environment. During this stage, the team experiences a state of chaos in which learning is virtually nonexistent. Members at this point still have not reached consensus on their new roles. They may not cooperate well with each other, may have conflicting agendas and priorities, may lack a clear understanding of their roles and the objective of the work team, and may be unable or unwilling to shift paradigms in how they view their work functions (i.e., to shift from individual to team responsibility). Some team members may be happy about the new work environment and exhibit interest in their new roles. However, when some team members are noted to be uncooperative and continue to function as if the work environment never changed, other members start to exhibit anger and frustration (i.e., storming stage) with the work team concept and the process-centered philosophy. The state of chaos of the work team becomes more complicated. During this stage of work team development, none of the members is conscious of the importance of work team learning or even willing to consider such activity. During this stage, learning is mainly the responsibility of the process owner. He or she plans the learning sessions. These learning sessions focus predominantly on the new work environment; that is, process-centered care, its objectives, member role clarification, and delineation of responsibilities and functions.

As work team members iron out the operational details of the team and process-centered concepts; determine and agree on acceptable behaviors, roles, and responsibilities; clarify their decision-making processes; and identify their goals, values, and performance objectives, the work team concept reaches a stage of normalization. During this stage, the opportunities for learning are clearer;

this allows team learning to begin. Although, it is minimal, some expert team members begin to mentor other less expert members. For example, a registered nurse shifts focus from being angry because of the change occurring in the work environment and starts to help a patient care associate learn how to perform an electrocardiogram on a patient. Thus, members begin to feel a sense of responsibility toward each other and toward learning and mentoring. However, not every member reaches such a state at the same time. The time during which work team members attempt to clarify their roles as they pertain to the process-centered environment is described as the norming stage in the team development process. Learning during this stage takes place through questioning and clarification where members question either the process owner or each other in pursuit of clear understanding of the new environment, the newly formed work team, and the team goals and performance expectations.

When team members become more comfortable with their roles and the process-centered work environment, the opportunities for team learning and member-to-member mentoring increase. Members become more helpful to each other and perceive member mentoring and learning as an obligation rather than a delegated activity. Accountability for self-learning and development becomes more evident in members' behaviors. As the team reaches the performing stage of its development, comfort in team learning is enhanced. Reliance on the process owner for learning decreases, while reliance on members of the work team increases. Comfort in learning is not achieved unless members are able to establish trusting relationships, open communication, and a sense of team purpose and common goals. Such achievements allow the work team members to feel more at ease in exchanging information and guiding and mentoring each other. When such a state of comfort dominates the work environment, work team cohesiveness becomes more evident.

When members of the work team become more cohesive, learning is maximized. Members are more open to verbalizing their learning needs, are better at approaching another team member for mentoring and learning, and do not feel threatened by doing so or by admitting their learning needs. Such performance is also coupled with a complete understanding of how a process-centered organization operates. The team then reaches a state of transformation; a true process-centered team wherein all the team needs, especially the learning ones, are tackled within the team in collaboration with the process owner as needed.

The importance of on-the-job-learning rather than learning in a classroom setting away from the work environment becomes the norm for the transformed team. As members are more successful at providing learning for each other, they become more willing to involve themselves in this type of learning. After recurrent successes at member-to-member mentoring and learning are experienced, team members feel a sense of accomplishment. When their mutual learning efforts are found to be beneficial to other members, the importance and necessity of team learning are confirmed. Therefore, team learning becomes a daily reality and an integral component of the team's performance. The work team then incorporates team learning and mentoring in its goals and values.

During this process of learning development (Figure 14–1), the responsibility for learning gradually shifts from the process owner to the work team (Figure 14–2). The process of work team learning may take up to eight months to become a daily reality of the team's activities; thus, the shift in responsibility may take a similar period of time. During this time, it is the role of the process-owner to provide the work team with an environment conducive to risk taking and to building a sense of accountability, responsibility, and independence. It is also the responsibility of the team members to be open to change, to experiment with team learning and mentoring, and to seek guidance and help from the process owner as indicated by the situations faced. The shift in responsibility for learning is made possible only if team members have a positive self-concept and attitude toward learning and are motivated, optimistic, trustworthy, sensitive to their own and others' needs, disciplined and determined, goal oriented, knowledgeable, consistent, responsible and professional, and frank and honest with each other.

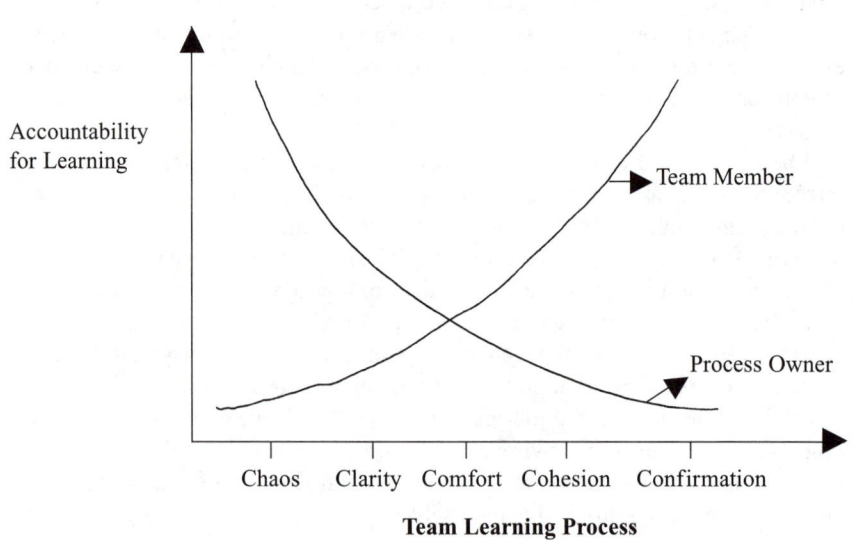

Team Learning Process

Figure 14–2 Accountability for Learning

STRATEGIES FOR SUCCESSFUL WORK TEAM LEARNING

To facilitate learning in the most efficient and effective manner, the process owner and team members must always minimize trauma from the learning experience and maximize its potential for success. The first strategy one must follow is to gain the inner freedom to consider new ideas, new possibilities, and creative learning strategies. This step is not as easy as it sounds. Most of the time, members of work teams do not allow themselves to try new ways of learning because they always felt comfortable with the status quo and are hesitant to leave their comfort zone. The process owner should help the work team members break the barriers they create around themselves and mentor them through the new learning innovations, encouraging them to take risks and attempt member-to-member mentoring and on-the-job-learning. He or she should support them intensively through the process until they develop an acceptable comfort level with it.

The next strategy in work team learning is to be able to verbalize one's learning needs (i.e., expression) and pursue meeting these needs. It is important for each team member to perform a self-evaluation and to identify the areas that require improvement. It is even more important to make these areas known so that other team members will have the opportunity to provide the needed learning as they are known to be competent in those areas. Such activities are usually reciprocal; that is, members exchange knowledge and information. Members must feel comfortable asking questions or requesting help from each other. Asking for assistance is not shameful. No one knows the answers to every question or possesses every skill, regardless of the years of experience or degrees of education one may have. In the process-centered organization, asking for help and seeking learning from work team members is an expectation.

The third strategy for work team learning is the ability to create. As team members are successful at freeing themselves of the obstacles they create, and are willing to express to others their deficient areas and their needs for learning, team members gain the opportunity to become creative in how to provide learning and mentoring. Work team members are then able to join forces and thoughts in deciding on the best way to meet the learning needs of the team. Together they are able to re-create themselves, to establish new ways of learning. They also end up seeing things differently because they are given the opportunity to uncreate the status quo or the past, to put it together again in a new way and re-create the present and imagine the future. This strategy works best if members of the team are cohesive and able to work collaboratively at resolving problems and making decisions.

Creativity allows action. Thus, the last strategy is the ability to perform. Action means realistic and successful learning. Action and performance are interrelated. If members are able to seek learning in an innovative and appropriate way, team performance and productivity should be enhanced. Over time, members' skills and knowledge are improved. These accomplishments usually strengthen teamwork, collaboration, team reliance, mutual trust and respect, and cohesiveness. Therefore, a cycle is created in which team learning feeds into team cohesion and performance and vice versa.

Based on the strategies identified above, the work team members are able to improve their learning abilities and increase the opportunities for mutual learning by:

1. freeing their work environment from the constraints, barriers, and boundaries they create around themselves
2. making their learning needs known to the process owner and fellow members
3. creating opportunities for mutual learning and mentoring, especially in the event of unfamiliar or unusual situations
4. actively pursuing learning to expand their knowledge and skills, and participating in learning activities that aim to build the knowledge and skills of others

IMPORTANT ASPECTS FOR HEALTH CARE WORK TEAM LEARNING

Multiskilling is a major result of reengineering of health care organizations. In the new environment of patient care delivery, health care professionals and technical staff are required to learn new roles, develop new skills, and acquire new knowledge as a result of their redesigned roles. They are asked to assume more responsibilities. Therefore, learning in the process-centered organization becomes a necessity. Learning also becomes an expectation rather than a voluntary activity. Since jobs are more complex and bigger after reengineering, a health care organization should be sensitive to the fact that not every needed skill could be learned at the bedside or on the job. Thus, the process owner must make sure that certain learning sessions are provided in a centralized place and then reinforced at the bedside as work team members perform their mutual mentoring activities. Some examples of topics that serve well in a centralized formal learning method are the following:

- customer relations
- objectives and goals of reengineering and the process-centered organization
- team responsibilities and expectations and individual member role changes
- teamwork and interpersonal dynamics

- telephonc courtesy and skills
- automation, information systems, and technology
- work management
- conflict resolution, decision making, and problem solving

The learning needs of members of the work team can be categorized into three different categories. These are nonclinical, clinical, and multidisciplinary. The nonclinical needs are defined as the administrative and clerical duties and responsibilities such as paperwork and reports. These needs are best learned via demonstration and practice. They may be learned on the job; however, some theoretical information should be shared first in a centralized setting. For example, decentralizing the process of admitting to the patient care unit level requires the work team to learn how to use the automated admitting system. Therefore, members of the team need to learn the process before they assume responsibility for it. Thus, a centralized learning session is helpful in this case before the actual practice occurs on the patient care unit.

The clinical learning needs are defined as the skills and knowledge required for effectively caring for a patient. They are focused on clinical care activities such as measuring a patient's vital signs or administering medications. These needs are not well met in a centralized learning environment. However, one may use centralized learning to provide members of the work team with the theoretical component of the clinical activity and then follow up with the application part at the bedside as members are working. Team members, then, mentor each other in this learning process, since membership of the work team is decided based on the needs of the patient population served and by ensuring that the skills and knowledge of the team members are complementary and meet the patient needs at any given time. Mixing and matching learning methods reduces costs and increases the opportunities for members to learn. Some members may learn more through lecturing; others may prefer demonstration and practice. Combining the two methods maximizes learning and allows the process owner to meet the needs and preferences of the work team members.

The multidisciplinary learning needs are those that address teamwork, dynamics, and interpersonal communication. They are best learned in an environment where all team members, regardless of role category, are present together. Exchange of information and knowledge through case study discussions enhances teamwork and allows the team members to start forming their teams and get to know each other on a personal level. Building such dynamics is essential for the team development and transformation, thereby enhancing learning.

The responsibilities of a newly formed work team may be varied, numerous, and overwhelming. Team members are not able to learn too many new skills in a short period of time. It is advisable to introduce the newly added responsibilities gradually. This process is called layered learning. Layered learning is a continual phasing in of learning. Instead of introducing all the required learning activities at once and over a short period of time, learning is phased in incrementally over a longer period of time. Layered learning allows work team members to gain a new skill and master it before another skill is introduced.[5] Therefore, this process provides a better learning environment and allows team members to concentrate on a few tasks at a time rather than being overwhelmed by the amount of required learning.

Layered learning allows the creation of an environment of constant learning. However, it requires careful planning and ongoing follow-up and review by the process owner. Centralized learning sessions must be planned so that knowledge and skills that are prerequisite to others are presented first. The process owner, in such situations, can plan a learning schedule for team members in coordination with what can be provided via member-to-member mentoring in the clinical area. The topics that are addressed first should be the ones that are considered of high importance to achieving the goals of the redesigned process. Usually the learning topics addressed first are the 20 percent that contribute 80 percent of the outcomes expected in the team performance.

While learning is gradually introduced via a centralized design, some learning activities could be introduced via interim designs; that is, in the patient care unit via member-to-member mentoring and coaching. However, the topics introduced via the interim design should be carefully selected based on their feasibility and appropriateness for such design. Mentoring a patient care associate in how to measure a patient's blood pressure is an example of a skill that can be introduced in an interim design. Combining centralized and interim designs is important because it enhances an expeditious multiskilling process. Members assisting other members in their learning pursuits allows the work team to transition into a process-centered team that is capable of attending to all patients' needs. Such teams are truly learning teams and are self-dependent, autonomous, and accountable for their duties, responsibilities, and learning needs.

CONCLUSION

Effective learning can prepare health care providers and organizations for success. Work teams that are able to function successfully as learning teams are considered an invaluable asset for the process-centered health care organization. This chapter presented some ideas, strategies, and insights regarding learning teams. Health care administrators championing the reengineering efforts in their institutions are encouraged to apply the concepts of the learning team discussed here to their environment of learning. This chapter also helps stimulate a healthy discussion regarding the futuristic approach to learning. In addition, it allows for an enhanced understanding of the effects of team learning on team performance and productivity, through which the professionalism of team members can be improved. An ultimate outcome of team learning is meeting the customers' as well as the organization's goals and expectations.

REFERENCES

1. Hammer M, Champy J. *Reengineering the Corporation: A Manifest for Business Revolution*. New York: Harper Business; 1993.
2. Hammer M. *Beyond Reengineering: How the Process-Centered Organization Is Changing Our Work and Our Lives*. New York: Harper Business; 1996.
3. Hendricks W. *Coaching, Mentoring, and Managing*. Franklin Lakes, NJ: Career Press; 1996.
4. Tuckman B. Stages of small-group development revisited. *Group and Organization Studies*. 1977; (12)419–427.
5. Leander W. Layered learning. *Patient Focused Care Assoc Rev*. 1994 (Summer):2–7.

PART II

Case Studies

CHAPTER 15

Team 2000: One Hospital's Initiative in Reengineering

Mary Lou Helfrich Jones, PhD, RN, CNAA
Dorothy Counts, MA, RN, CPHQ

Health care organizations and systems are daily creating their future. They are reinventing themselves to meet the onslaught of challenges in volatile health care environments brought on by economic, social, organizational, political, and community upheavals. This chapter describes one health care organization's approach to institutionwide reengineering. Included is an illustration of the phases of transition from reengineering design to implementation and integration to a process-centered infrastructure for ongoing organizational improvement.

ENVIRONMENTAL AND HISTORICAL PERSPECTIVES

Pennsylvania Hospital is a 505-bed, nonprofit tertiary teaching acute care facility located in Center City Philadelphia, with approximately 2,500 employees and 850 physicians and allied health staff. It is the oldest running hospital in the United States, founded by Benjamin Franklin and Thomas Bond, MD, in 1751. History and tradition abound in the original Pine Building that housed the first hospital pharmacy, first outpatient clinic, first medical library, and first surgical amphitheater. *Christ Healing the Sick in the Temple,* an oil painting donated by Benjamin West in 1817, is prominently displayed and viewed daily by both staff

Acknowledgments: The authors acknowledge the contributions of John R. Ball, MD, JD, President; Charles Wolf, MD, President, Professional Staff; and William Grice, Vice President, Quality and Outcomes Management, all of Pennsylvania Hospital, for their leadership during this reengineering initiative. Additionally, appreciation is extended to Robert Campbell, MD, Chairman, Department of Radiology, Pennsylvania Hospital, for the leadership of the General Services Team and the achievements realized through the team-building activities encouraged during this initiative.

and visitors. The original mission, as stated by Benjamin Franklin, was to serve the sick and miserable.[1]

Health care delivery in the Philadelphia area and across the nation has changed dramatically in the last decade as costs have increased and managed health care has shifted the care provided to the outpatient setting. Moody's Investors Services has characterized Philadelphia's health care market as one of the most explosive and competitive in the country.[2] Hospitals in the Philadelphia area have been organizing around four major academic medical centers, with individual hospitals joining systems as a way to survive in the fiercely competitive marketplace. In 1997, Pennsylvania Hospital board of managers made a strategic decision and voted to join the University of Pennsylvania Health System.[2]

The hospital's reengineering project illustrates one process to improve efficiency while maintaining and actually enhancing the quality of care provided. Hospitals need to provide care as efficiently as possible to survive and prosper in preparation for the 21st century. Pritchett stated that the only way for an organization to survive in this fiercely competitive environment is to keep reshaping, shifting, and flexing to fit the rapidly changing world.[3]

REENGINEERING INITIATIVE

Based on the institution's mission, vision, values, and strategic priorities, six guiding principles and five service standards were developed to frame the institutionwide reengineering initiative and serve as decision drivers. The six guiding principles are displayed in Exhibit 15–1. They reflect a set of first principles articulated by Hammer that assert (1) that the mission of a business is to create values for its customer; (2) that it is a company's processes that create value for its customers; (3) that business success comes from superior process performance; and (4) that superior process performance is achieved by having a superior process design, the right people to perform it, and the right environment for them to work in.[4] The service standards adopted address interactions with patients and families to create the environment for delivery of patient care services. The behaviors expected include courtesy, friendliness, and compassion; confidentiality and respect; consistent, reliable, skillful care; sound judgment and competent decision making; and professional pride.

Principles of high-performance work systems were delineated. Hammer elaborated on the concept of processes by explaining that processes occupy center stage and influence the structure and systems developed in an organization. The organization starts with the customers and what they want then works backward to design the service. Then the employees of the organization center on a common goal for patient care. The activities then lead to the design of patient care

Exhibit 15–1 Six Guiding Principles

1. Patients and their families are the central focus of the work we do. Services hospitalwide are designed and coordinated in their best interests.
2. We ensure that patients and families understand their rights, that we educate them about their condition and treatment, and that we involve and support them in decisions about their care. We also provide resources for health promotion to our patients and their families, as well as members of the community.
3. We treat patients as individuals, each with his or her own set of physical, psychological, spiritual, and cultural needs.
4. We provide a safe, secure, and comfortable health care environment.
5. As a cohesive team, we provide service in a positive atmosphere that fosters mutual respect and open communication.
6. We strive to promote innovative, efficient, and fiscally responsible use of resources.

Source: Courtesy of Pennsylvania Hospital, UPHS, Philadelphia, Pennsylvania.

processes that shape how people work, think, and develop their attitudes.[4(p.6)] In this reengineering initiative, the focus was on patient care processes.

A commitment was made to undergo a three-year institutionwide reengineering initiative, beginning in fiscal year 1996 and ending in the year 2000; hence, the name given to this effort was Team 2000. To provide expertise with the design phase of the reengineering initiative, an external consulting firm was chosen through a rigorous selection process in fall 1995.

DESIGN PHASE

The structure created for this reengineering initiative included a steering committee, composed of senior hospital administration and medical staff leadership, and the consulting firm. Six multidisciplinary design teams were organized and led by a medical staff leader and a hospital administrator, who served as chair and cochair. The design teams were general administrative services; general services and centralized ancillaries; patient care; admitting, billing, and revenue generation; materials management; and quality and service targets. More than 700 grassroots employees were members of these design teams.

The roles in this design phase team structure were consistent with Hammer's operational definitions delineating the change in manager roles. The steering committee served as the business leaders; that is, they shaped the firm's vision and inspired workers with a transcendent view of the meaning of their work.[4(pp.133–134)] The design team chairs and cochairs were process owners and coaches. In this process-owner management role, they were responsible for the design of the processes: creating them and developing the measures to evaluate performance of the system process.[4(pp.75–76)] Moreover, in the coach role, they developed the employees (process workers) through guidance, mentoring, and intervening to resolve conflicts.[4(pp.120,129)] The design team members were both professional and traditional process workers. In these roles, they participated in the design of the work, and some of them would also be actually performing the work during the implementation phase.[4(pp.44–46)]

The consultant firm worked in collaboration with hospital employees (financial, education and organizational development, clinical, marketing, and managers) dedicated to the project to support the work of the design teams. In the design phase, four elements of process centering were a part of the design teams' work. The teams recognized and named the processes involved in the scope of their redesign area of responsibility. All members of these interdisciplinary teams were made aware of (1) the processes and their importance to patient care; (2) the process measurements, such as yardsticks and benchmarks, that were to be developed; and (3) the method of process management, that is, ongoing monitoring and evaluation, to be established during the transition to implementation following the design phase. These process management activities would become a way of life within the hospital that would result in the creation of a learning organization.[4(p.12)]

The methodology used in the design phase included assessment and idea generation followed by an analysis. During idea generation, the first step was to examine all work processes for the services included in the scope of the assigned team. A consultant and project support staff member assisted the team chair and cochair initially to perform this idea assessment and to set priorities. Tools used were budget, financial performance, productivity, management engineering, and other management reports. Focused attention was then given to those areas of salary and nonsalary expenses that were at financial variance and those with major expenses. Changes in work processes were explored. Internal solutions were considered and expertise was sought from external vendors. The decision-making rationale was to examine the most effective solution yet to maintain consistency with the six guiding principles.

Team members, called process workers, were organized into action groups and worked with project support staff to study specific ideas. These process workers interacted with individuals and managers in departments across the organization to assess the opportunities presented from the ideas. Then these ideas led to the development of recommendations for approval and implementation.

Subsequently, recommendations were presented and discussed in the design team. After review and revision, followed by endorsement, the design team chair and cochair made recommendations to the steering committee. If approved, implementation planning for scheduling the immediate or designated change over the next three years occurred. Implementation of changes was organized to maintain a balance with regard to the enormity of the institutionwide change.

IMPLEMENTATION

At the completion of the design phase in May 1996, the structure for implementation was decided. A decentralized structure was chosen to implement recommendations, which were disseminated to the appropriate department for all teams but the patient care team. The patient care team remained centralized to implement the newly designed patient care delivery model. The steering committee transitioned to become the operations executive council, without the consultant group and medical staff leadership, as an approval body. A newly designed and implemented institutionwide committee structure was used to support clear communication patterns, facilitate ongoing monitoring functions, and enhance feedback on organizational performance.[5,6]

Application of Hammer's operational definitions for the implementation structure provides clarity to the commitment for ongoing process improvement. The operations executive council members' roles were to function as business leaders. Department managers became process owners, coaches, and advocates, while the employees became professional and traditional process workers.[4(pp.44–46)]

The work of the general services team illustrates the reengineering initiative in this organization. The chairman of the department of radiology and the author, Mary Lou Helfrich Jones, an administrator at the time of this initiative, were the process owners of this team. The team's scope of services included the work processes in the engineering department, environmental services, food and nutritional services, and laundry and linen services. This design team was targeted for 17 percent of the overall 20 percent in expense reduction of this institutionwide reengineering initiative to be achieved over three years. Design team members as process workers joined action groups to study the four areas.

A careful assessment was conducted to examine the expenses in each area. Department managers and workers conducted an orientation and observation of the work performed in some of these general services departments. Multiple ideas were generated based on priorities identified related to inefficient processes and redundant, duplicative, and overlapping workloads. Consultation was sought from external vendors to consider outsourcing some of the various services under study. With the help of the Team 2000 project support staff, financial analyses of all ideas generated were included to present objective recommendations based on sound principles.

Exhibit 15–2 shows multiple results of recommendations implemented in the four areas (action groups). Engineering department savings resulted from labor savings in two areas: management restructuring (closure of one campus of the institution, thereby reducing workload) and redesign of roles, which included cross-training for multifunctional workers. Nonlabor costs were realized in utility

Exhibit 15–2 General Services Team Reengineering Results

Action Group	*Results*
Engineering Department	• Management restructured • Engineering roles redesigned with cross-training • Department at the top of the nation for being low cost (benchmarked)
Environmental Services	• Employees decentralized to patient care units where redesigned patient care delivery model implemented
Food/Nutritional Services	• Employees decentralized to patient care units where redesigned patient care delivery model implemented • Specialty restaurant outsourced • Policy changes made for catering, menu selection
Laundry/Linen Services	• Laundry closed and linen services outsourced: – Laundry costs reduced by 42 percent of pounds per patient day – Reduced linen distribution staff by 3.5 employees • Reengineered laundry and linen operations: – Uniform and scrub policy introduced – Scrub exchange system implemented – Improved availability and service to patient care units – Constructed and placed an OR pack room into operation

Source: Courtesy of Pennsylvania Hospital, UPHS, Philadelphia, Pennsylvania.

savings and paper product cost renegotiations. Environmental services and food and nutritional services decentralized employees to patient care units and redesigned roles to include multiple activities, leading to more efficient service at the point of care.

Laundry and linen services savings were achieved by closing the laundry on an institutional campus that was sold. With the laundry closed, linen services were outsourced, which resulted in a 42 percent reduction in the cost of linen per pound per patient day. The number of laundry and linen department staff was reduced to correspond to the decrease in workload. Laundry and linen operations also were reengineered with the introduction of a uniform and scrub policy, resulting in significant scrub uniform savings (over $75,000), because personnel who needed to wear institutionally provided scrub uniforms were identified. A scrub exchange system was implemented, which led to further savings on scrub uniforms (over $75,000). An operating room pack room was constructed and placed into operation. Improved availability and service to patient care units was provided by implementing a full day's par level and providing space for adequate backup supply. A work order approach was established to address problems.

For ongoing process improvement, the implementation of some of the ideas related to laundry and linen services were delegated to a linen value analysis committee. This was one of several value analysis committees created to establish a systematic process for the selection of equipment, products, services, and contracts to support the institution's work. These committees were formed as part of the newly designed and implemented institutionwide committee structure illustrated in Figure 15–1.

EVALUATION

Hammer claims that after reengineering, the organization will progress to become process centered; become very focused on its processes; and center most organizational activity on identifying, reengineering, and strengthening the organization's processes. A process-centered organization generally moves to a multidisciplinary team focus.[4] What were the organizational realities at Pennsylvania Hospital? How did structure shift? How did employees view their work? Did the work provide opportunity for fulfillment and meaning?

As the reengineering project shifted the focus from design to implementation, the revised organizationwide committee structure was rolled out. Each multidisciplinary committee had clearly defined goals and objectives. The chairs were physicians, with administrative cochairs, similar to the Team 2000 structure to continue the collaboration between administration and physicians. This structure provided a framework for organizationwide communication and reporting of committee activities. Standardized minutes and agendas were provided, and a

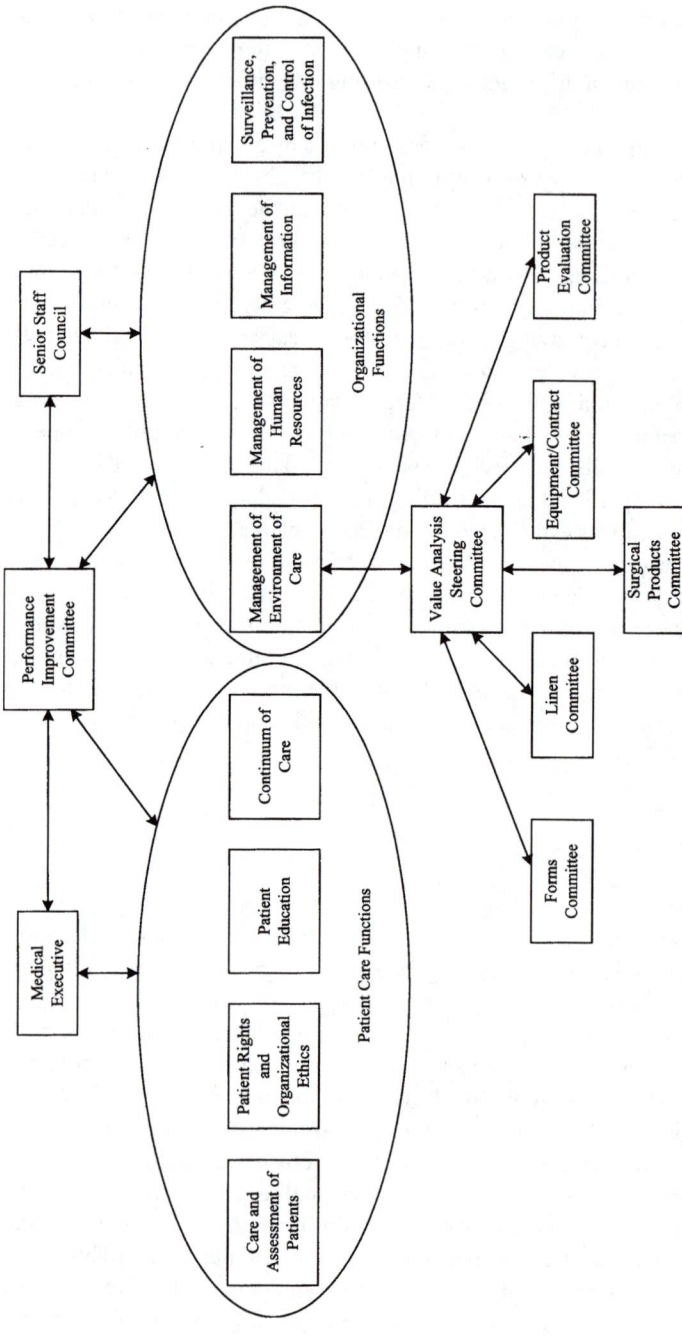

Figure 15–1 Organizational Committee Structure. *Source:* Courtesy of Pennsylvania Hospital, UPHS, Philadelphia, Pennsylvania.

summary report of the minutes was distributed. The goal was to continue meetings that were focused and productive.

The majority of the redesign implementation responsibilities were delegated to the specific department managers, staff, and key representatives from other areas. For each initiative, work plans were developed that defined objectives, resources, responsibilities, and timelines. Projects that required construction or installation were coordinated with facilities planning. As construction proceeded, costs were monitored against the capital budget and timelines were established.

Information systems integration was key to moving into the 21st century. Planning included system costs, training needs, and the timeline for purchase, installation, and implementation. The information management steering committee (part of the organizationwide committee structure) transitioned as the strategic multidisciplinary team to define the system needs, incorporating identified priorities into a request for proposal (RFP), then evaluated vendors and eventually selected the best choice. Both process owners (physician and administrative chairs) and process workers (committee members) were integral to the success of the project redesign implementation phase.

HUMAN RESOURCE CONSIDERATIONS

The reality of all reengineering endeavors to increase efficiencies and contain costs in a rapidly changing health care market is that people need to adjust to new roles and responsibilities. This corresponds to two of Hammer's "rethinking" strategies: intensification, which is improving processes to serve current customers better, and augmentation, which is expanding processes to provide additional services to customers.[4(pp.198–199)] In some patient care areas, positions were restructured and job descriptions were revised, which led to redeployment of personnel and, in some cases, elimination of jobs. Opportunities were made available for either retraining or reassignment of employees in affected departments. Information was provided related to all redesigned roles, and competency criteria were established. Both classroom and on-the-job training were provided, as appropriate. The delivery of care in the most efficient and effective manner was incorporated into the training program. Training was provided for every displaced employee who expressed the willingness and possessed the skills and abilities to meet the requirements of the redesigned positions.

Change within an organization affects individuals differently depending on each individual's perspective and personality traits. According to Pritchett, pinning down your job during change can be like trying to nail Jell-O to the wall. People who have a high need for structure have difficulty dealing with new expectations, shifted priorities, and different reporting responsibilities. Those who have the ability to tolerate ambiguity and uncertainty, and are able to improvise, will be prepared to handle the future.[3]

COMMUNICATION

Various methods of communication were used throughout the Team 2000 design and implementation phases. Frequent newsletters gave regular updates on all the teams' activities and progress. Open forums (town meetings) were held to provide updates and allow time for employee questions and answers. The meetings were repeated at times convenient for all shifts to attend. Updates were provided at service director and management meetings and communicated to staff by either managers or unit directors at routine staff meetings. Pritchett noted that communication is the crucial element in keeping the program moving forward.[7] As people questioned the need for change, they were reminded of the logic behind the effort. When they complained about all the problems, they were informed of the benefits. Communication at Pennsylvania Hospital was open and honest at all times, and rumors were dispelled while changes were occurring. Ongoing communication continues to be forthcoming and timely as the implementation phase progresses.

MONITORING QUALITY AND OUTCOMES

The service and quality targets team met during the design phase to assist the teams in defining clinical outcomes and satisfaction measures. The overall goal was to make certain that service and quality were sustained or improved over the course of reengineering. Baseline measurements were obtained or developed to assist the design teams in evaluating current practices prior to introducing changes. Ongoing measures were used to evaluate whether the change resulted in the desired improvement. The organizationwide process improvement methodology is the plan, do, check, act (PDCA) system conceived by Shewhart and promoted by Deming.[8,9]

At the completion of the design phase, quality and outcomes monitoring became the responsibility of the committees on care and assessment of patients and organizational performance. The performance improvement committee, composed of physician and administrative leaders, became the oversight body. An ongoing clinical quality improvement effort directed by physician leaders was implemented to focus on improving clinical efficiency and quality of health care within specified processes. The physicians led multidisciplinary teams that analyzed, evaluated, and assessed data such as clinical outcomes, resource utilization, cost, and customer satisfaction from multiple and varied sources. A methodical approach was used to identify performance improvement priorities that would affect customer satisfaction, care processes, and appropriate resource utilization. The PDCA method was used to implement the change concept, using benchmarking for identification of best practice, multidisciplinary teams, and other related performance improvement tools.

CONCLUSION

Life after reengineering at Pennsylvania Hospital is one in which employees and professional staff (the health care team) remain focused on patient care processes and processes that support the work of the organization. The reengineering initiative marked the beginning of a cultural transformation for this organization, which is now a more collaborative, consensus building environment with a focus on the mission, vision, values, and guiding principles outlined in this chapter. Today, this organization is positioned for survival and growth in an evolving health care system—to go forward while continuing to examine and change its processes, where appropriate, and to serve patients and families as Benjamin Franklin originally envisioned when this institution was built some 247 years ago.

REFERENCES

1. Morton TG, Woodbury F. *The History of Pennsylvania Hospital—1751–1895*. Philadelphia: Times Printing House; 1895.
2. Savage T. Oldest living hospital tells all. *Hosp & Health Networks*. 1998; 72(13):49–52.
3. Pritchett P. *The Employee Handbook of New Work Habits for a Radically Changing World*. Dallas, TX: Pritchett & Associates, Inc; 1994:2.
4. Hammer M. *Beyond Reengineering*. New York: Harper Business; 1996.
5. Ball JR, Counts D, Jones MLH, Vinci C, Winn C. An organization-wide approach for an effective communication system, Part 1. *J Nurs Admin*. 1998; 28(3):28–34.
6. Jones MLH, Counts D, Vinci C, Winn C, Ball Jr. An organization-wide approach for an effective communication system, Part 2. *J Nurs Admin*. 1998; 28(4):27–30.
7. Pritchett P. *Resistance: Moving beyond the Barriers to Change*. Dallas, TX: Pritchett & Associates, Inc.; 1994:17.
8. Shewhart W. *Economic Control of Quality Manufactured Product*. New York: Van Nostrand; 1931.
9. Deming WE. *Out of Crisis*. Cambridge, MA: Massachusetts Institute of Technology, Center for Advanced Engineering Study; 1986.

CHAPTER 16

Creating a Process-Centered Organization

Mae Taylor Moss, MS, MSN, RN, FAAN

This chapter looks at the process-centered reengineering that occurred at a 950-bed, full-service U.S. health care facility with a level-two trauma center. In retrospect, this organization's lengthy reengineering journey produced remarkable efforts to streamline services without sacrificing outcomes, insightful ways of looking at core processes and business structure, and profound changes in organizational culture. This institution's reengineering effort began in 1989 and has become an evolutionary process that continues today. While the massive initial changes of yesterday have been replaced by the more subtle refinements of today, change itself has become a way of life.

The reengineering effort at this organization progressed through three distinct phases, as presented in Figure 16–1. They were:

1. analysis and measurement of existing processes
2. redesign of core processes
3. implementation and measurement of each reengineered process with built-in continuous monitoring

The built-in continuous monitoring of the final phase of reengineering makes this a reiterative process. Each time the hospital administration introduces a reengineered process, staff monitor, evaluate, and refine the redesigned process as needed. This reiteration forces the organization to perform continuous improvement and function as a learning organization. Employee education occurs throughout all three phases.

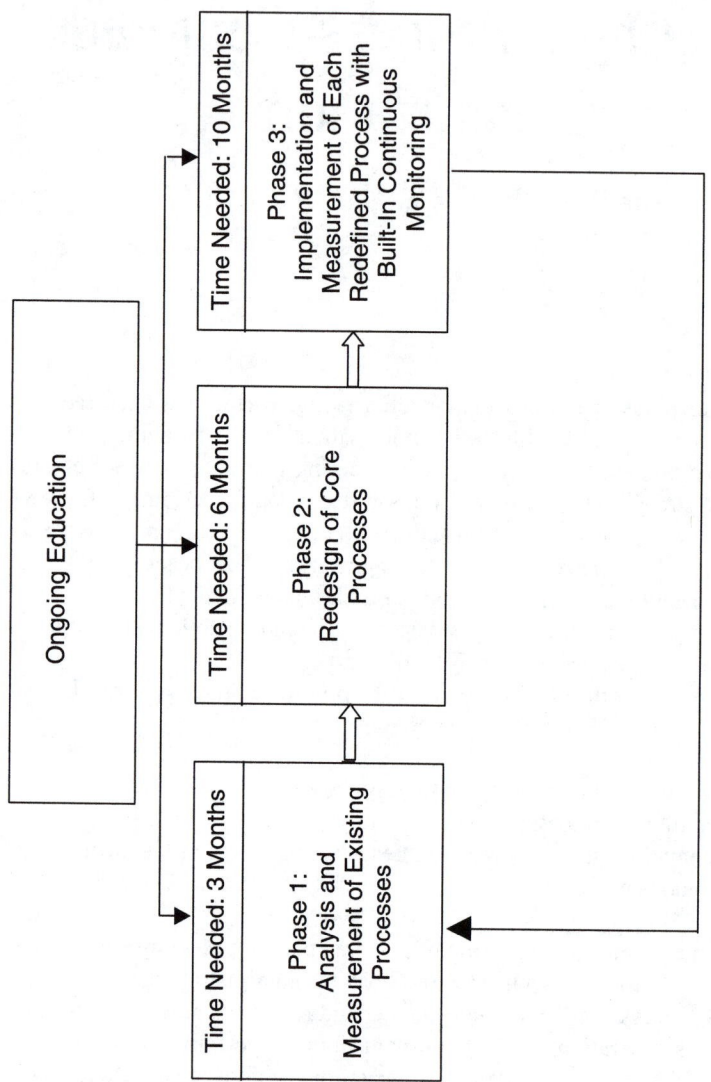

Figure 16–1 The Three Reiterative Phases of This Reengineering Effort

THE NEED TO REENGINEER

In 1989—four years before the publication of Hammer and Champy's landmark manifesto, *Reengineering the Corporation*[1]—those of us working to improve hospital conditions in response to pressure from managed care were already knee-deep in reengineering. Along the way, we were discovering the value of defining core processes and streamlining operations around these core processes.

The goal was to diagnose what was wrong with the way in which an institution operated and to correct it. The starting point was to look at processes. With hindsight it is easy to see that these reengineering efforts resulted in the creation of a process-centered organization. But it was much like driving without a map, or cooking without a recipe. The output was a process-centered organization, but the original intent was not specific enough to identify this output as the goal.

Several immediate clues to the depth of this organization's problems were:

- a hierarchical organizational structure burdened by too many layers of management
- a high turnover rate
- an unwieldy and expensive inventory of supplies
- underutilized surgical services

Reengineering efforts were aimed at solving these problems while introducing a new work ideology that would enable the seamless delivery of services to patients, payment to vendors, and invoices to payers. This seamless delivery was accomplished by looking at processes and forming teams to perform all of the individual steps required by these processes.

EMPLOYEE CULLING AS A BYPRODUCT OF REENGINEERING

Like most, this reengineering effort was not without casualties. Many employees who could not cope with the new organizational landscape left the institution by self-selecting themselves out the door. Employees realized quickly that "as organizations focus themselves on processes, job requirements, measurements, and rewards all change."[2(p.53)] In spite of educational efforts to explain the reengineering process and its outcomes to employees, as well as a forthcoming attitude regarding changes to the organization and work environment, certain individuals just could not change to conform to the new methods and ideas. This did not make them unsatisfactory employees, but revealed that at that time they just could not fit into a reengineered organization. The reengineering team

(Figure 16–2) found that by including all workers in the reengineered organization, those who were not comfortable with working under these conditions would cull themselves from the group by leaving the organization. It was not necessary to perform layoffs or terminations. Those whose values do not match the reengineered organization often leave on their own without any pressure from the organization. It is important to provide education and information on the reengineering of the institution early in the process, however, so that employees are not leaving the organization misinformed or fearful of situations that will exist only in the rumor mill. When possible, it is also useful to illustrate the new

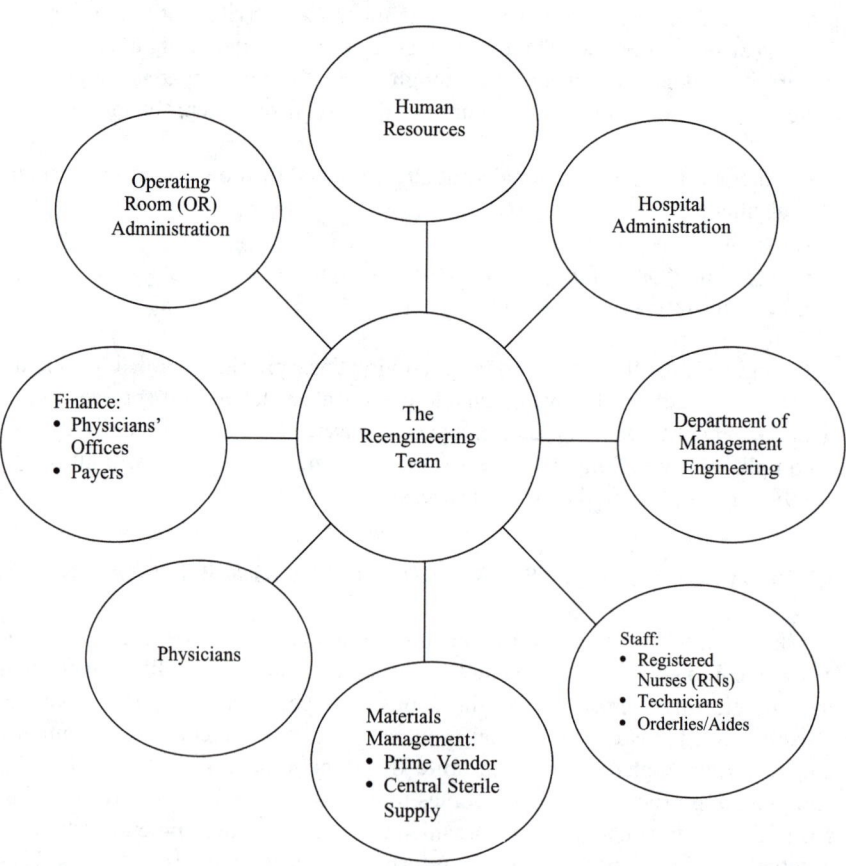

Figure 16–2 Composition of the Reengineering Team

order through success stories at other institutions. If all of that fails to retain employees, then those who leave the organization truly know they are not suited for their jobs after reengineering has been instituted.

PHASE 1: ANALYSIS AND MEASUREMENT OF EXISTING PROCESSES

Before this organization could redefine processes, the reengineering team needed to first analyze and measure the existing processes. In this way, the team created a baseline from which changes could be made. When this phase began in 1989, reengineering core processes was not the accepted discipline it is today. In fact, "core processes" was not the buzz phrase that it is today. The reengineering team knew which processes were "core" processes, but in those days we referred to them as "critical" processes. Semantics aside, in 1989 we were on the frontier of process-centered reengineering. With no previous success stories to assuage fears, the environment was hostile toward changes that were unproven, and fear of the unknown was rampant.

In response, the reengineering effort focused on educating the entire organization about the team's reengineering work and the changes that were to take place. The whole mind-set of the organization needed to change. Changing attitudes was high on the team's priority list. The reengineering team achieved this through education and by being visible to administration as well as other departments. Suddenly, operating room (OR) representatives were on hospital committees for the first time. During Phase 1, the department of management engineering helped the team look at individual processes through time-in-motion studies that measured the time associated with each process in its current state. The team used these studies to show employees the depth of existing organizational problems as well as the cost, in time and money, that it took the organization to operate in this manner. From this point, the team could project how the organization would function with reengineered processes. The team's education effort was twofold: (1) Give an accurate representation of life in the reengineered organization, and (2) prepare staff for life after reengineering by teaching them the skills that they would need to work in this new organization.

The gap of understanding that existed when restructuring began was incredibly large. Employees did not appreciate what restructuring meant, nor did they understand what the process of reengineering entailed. They were just concerned about themselves and their careers. Titles were important to them, as they had been used to titles. They were afraid of losing their titles—which meant power to them—and felt work could not get done without using the power of a title.

Each member of the perioperative staff took a 16-hour course to learn all about team building, the first step toward a reengineered work force. Working in teams was an essential part of the reengineering effort. Without the ability to work in teams, the perioperative staff had no chance of adjusting to the upcoming changes. Following this phase, each worker knew his or her role and responsibilities as staff began to work on the redesigned processes in their new teams.

PHASE 2: REDESIGN OF CORE PROCESSES

Redesigning Processes

The reengineering process was a hospitalwide effort in which the author participated in reengineering the perioperative services, including the central sterile and materials areas. The reengineering of perioperative services discussed in the remainder of this chapter began by looking at any systems that affected patient flow, supplies, and equipment and examined the path that these items took to get to their destination. During this phase, the reengineering team measured each process by looking at the overall process and then breaking it down into all of the individual components that made up the whole. For each process, the team developed two flowcharts (Figures 16–3 and 16–4): one that detailed the existing process and a second that presented the team's view of the ideal process as it would operate in this specific organization. For example, in reengineering the patient flow process the reengineering team formed teams that performed preadmitting duties (including calling patients before they came to the hospital, rectifying insurance and financial issues, and answering admissions questions); provided intraoperative care; transported patients; turned over patient rooms; and performed blood and other testing. In other words, instead of moving patients throughout the hospital, the team changed the process (as much as possible) so that services were brought to the patient and that the same team stayed with the patient throughout the patient's hospital experience from preadmission to discharge.

All colleagues that touched a patient in some way were included in the restructuring (i.e., physicians' office staff, physicians, finance department workers, admitting personnel, pathology and lab technicians, anesthesiologists, radiologists, medical records personnel, and risk management and quality management staff).

In addition to looking at the redesign of these core processes, the institution also looked at the top-heavy hospital organization and how the processes of each department and unit interacted with each other, as well as with hospital administration, physicians, and payers. The analysis of Phase 1 enumerated 11,000 separate tasks (e.g., making a bed, mopping a floor, transporting a specimen, etc.) performed by members of perioperative services. It did not take long for the team

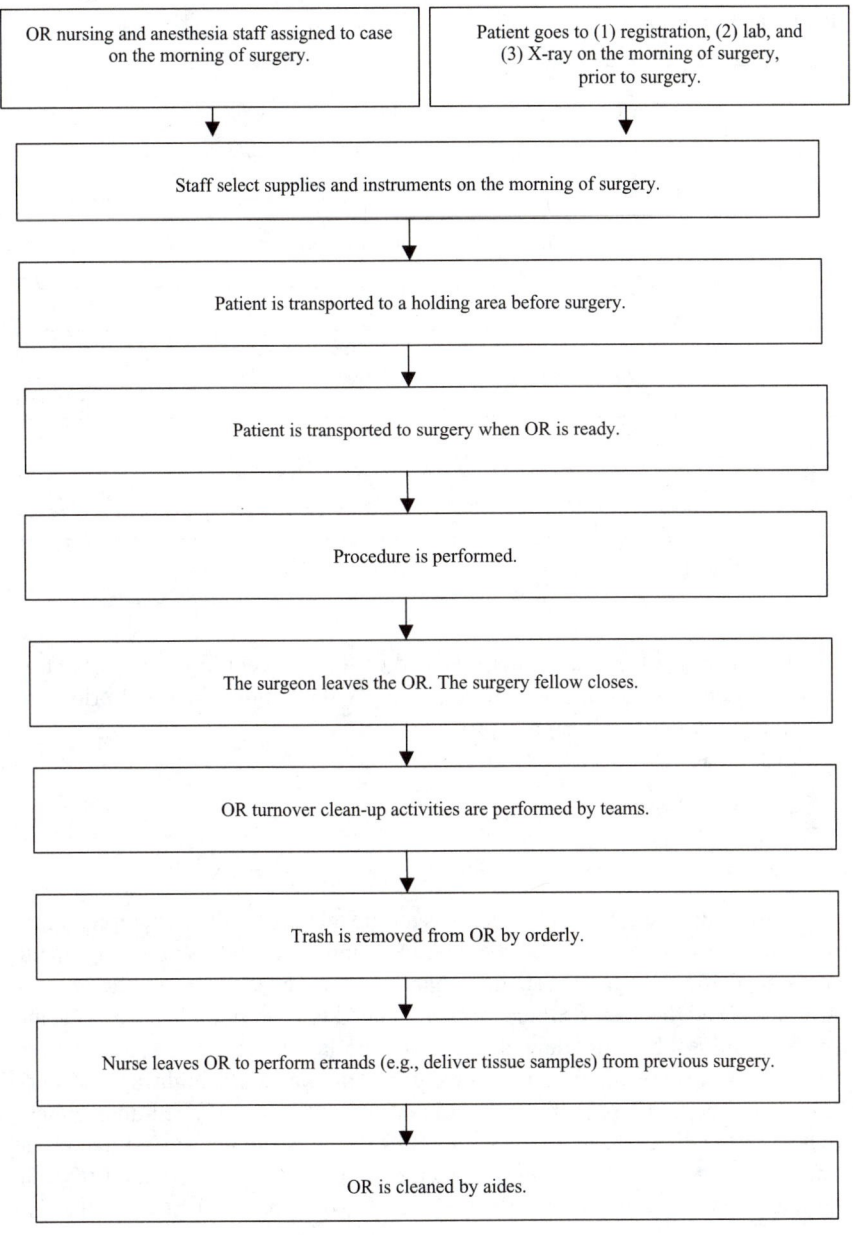

| OR nursing and anesthesia staff assigned to case on the morning of surgery. | Patient goes to (1) registration, (2) lab, and (3) X-ray on the morning of surgery, prior to surgery. |

Staff select supplies and instruments on the morning of surgery.

Patient is transported to a holding area before surgery.

Patient is transported to surgery when OR is ready.

Procedure is performed.

The surgeon leaves the OR. The surgery fellow closes.

OR turnover clean-up activities are performed by teams.

Trash is removed from OR by orderly.

Nurse leaves OR to perform errands (e.g., deliver tissue samples) from previous surgery.

OR is cleaned by aides.

continues

Figure 16–3 Flowchart of Existing Process: Intraoperative Care for Surgical Patients

Figure 16–3 continued

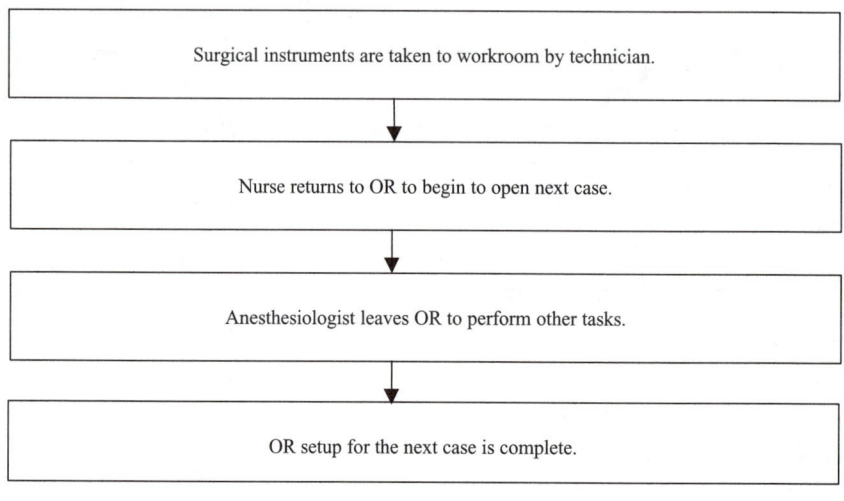

to realize that all of the problems revealed by Phase 1 could not be solved in Phase 3. In Phase 2, the team needed to identify the major issues and prioritize the implementation of redesigned processes.

Identifying the Issues

Organizational Structure

Prior to reengineering, this facility was a rigid, hierarchically structured, traditional hospital that operated with very limited input from staff. While equipment and medical advances had drastically changed over the last 50 years, the organization itself and the way in which workers related to each other had grown stagnant. The philosophy promulgated by the autocratic leaders of this facility's over 30 surgical suites was often best summed up as "my way or the highway." Leadership was not culturally sensitive and did not invite any sort of open-door policy. Frequently, the director did not know the staff by name. An unsuccessful attempt at decentralization produced very segmented departments that resulted in each unit individually dealing with staffing, lunch breaks, absenteeism, and other issues. Consequently, no department helped another department. The OR was very closed to other departments. No one knew who the OR staff members were or what they did.

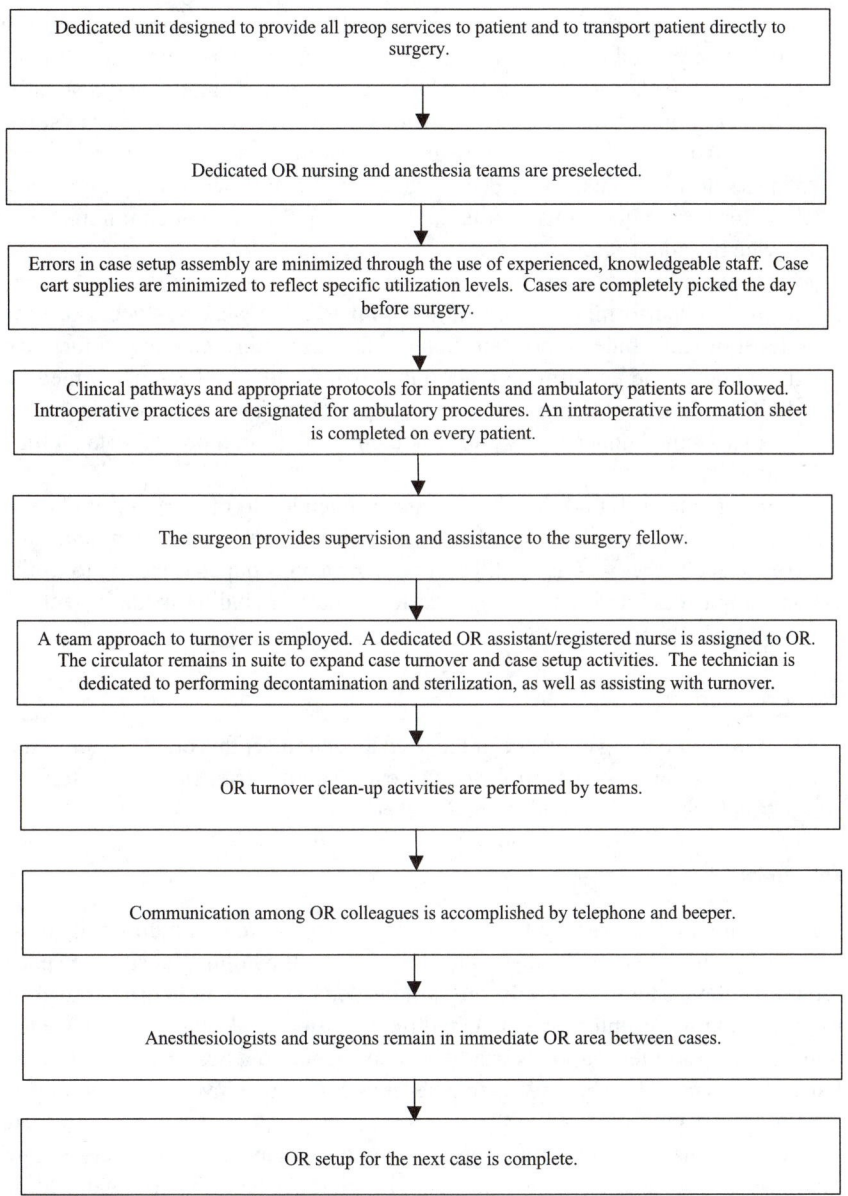

Figure 16–4 Flowchart of Ideal Process: Intraoperative Care for Surgical Patients

Far worse was the reality that whenever a staff nurse raised a question regarding a policy or procedural issue, this question would take a long and slow trip up the administrative ladder (Figure 16–5) before it would get an official response. In reality, staff nurses were making decisions without authority in order to solve immediate issues that required immediate attention. The level of management with the authority to make these decisions was ineffective because it simply took too long for formal questions to filter all the way up the chain of communication to the vice president/director of OR.

Non–value-added work was also a problem. The team looked at non–value-added work by performing a task analysis to determine what was necessary for each level of staff. Indeed the team found that nurses were mopping floors, answering phones, and performing other duties that could have been performed by less skilled workers. Nursing staff also were performing repetitive duties—busy work—that seemed unnecessary and took them away from more important clinical duties.

Overall, the team found that the changes it intended to bring about in the organizational culture were so vast that even changing how management and staff referred to each other was helpful. Therefore, the team stopped referring to workers as "employees" and instead referred to all staff, including management, as "colleagues."

Turnover Rate

The most compelling evidence of the need to reengineer this organization came from the team's analysis of employee turnover. The turnover rate at this facility was astronomical and disruptive at 38 percent.

Inventory

Carrying an unnecessarily large inventory is expensive in a number of ways. There is the initial cost of the supplies themselves, the holding costs (the space required to house these materials, the staff needed to keep it all in order, the need to perform large inventory checks), and the lost time it takes to retrieve needed items. Having too few supplies can be as detrimental to a health care facility as having too many. The objective is to determine how much inventory is appropriate and to trim the excess.

The team analyzed how many instruments the organization had versus how many were needed. It examined how supplies and par levels were organized. It looked at the weekly deliveries the organization was getting versus a just-in-time (JIT) inventory concept that would require daily deliveries. The team also looked at the value of paying face value for all supplies instead of entering into contract negotiation with vendors.

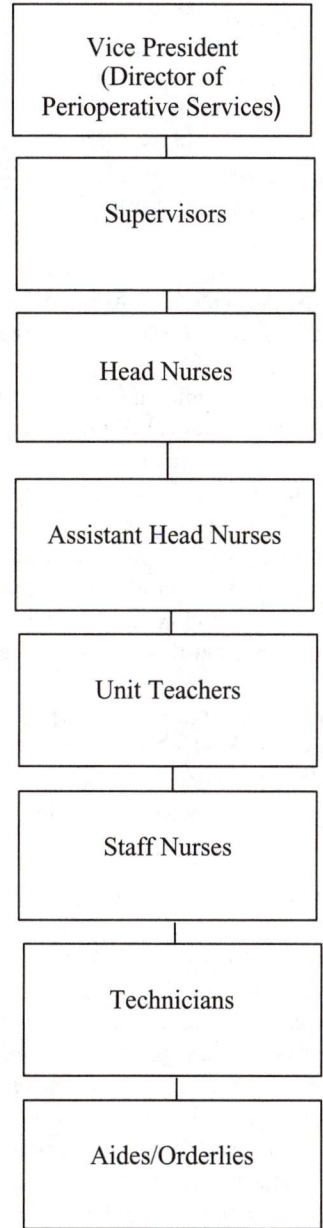

Figure 16–5 Perioperative Services Organizational Chart—Before Reengineering

Utilization of Surgical Services

In 1988, prior to reengineering, this hospital realized $28 million in surgery revenue. Unfortunately, 50 percent of that sum was allocated to expenses. This facility had plenty of ORs, but did not use them efficiently. The OR turnover rate (the amount of time it took to disinfect an OR, sterilize instruments, and be ready for the next surgery) was so high that it was an enormous burden.

PHASE 3: IMPLEMENTATION AND MEASUREMENT WITH CONTINUOUS MONITORING AND IMPROVEMENT

The team performed the initial implementation of reengineered processes in stages over a 10-month period. The team's implementation plan set out a time-table for the deployment of redesigned processes. Some processes took longer to implement than others. In general, the team attempted to implement the easy items first, then worked on longer-term implementation of complicated processes.

The team learned quickly that this is the stage in which many organizations lose their redesign. There are many pitfalls, for example, balancing the day-to-day work that needs to be done with implementation of a new process, having the patience to see the implementation through, and investing the time to refine a redesigned process that does not work well.

In the implementation phase, the team implemented all plans and waited to see the results of these process-centered reengineering efforts. Once the initial imple-mentation was complete, the team began to measure and monitor each redesigned process. Continuous improvement began at this time and continues today.

Organizational Structure

In all, management decreased from five levels (vice president, supervisors, head nurses, assistant head nurses, and unit teachers), as illustrated in Figure 16–5, to two levels (vice president and nurse manager) in the reengineered organiza-tion (Figure 16–6). The role of management changed from focusing on day-to-day activities to performing the broader duties of coach and facilitator. Managers, now at the bottom of the organizational chart because they exist within the or-ganization solely for the benefit of those who work in each unit, became servant leaders. "Servant leaders listen and learn from those they lead. They work at mak-ing themselves available.... As they listen, they learn. They become frantic learn-ers and avoid the trap that so many so-called successful leaders experience—the arrogance of ignorance."[3(p.245)]

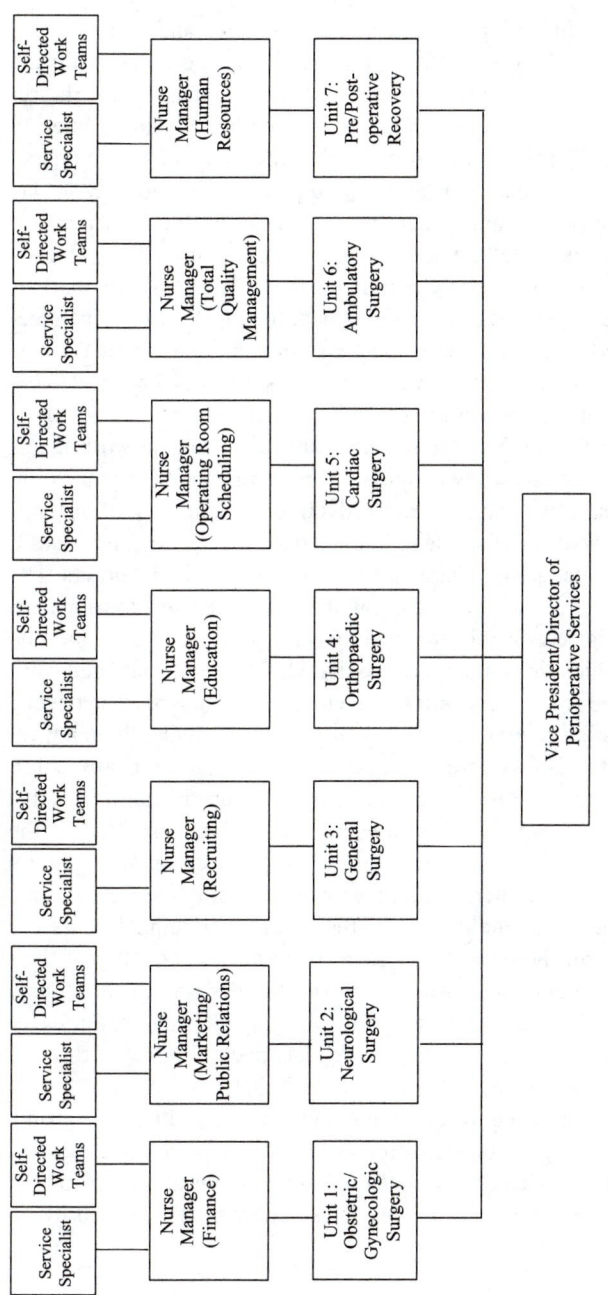

Figure 16–6 Perioperative Services Organizational Chart—After Reengineering

In this reengineered organization there is more cooperation and less competition among units. Each unit's nurse manager now performs one function for the entire perioperative services department. One nurse manager may have the responsibility for recruiting new perioperative staff, another for administering perioperative education. The significant difference is that each nurse manager is now a member of a team that performs all of the duties required for day-to-day functioning of all perioperative units. There is no need for each unit to perform the same administrative tasks that are performed in all other units. Instead, each nurse manager becomes a specialist in one functional area (i.e., finance, marketing/public relations, recruiting, education, OR scheduling, total quality management, postop/preop recovery, or human resources). An additional benefit of this new organizational structure is that the units are not as isolated as they used to be. Each unit helps out the other, and working together fosters success.

Reporting directly to the unit's nurse manager are self-managed work teams composed of colleagues with a variety of skills. In the reengineered organization, titles of these team members changed from reflecting the authority of an individual to describing the activities that the individual performs. For example, aides and orderlies now are called patient care assistants or multiskilled workers. The reengineering team also added the new position of service specialist to each unit. The service specialist is responsible for dealing with the specifics of the one surgical discipline to which this colleague is assigned. These self-managed work teams were implemented first on one unit and eventually on all units. Whenever a colleague raises a question regarding a policy or procedural issue, the team resolves the issue. These teams take care of their own problems, patient care issues, and physician issues. There are no more long, slow trips up the administrative ladder for answers. The colleagues are responsible for solving a problem for the customer, whether that customer is a patient, peer, surgeon, or supplier. All are considered and treated as customers, and a response regarding the status of the problem and the expected outcome is given to the customer within 24 hours.

The teams also perform the important task of improving the quality of their processes after measuring and monitoring. Non–value-added work is less likely to occur with members of a team capable of performing a wide range of duties for which they were trained and hired. "Busy work" has been eliminated through innovative means such as charting by exception and charging by exception. A peer review committee is in place to review nursing practices within this group. The colleagues' work and behavior are different now that restructuring is complete. The organization established a colleague-of-the-month award for physicians as well as an award for nonphysicians. These awards are voted on by all colleagues.

Every colleague is encouraged to offer suggestions and ideas; each individual is recognized as a valuable member of the team. Colleagues also are encouraged to:

- Try improvements without fear of failure or the need to get approval from a cumbersome hierarchy.
- Achieve certification in their respective areas.
- Be problem solvers rather than drones that just follow directions.

The organization also initiated shared leadership through committees and councils that fit in with the overall structure of the organization. The shared leadership committees are education/continuous quality improvement (CQI), products/services, patient care, and professional activities. These actively working committees were structured so that issues are addressed in a timely manner. Committee members form ad hoc task forces as needed to deal with specific, intense issues and policies. Although shared leadership initially was viewed as increased work and responsibility in the absence of increased pay, and was greeted with employee hostility, eventually colleagues realized that shared leadership enabled them to have a say in the reorganized organization. In stark comparison to this institution before reengineering, when the director barely knew the names of staff members, the director now actually sits at the table and is a part of the new leadership structure.

The attitude of "I'm just doing my job" has changed. Colleagues are responsible for performing their tasks as well as ensuring that each task is successfully completed. Nurses are responsible for specific activities within their services (i.e., orthopaedic nurses are responsible for making sure they have the appropriate supplies for their cases, as well as for reordering and charging correctly for these supplies). Merit pay increases for outstanding performance now motivate and reward colleagues, who no longer feel that the only path to success is by climbing an organizational ladder that leads to a management position.

Turnover Rate

The first 18 months of the reengineering effort saw the stabilization of the turnover rate to a below-industry norm of two percent and relied heavily on the introduction of staff involvement initiatives, such as an education program, innovative staffing, and increased communication.

The education program began as a formalized nine-month program for registered nurses, which was changed to a six-month program during the nursing shortage of 1989. Nurses new to the OR received intense training in perioperative nursing. Also, in the reengineered organization the team planned to use cross-trained staff. With this in mind, the reengineering team designed components of the education program to enable staff to perform equally well in the unit they were assigned to as well as on another unit in which they would cover for staff, as needed.

Since registered nurses were not readily available and were difficult to recruit, the organization had no choice but to become innovative in recruiting and offering different options for nurses. For example, the team instituted mothers' hours for shifts from 9:00 A.M. to 2:00 P.M. to attract nurses with school-aged children.

Communication among administrators, physicians, nurses, and staff was nearly nonexistent. The team fostered communication among these groups through a newsletter, bulletin board postings, and weekly staff meetings; open forums for all staff and physicians; and the use of staff input on how to improve the OR environment.

Inventory

The results of the team's inventory analysis enabled this facility to reexamine its needs and decrease its $5 million inventory to less than $1 million in inventory. The team implemented JIT inventory methods and now the institution receives supplies daily instead of weekly. Where the organization once paid face value for supplies, it now enters into contract negotiations with suppliers who submit competitive bids to win the organization's business. The reengineering team streamlined supplies and implemented modified case carts so that the professional staff did not have to pull supplies and spend time looking for items. While the reengineering team reduced inventory in many areas, it found there was a need to increase the number of surgical instruments. The team appealed to the hospital's chief executive officer (CEO) to invest over $500,000 of unbudgeted money on more instruments. This lack of instruments affected turnover time, and time is money in the OR. Prior to reengineering, the OR turnover rate varied depending on the specific surgery performed but nonetheless ranged from a minimum of 110 minutes to 300 minutes, an overly lengthy time that caused case delays. By showing the CEO the time-in-motion studies, the team justified the out-of-budget expense for more instruments to bring instrument trays up to standard and reduced OR turnover time dramatically. During Phase 2, the goal was to bring OR turnover down to an average of 20 minutes. In Phase 3, the average OR turnover rate was reduced to 34 minutes—not as good as the goal, but greatly improved. Eventually, the team developed turnover times by specialty.

Utilization of Surgical Services

In 1994, five years after reengineering efforts began, surgery revenue had risen to over $90 million and expenses, despite inflation, had risen only to $15 million. The profitability of perioperative services increased as a benefit of the reengineering effort. This was accomplished in two ways: by trimming expenses and by improving the institution's reputation enough to bolster surgical admissions. Fewer expenses also meant that the organization could afford to actively recruit managed care surgeons before the competition had these surgeons under contract in their facilities. Reengineering efforts transformed expensive, underutilized surgical services into an organizational cash cow (Figure 16–7).

CONCLUSION

To this day, managing the core processes is a continuous project. Improvements are made all the time. This health care facility, no longer the tradition-laden hospital of the past, is an evolving organization that changes to meet the continually changing needs of its customers and to remain successful in the competitive health care industry.

In the same way that looking at processes changed attitudes toward tasks, looking at teams changed attitudes toward workers. Now, colleagues are responsible for achieving a result rather than the actual task itself. After the organization implemented teams, all of the busy work went away. All colleagues knew their roles in the team as well as their contributions to patient care and their customers.

Learning and development take place in a big way. Money is budgeted for colleagues to continue their professional development. All levels of colleagues are given time for formal and informal education. The organization recognizes colleagues for their intrapreneural work. For example, one colleague was recognized for getting a large manufacturer to change a labeling system. The organization gave its full support to this professional as she worked to change the process with the manufacturer. Due to her efforts, the manufacturer changed the labeling system and improved the overall process.

In the transition to a process-centered organization the team went from not monitoring anything to monitoring and selecting pertinent core processes for improvement. A comprehensive total quality management (TQM) program was developed hospitalwide for process improvement. Shewhart and Deming's Plan-Do-Check-Act (PDCA) cycle is a routine part of the overall organizational process.

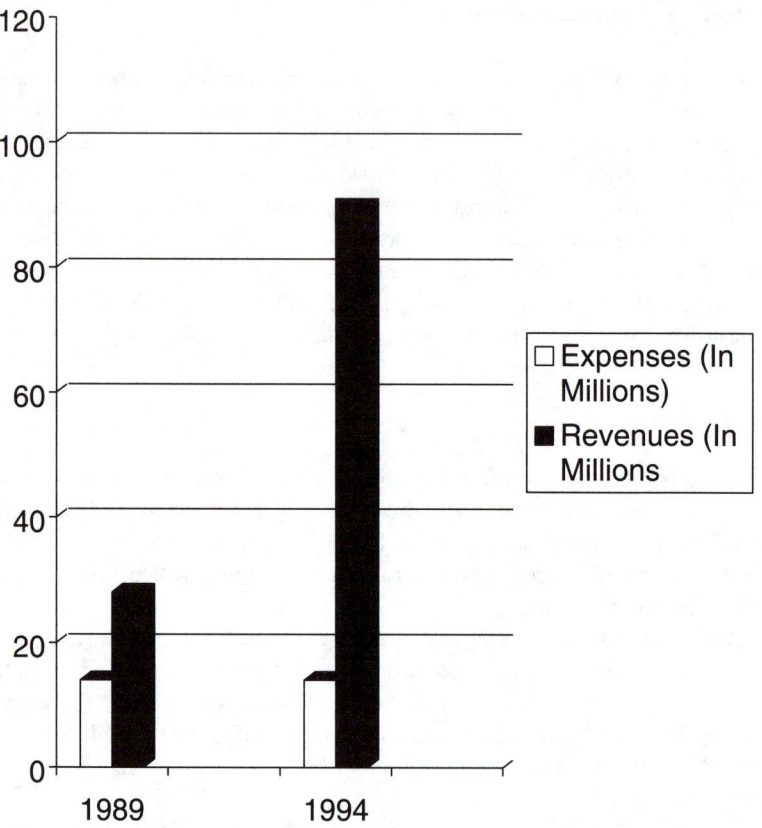

Figure 16–7 Reengineering's Impact on the Expenses and Revenue of Perioperative Services

---

Years after the initial reengineering effort began, employees who were once fearful and angered by the coming organizational revolution each play a role in the continuous redesign and refinement of processes. They have become teachers of this learning organization. There is a widespread recognition that their destinies are tied to those of the institution where they work, and this is motivation enough for performing continuous monitoring and improvement. They realize that in the fierce competition for health care customers, "there are no winners on a losing team."[2(p.65)]

REFERENCES

1. Hammer M, Champy J. *Reengineering the Corporation: A Manifesto for Business Revolution.* New York: Harper Business; 1993.

2. Hammer M. *Beyond Reengineering: How the Process-Centered Organization Is Changing Our Work and Our Lives.* New York: Harper Business; 1996.

3. Pollard CW. The leader who serves. In: Hesselbein F, Goldsmith M, Beckhard R, eds. *The Leader of the Future.* San Francisco: Jossey-Bass, Inc. Publishers; 1996.

CHAPTER 17

The Patient Care Documentation Process: The Infrastructure to Support Outcome–Based Standards of Care

Lana S. Peters, MHA, MBA, RN
Myra Mengwasser, MHA, RN
Curt Kretzinger, BSN, RN

Despite previous reengineering efforts to move to a more patient-centered, team approach to care, many health care organizations are finding that caregivers do not have the tools to support and enable the interdisciplinary communication aspect of their model of care. As the health care continuum expands, these challenges are requiring many organizations to again redesign processes to enable all disciplines throughout an episode of care to communicate and collaborate in providing patient-centered, outcome-based care. As information technology advances, automating clinical documentation is receiving more attention as a viable solution to this demand.

Heartland Health System (Heartland) wanted to improve its documentation system to facilitate an interdisciplinary care process. Although it was already using an automated system, the organization realized it was necessary to redesign the process first. Heartland integrated interdisciplinary standards of care, clinical pathways, and a new documentation approach to increase the continuity and coordination of care for patients across the continuum. As Heartland now prepares for automation, it has found both benefits and pitfalls in redesigning documentation and linking standards of care to that system.

In 1993, Heartland, an integrated delivery and financing system located in St. Joseph, Missouri, developed a patient-centered model of care called CARING. Their goal was to take the concept to a new level and institute an interdisciplinary practice model and interdisciplinary standards of patient care. The leadership team members realized from previous reengineering efforts that interdisciplinary standards of care required mechanisms or tools to reinforce the standards in everyday practice or the cultural changes would be difficult to achieve and sustain. They needed a method to bring all disciplines together in team formation with a focus on patient care outcomes. Having gone through reengineering of the patient care processes, Heartland found its documentation and communication of information to be nonsupportive of such a model. It wanted to develop an infrastructure to support and enable reengineered processes versus functions. Heartland began a redesign process to develop standards of care to standardize care functions performed by multiple disciplines and departments across the continuum through a project that came to be known as the Interdisciplinary Standards of Care and Documentation (IDS) project.

The goals of the IDS project were to (1) reduce fragmentation of care across the continuum, (2) increase interdisciplinary collaboration and communication, (3) decrease charting time, and (4) reduce redundancy of documentation and interdisciplinary work efforts. Heartland envisioned a cutting-edge solution to many of the challenges integrated delivery and financing systems (IDFSs) face with promoting patient-centered care that is consistent among all disciplines and in all venues (Figure 17–1). As a result, it developed a system that drives interdisciplinary, evidence-based care and supports better patient outcomes; standardizes care across the continuum for episodes of care; streamlines documentation and communication; and uses clinical pathways as a support tool to enhance this process.

Historically, Heartland operated in a system built to support acute patient care delivery, as did many integrated health care delivery systems across the country. Such a system encouraged health care providers to treat their patients as individual encounters rather than within a continuum of care. Although strategies to move patients across multiple venues were developed, there was not a mechanism or tool in place to proactively move patients across the system while ensuring continuity of care and information. Health care organizations talk about providing interdisciplinary care after reengineering efforts, but each department and discipline often operated independently (from its own representative professional perspective and departmental functions) to provide care to the patient, creating a department-focused rather than a patient-focused model of care. This often results in patient care and education being inconsistent between disciplines, which leads to fragmented care as patients move across the continuum.

In response to growing competition, an intense cost-conscious focus, a changing health care market, and a movement away from acute care in the 1980s, Heartland again saw an opportunity to improve its care delivery and better compete in this challenging environment. In 1993, Heartland redesigned its patient care model to provide the framework for patient-centered care and a stronger team approach to care. However, Heartland was disappointed to find that with a new, reengineered

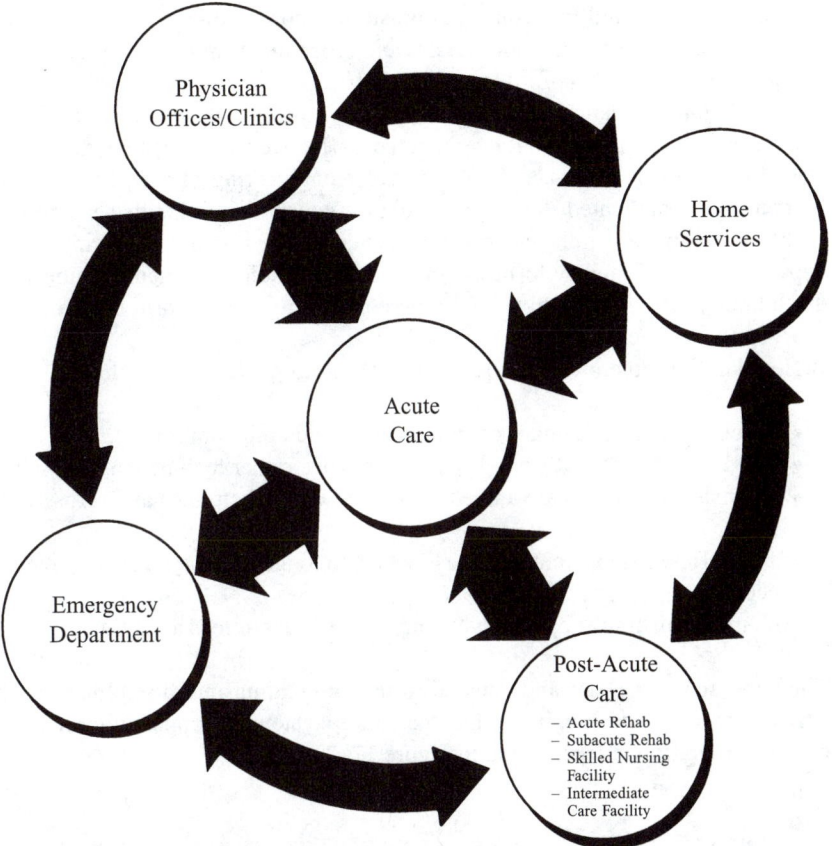

Figure 17–1 Heartland Health System's Continuum of Care. *Source:* Courtesy of Heartland Health System, St. Joseph, Missouri.

---

team approach to care, there was a lack of communication and coordination as patients moved across the continuum. Although reengineering initiatives at that time were visionary and cutting-edge for improving patient care delivery and efficiency, disconnects in day-to-day processes still existed, and there was a lack of clear, well-defined standards to support cohesion across disciplines and departments. Like many organizations in the post-reengineering era, it seemed that the organization was still focused on independent functions of patient care rather than the process of providing patient care to achieve optimal outcomes. Each discipline and each venue of care still operated independently. This resulted in too many policies and procedures, confusion in how standards are defined, an inadequate approval process for policies and procedures, and a lack of coordination and communication of information.

Heartland found that its automated documentation system, which exists to support patient care delivery, no longer met the staff's needs. The system, developed prior to care management and patient care reengineering efforts, had become burdensome, fragmented, duplicative, and time consuming rather than supportive to the care team. When the current documentation did not meet a discipline's or department's needs, a new form was created. As a result, documentation became discipline-focused, duplicative, and time consuming, with a form or screen for everything and everyone.

Heartland's problems, like those of many other organizations, included

- a lack of interdisciplinary communication and collaboration
- standards of care that were discipline specific rather than patient focused
- inconsistent patient care and education between disciplines and across venues
- an inefficient documentation system that no longer met patient care provider needs
- no mechanism to support the patient care process across a continuum

The approach that Heartland decided to use in creating interdisciplinary standards of care and developing a documentation system to support interdisciplinary collaboration is represented in Figure 17–2.

ESTABLISHMENT OF FOUNDATION FOR INTERDISCLIPLINARY STANDARDS

To begin the process redesign project, a leadership team with representatives from disciplines across the continuum was formed to develop interdisciplinary standards of care and documentation. Their challenge was to develop a vision and guiding principles and to lead the design teams through the development process. The vision for care delivery and standards for how care would be delivered were developed first (Exhibit 17–1).

Next, this group developed a framework for interdisciplinary standards of care and a common set of definitions for the system. Although previous work had been done on developing a framework for standards of care,[1,2] it was important for Heartland to adopt a framework that not only was nursing focused but that also supported interdisciplinary care. The team determined that the concept of structure, process, and outcomes would provide the framework for interdiscipli-

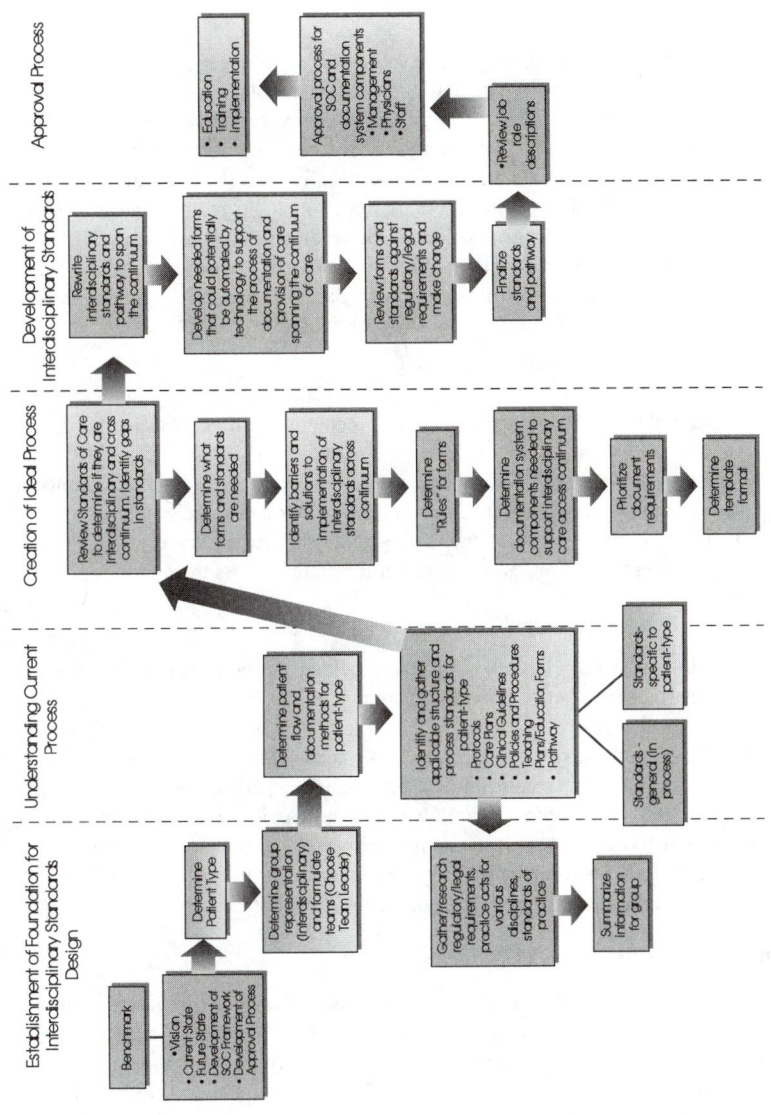

Figure 17–2 Process Overview. *Source:* Courtesy of Heartland Health System, St. Joseph, Missouri.

Exhibit 17–1 The Vision for Interdisciplinary Standards of Care and Documentation

Standards of Care

In the future at Heartland, health care providers will be committed to and accountable for interdisciplinary standards of care. These standards are inclusive of all disciplines and will be clear, measurable, evidence based, results driven, and based on the patient's needs. Policies and procedures, guidelines, regulatory and professional standards, standing orders, protocols, medical bylaws, and other resources will be reflected in the standards. A common language to define standards will be established with a congruent format for development. These standards (i.e., process and outcomes) will be incorporated into clinical pathways. Our documentation process will support interdisciplinary standards of care and the flow of information between disciplines and through the continuum.

Venues of Care

Interdisciplinary standards of care and documentation will assist us in providing seamless care across all venues. Holistic patient profiling (e.g., home assessment) will occur at the front end of patient care in order to predict patient needs. Patient progress will follow phases of care determined by outcomes rather than by days of care. Documentation will support interdisciplinary standards of care, and technology will enable entry and access to patient information across the continuum.

Disciplines: Roles and Impact

Interdisciplinary care at Heartland will be provided across the continuum. Disciplines will partner together in providing care that is patient focused. The patient's needs and expectations will be first and foremost, and health care providers will understand their unique roles in meeting these needs. The interdisciplinary team will value each individual's contribution and his or her knowledge or expertise in providing the best care to the patient. Overlaps and barriers will be minimized as the care team works toward goals. Documentation will reflect and support this integrated care process. Health care providers will spend less time on documentation, allowing more time for processes that positively affect patient care.

Patient and Family: Roles and Effects

Patients and families will experience a seamless flow of care without fragmentation. They will take ownership and make decisions regarding their care, which will allow them to know that their expectations of care have been met or exceeded. Patients and families will receive consistent information and education from interdisciplinary team members.

Source: Courtesy of Heartland Health System, St. Joseph, Missouri.

nary care. Its adaptation was thought to be facilitative of an outcomes focus and to fit into the overall organizational objectives. The interdisciplinary standards of care framework was divided into three components: structure standards, process standards, and outcome standards (Figure 17–3). These standards are not nursing focused but include all disciplines involved in patient care (i.e., physical therapy, occupational therapy, speech therapy, recreational therapy, respiratory therapy, spiritual health, case management, social services, dietary, etc.).

The three components of the interdisciplinary standards of care framework can be explained as follows:

1. *Structure standards* are those standards that define all the conditions and mechanisms needed to operate Heartland Health System. For example, these might include job descriptions or performance standards, or they might be the types of patients a unit takes or the hours of service for the physical therapy department.
2. *Process standards* define the actions, knowledge, and skills needed by all staff in performing job functions and/or carrying out care, as well as what constitutes that care. Some examples might include a Foley catheter insertion procedure, a Coumadin teaching protocol, a clinical pathway, or documentation instructions.
3. *Outcome standards* specify what patient goals are to be accomplished. An

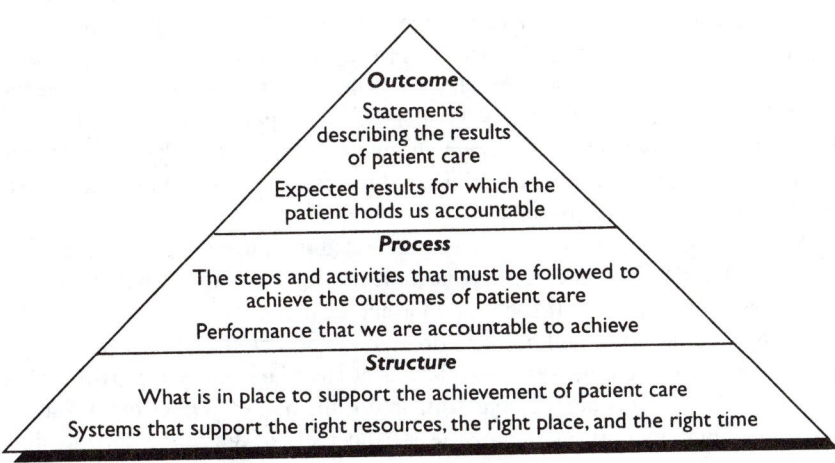

Figure 17–3 The Interdisciplinary Standards of Care Framework. *Source:* Courtesy of Heartland Health System, St. Joseph, Missouri.

example might be "a patient will be able to return to work within two weeks after discharge from the hospital."

Once the interdisciplinary standards of care framework was defined, Heartland was able to focus on the actual design of the documentation process. Documentation is a significant part of patient care delivery, and many organizations spend a great deal of resources to improve this process. Evidence of a system that supports a process-centered organization is lacking. Heartland researched what types of documentation were currently being used by other organizations across the United States. Current literature was reviewed and other organizations were interviewed. In discussing IDS with organizations across the country, it was found that very few organizations truly have interdisciplinary documentation and that even fewer have tried to link interdisciplinary standards of care to that system.[3–5]

UNDERSTANDING THE CURRENT PROCESS

A thorough assessment of the current care delivery and documentation processes was conducted. Interviews and focus group sessions were conducted with approximately 100 staff, managers, and physicians. Patient feedback was also analyzed to better understand the patients' perception of communication, education, and coordination of care. Heartland found staff and physician dissatisfaction with communication between disciplines and across venues. Staff felt the care and education they provided was at times contradictory and felt disconnected. Disciplines were unsure of how their practice contributed to the final patient outcome. They identified concerns about the amount of time they spent documenting and away from patients and about times when collaboration between caregivers, other departments, and other disciplines was not smooth. They could not see the benefit of documentation and how it better served the patient care process; it was merely a "required function." During interviews, patients stated that they felt they were being asked duplicative questions and indicated that they had seen and experienced disconnects between different disciplines.

Time-and-motion studies were also performed with nurses and other professional staff as they documented routine patient care. Heartland found that nurses and other professional staff spent an inordinate amount of time on documentation. This is time that could be spent doing other activities that positively affect patient care. For example, registered nurses at Heartland spent approximately 4 hours and 50 minutes per 12-hour shift in documentation. Other organizations have also found that nurses spend at least 30 percent of their time documenting patient care.[4]

There was also an excessive number of forms being used. Approximately 3,500 forms existed, both as part of the permanent medical record and as communication tools between care providers. Each department had its own forms and screens, and pertinent patient information was being recorded in multiple places and usually not being reviewed by any other care providers. For example, four different admission forms were being used in different areas across the continuum. Information on these forms was redundant and recorded on other forms during the patient's stay.

Current policies and procedures were also reviewed across the system. Although Heartland operated as an integrated care system, multiple policies and procedures were found that were not standardized between departments. For example, 11 different policies and procedures were found for Foley catheter care within the system. Patient education protocols were also reviewed. No standardized patient education instructions were found between departments. The implication of all this was fragmentation and gaps in care delivery, resulting in health care providers spending too much time on documentation and redundant work efforts.

The current-state analysis confirmed that there existed a need to:

- Streamline the documentation process and reduce the number of forms used.
- Reduce the time it takes to document on the computer.
- Create a documentation system that encourages disciplines to communicate together and supports the coordination of care across venues.
- Standardize the care and education provided to patients across the continuum.
- Build an infrastructure for the development of standards of care for the entire system.

CREATION OF THE IDEAL PROCESS

Based on the current-state analysis and the identified gaps to achieving the desired future-state processes, Heartland built a case for changing not only how it documented but also how care is defined and delivered across the organization. To do this, the new documentation process must support and enable interdisciplinary patient care delivery and facilitate the flow of information through the system.

Because Heartland had many clinical pathways in place, it chose to further develop clinical pathways to span the continuum and to use them as the primary documentation tool, as well as a tool to enhance care management functions. Heartland incorporated a methodology for exception-based charting on clinical pathways and called it "Charting against Standards." Charting against standards is a format or methodology used to streamline the documentation of interdisciplinary care delivery and patient outcome achievement as defined by a preestablished care plan (pathway) and standards of care. Narrative notes are used to document exceptions from standards and outcomes. The goal of this is to allow easy visualization of patient outcomes, goals, and pertinent problems (Exhibit 17–2). With this system, standards of care drive not only documentation but also interdisciplinary collaboration and standardized care as well.

Because Heartland had many problems with the current automated documentation system, a key decision point in redesigning the process was whether to create it as a manual system or to redesign the automated system. Because documentation is such an important part of patient care, Heartland wanted to ensure that the manual process was perfected prior to automation. One lesson Heartland learned, and a lesson many organizations learn as they move to automation, is that computers only automate documentation. If the process itself is "broken" in the manual form, organizations will only automate the broken process. Although Heartland had already moved to computerized documentation in 1992, it elected to design this system in a manual template first with the potential for automation in the future.

Design of the new system began with the selection of two patient populations and the formation of two interdisciplinary teams. The teams created the documentation templates on two clinical pathways. The pathways selected were elective total hip replacement and cerebral vascular accident (CVA). A design team was formed to develop the standards of care and the documentation forms. Members of the design teams represented multiple disciplines and different areas of patient care from across the continuum.

Over an eight-week period, team members worked diligently to conduct research, gather information, and design new forms and new interdisciplinary standards of care. Work group members researched internal policies and leading practices, external legal and regulatory requirements, practice acts, and standards of practice as a basis for their interdisciplinary standards of care. Using current (medical model) clinical pathways, they redesigned the pathways to include such components as patient outcomes, patient teaching, therapies, activities of daily living, and discharge planning and developed them to span the continuum. Members of the work groups rewrote current policies and procedures and developed them into interdisciplinary standards of care. For the first two patient types, over 170 policies and procedures were developed into approximately 90 standards common for all venues and disciplines. In addition, new standards of care and teaching protocols were also developed to support a more outcome-focused, interdisciplinary model of care.

The work groups developed a set of core forms to be used for all patient types, as well as clinical pathways for each specific patient type for the entire episode of care (Figure 17–4). These core forms, for the first time, would move with the patient to different venues to reduce redundant questioning, facilitate information flow regarding the patient's care, and provide a smoother transition for the patient. For example, the work groups deleted four different admission profile forms and developed a joint admission form that is completed upon admission to the system and is used by all disciplines across the continuum.

Exhibit 17–2 Charting against Standards

LOCATION OR LEVEL OF CARE: ACUTE CARE

POTENTIAL PATIENT PROBLEMS	DATE IDENTIFIED AS ACTUAL		DATE RESOLVED		INTERDISCIPLINARY NOTES
	Date	Initial	Initial (Y/E)	Date	
1. Nutritional status			__/__	__/__	
2. Knowledge deficit of disease process			__/__	__/__	
3. Dysphagia			__/__	__/__	
4. Impaired mobility			__/__	__/__	
5. Impaired auditory/ comprehensive			__/__	__/__	
6. Impaired expressive skills			__/__	__/__	
7. Impaired cognitive/ problem-solving			__/__	__/__	
8. Impaired perceptual function			__/__	__/__	
9. Alteration in bowel/bladder elimination			__/__	__/__	
10. Health maintenance			__/__	__/__	
11. Safety knowledge deficit			__/__	__/__	
12. Pain			__/__	__/__	
13. Alteration in skin integrity			__/__	__/__	
14. Safe living arrangement at time of discharge			__/__	__/__	
15. Impaired socialization			__/__	__/__	
16. Impaired ADL function			__/__	__/__	
17. Impaired psychosocial function			__/__	__/__	
18. Spiritual distress			__/__	__/__	
19. Other _____			__/__	__/__	
20. Other _____			__/__	__/__	

Signature/Title	Initials	Shift	Signature/Title	Initials	Shift
_____	___	___	_____	___	___
_____	___	___	_____	___	___
_____	___	___	_____	___	___
_____	___	___	_____	___	___

Documentation Key: Y = Yes E = Exception
* Initial "Y" column when completed according to standard of care.
* Initial "E" column for exception to standard of care of activity not completed and write explanation in Interdisciplinary Notes column.

HEARTLAND REGIONAL MEDICAL CENTER
St. Joseph, Missouri 64501
CVA CLINICAL PATHWAY DRG 14

continues

Exhibit 17–2 continued

ACUTE CARE

Day or Phase		POD #2	
Location of Level of Care		Floor	Interdisciplinary Notes
	Time	Date_____	
Individual Considerations (completed)	____ ____ ____	__/__ Other _____ __/__ Other _____ __/__ Other _____	
PT/CAREGIVER CONCERNS/GOALS (identified)	____ ____ ____	__/__ Other _____ __/__ Other _____ __/__ Other _____	
INTERMEDIATE PROGRESSION TOWARD NEXT LEVEL OF CARE/DISCHARGE (goals met)	____ ____ ____ ____ ____ ____ ____ ____	__/__ Time ___/___Time___/___Problem list/outcomes reviewed __/__ Minimal assist from bed to chair __/__ Ambulate with walker with minimal assistance for 25 feet __/__ Patient/caregiver verbalize understanding of S&S of infection Minimal assistance for 25 feet __/__ Patient obtains pain relief __/__ Patient (PO) meds are initiated __/__ Patient demonstrates adherence to hip precautions with verbal cues __/__ Wound site demonstrates healing __/__ Other _____ __/__ Other _____	
CONSULTS (contacted to see)	____ ____	__/__ Other _____ __/__ Other _____	
TESTS/DIAGNOSIS (completed unless otherwise stated)	____ ____ ____	__/__ Protime results obtained __/__ Platelet count if on Lovenox, for post-op day #3 (ordered) __/__ Other _____	
MEDICATIONS/IVs/ BLOOD (to be used ONLY as a guide)	____ ____ ____ ____ ____ ____ ____	__/__ Coumadin as per physician order __/__ _____ mg __/__ Lovenox administered as ordered __/__ Laxative if no BM __/__ Pain medication IM/PO __/__ Other _____ __/__ Other _____	

Signature/Title	Initials	Shift	Signature/Title	Initials	Shift
_____	___	___	_____	___	___
_____	___	___	_____	___	___
_____	___	___	_____	___	___
_____	___	___	_____	___	___

> **Documentation Key: Y = Yes E = Exception**
> * Initial "Y" column when completed according to standard of care.
> * Initial "E" column for exception to standard of care of activity not completed and write explanation in Interdisciplinary Notes column.

HEARTLAND REGIONAL MEDICAL CENTER
St. Joseph, Missouri 64501
CVA CLINICAL PATHWAY DRG 14

Source: Courtesy of Heartland Health System, St. Joseph, Missouri.

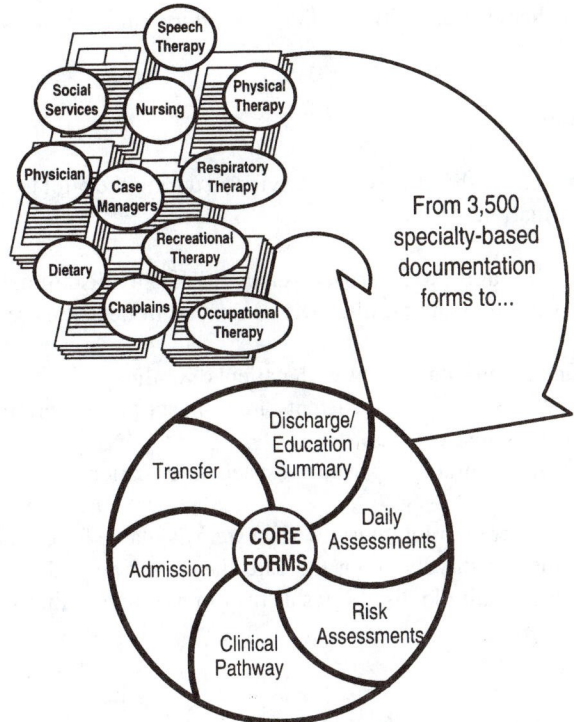

Figure 17–4 Forms Reduction. *Source:* Courtesy of Heartland Health System, St. Joseph, Missouri.

PILOT IMPLEMENTATION

Prior to automating this new system, it was necessary to pilot the system in the manual form and test the designs. After educating over 600 staff from across the continuum, a pilot of the IDS templates was initiated in patient care areas and with disciplines associated with the CVA and elective total hip replacement patients. Although fewer patients were seen than expected during the pilot, many of the patients in the pilot did move across the continuum from acute care to acute rehabilitation, subacute rehabilitation, skilled nursing, and/or home health.

During the six-week pilot, patient and staff satisfaction information was collected, a language assessment of consistent use of terms in interdisciplinary care was completed, chart audits were performed, and financial impact was analyzed to identify both benefits and pitfalls of the system. Preliminary analysis indicated the following.

Patient Satisfaction

Patients involved in the pilot were interviewed during the pilot to determine the following information:

- whether information was verified versus reasked by disciplines
- to what extent patients/families were involved in decisions regarding their care
- the amount of time staff spent with patients/families
- whether patients received consistent care from staff (e.g., gait training, home oxygen therapy instructions)
- whether patients/families received consistent information from their caregivers

Although no direct prepilot interview data were available for comparison, pilot patients responded positively about the care they received and the information they were given by multiple disciplines as they moved across the continuum.

Staff Satisfaction

Analysis of staff satisfaction and perception of how the system affects care delivery was important to the overall objective of the project. To assess staff satisfaction, surveys were distributed to staff involved in the pilot. Staff indicated that the system allowed them to follow the patient through the system more easily, review other disciplines' documentation more easily, focus on patient outcomes, and plan care for their patients. However, after only six weeks, they were still finding the manual documentation system to be time consuming, redundant, and difficult to learn. This may be attributable to staff having to adjust to using a manual chart rather than the computer, low pilot patient volume or contact, or using dual systems during the pilot (charting on the current computerized system for some patients and on the manual pathway for others). The more the staff used the new documentation tools and standards, the more they felt the system supported the care they provided and met their documentation needs.

Chart Audit

A retrospective chart review was performed on patient charts for CVA and elective total hip replacement patients prior to the pilot and then audited again at the end of the pilot to measure compliance with standards of care and regulatory/ accrediting requirements, as well as planned use of the new documentation forms. The audit of pilot charts showed improvement in admission assessments being completed within 24 hours of patient admission, functional status being assessed when indicated by criteria, reassessments completed according to standard, and an increase in individualization of pathways/plans of care.

For both patient types, signing the pathway and avoiding duplication of documentation on the pathway and in the computer are areas that still need improvement. This could be attributable to staff moving from an automated documentation system to a manual documentation system and to staff using dual systems based on patient diagnoses.

Language

One of the objectives of the IDS project was to establish a common language between disciplines and to develop an understanding of terminology used during this project. A pretest was given to staff during the education sessions and again at the end of the pilot to assess staff's understanding of terms basic to the interdisciplinary standards of care project (i.e., standards of care, interdisciplinary, etc.). The average test score improved by 25 percent during the pilot.

Financial Impact

Although the number of patients seen during the project in all of the venues was much lower than anticipated, some of the benefits of disciplines working together and providing standardized care along clinical pathways was evident. In all applicable venues (acute stay, acute rehab, subacute rehab, skilled nursing, and home health), average length of stay and cost per case decreased. For example, during the six-week pilot, total cross-continuum average length-of-stay reductions of approximately 11 days for elective total hip replacement patients and 23 days for CVA patients were experienced. These findings are being further studied.

Summary of Pilot Study

From the pilot, Heartland was able to demonstrate some of the benefits of using interdisciplinary standards of care and streamlining documentation across venues of care. Because a larger pilot sample size was needed to further measure the benefits and give staff the opportunity to use the new system, Heartland chose to continue the manual pilot and to further measure its impact while planning for

automation, selecting and developing the next clinical pathways (based on patient type), and working toward its "Next Steps" (Exhibit 17–3).

Heartland has expended a tremendous amount of time and effort in developing
interdisciplinary standards of care and documentation templates. With much of
the groundwork completed and many benefits of the system already realized
through pilot implementation, further steps and analysis are needed to move Heartland toward attaining its complete vision for interdisciplinary standards of care
and documentation.

CONCLUSION

Further work and study are needed in the area of clinical documentation and
the integration of standards of care to achieve interdisciplinary care across the
continuum. However, Heartland has learned what many organizations have learned
in the post-reengineering era. Reengineering has acknowledged the need for organizations to focus on their process and integrate tools and mechanisms to support the communication and collaboration of disciplines in achieving the final
patient outcome as the patient moves along a continuum of care. As technology
advances in the area of information systems, documentation is becoming a key
process that can be enhanced to achieve those results.

Exhibit 17–3 Next Steps and Expected Benefits

- Automation of IDS to increase staff satisfaction and reduce overtime
- Ability of staff to move from one venue of care to another following interdisci-
  plinary standards for patients along a disease process
- Preparation for skilled nursing and home health care prospective payment
  system (PPS)
- Measurement and monitoring of the outcomes of a population of patients from
  a clinical process and cost benefit perspective
- Prediction of workload for all care processes in the entire system
- Opening of continuous quality improvement process for care across the entire
  episode
- Measurement of clinical and financial impact, patient satisfaction, and service
  impact for internal and external audiences

Source: Courtesy of Heartland Health System, St. Joseph, Missouri.

Organizations redesigning their documentation or automating their systems should consider the following guidelines before proceeding:

- Include all departments or disciplines in the effort.
- Redesign the process before automation. Don't computerize a broken process.
- When selecting a computer software vendor, first clearly outline what capabilities the organization wants in a system.
- Make on-site visits to other organizations that are using a software vendor the organization is considering.

As organizations merge and reengineer to seek the benefits of coordinating and collaborating in health care delivery, care providers will need the tools to support and enable these processes to take hold. Documentation and standards of care are two examples of tools that health care organizations can use to support interdisciplinary care across the continuum. However, these tools will not be effective unless the process is designed to work within the infrastructure of the individual organization.

REFERENCES

1. McAllister M. A nursing integration framework based on standards of practice. *Nurs Management.* 1990; 21(4):28–31.
2. Corpuz LS, Conforti C. Organizing and documenting clinical standards. *Nurs Management.* 1994; 25(5):70–76.
3. Krause CR, Westdorp JM, Coonen DA, Jenks DL. Forming an integrated documentation system. *Nurs Management.* 1996; 27(8):25–26.
4. Short MS. Charting by exception on a clinical pathway. *Nurs Management.* 1997; 28(8):45–46.
5. Gage M. The patient-driven interdisciplinary care plan. *J Nurs Adm.* 1994; 24(4):26–35.

CHAPTER 18

The Outcomes Management Process: A Three-Year Experience

Celine Peters, MN, RN
Markie Cowley, MSN, RN, CHE
Jill Donaldson, MSN, RN, CCRN

Changes in health care reimbursement in 1994 were projected to reduce earnings of Mission Hospital Regional Medical Center (MHRMC) by $9 million over the next five years. This projection in decreased reimbursement drove the organization to change its approach in operations, since projections were alarming even though strong profit margins were seen. The vice president of patient care services was faced with the dilemma of decreasing the cost of care. The same approach in patient care would result in losses due to changes in reimbursement systems. Three clinical nurse specialists were employed by the facility. The goal was to retain this valuable resource; however, a change in role and accountability was paramount.

An outcomes management department was established in 1995 at MHRMC, a 271-bed, acute care, community hospital in Orange County, California. The development of the outcomes management program would affect all departments and personnel of the organization and result in a change in the patient care delivery approach. This chapter presents the reengineering of the clinical nurse specialist (CNS) role to outcomes manager to lead the change process, the outcomes management process, integration of the process in the organization, and developments in the organization three years postimplementation.

HISTORICAL PERSPECTIVE

California is a densely populated state with 33 million people, 2.7 million in Orange County alone.[1] The rapid change in the health care environment was precipitated by the following factors[2]:

- California's health care market is highly competitive.
- California experienced accelerated consolidation and integration of hospitals into systems (65 percent of all hospitals are part of a system).
- The unemployment rate in California was 6.1 percent; the national rate was 4.8 percent.
- The uninsured population in California was 24 percent; nationally, the uninsured population was 17 percent.
- California saw a shift from full-time to temporary employees.

California was and continues to be a mature managed care market, with 43 percent of the population enrolled in a health maintenance organization (HMO). Another 24 percent of the population belongs to a preferred provider organization (PPO) plan, which means that two out of every three Californians belong to a plan requiring some gatekeeper or authorization for treatment.[3] Further restrictions in 1994 were realized from Medicaid for undocumented resident care. In this area, California shares with Texas a disproportionate impact, accounting for 40 percent of the illegal immigrants seen in the nation.[2] Orange County itself experienced a population growth of 1.2 percent per year, with hospital discharges increasing by nine percent and a continued decline in length of stay.[4]

The five-year projection was for revenues to increase at the rate of 1.4–1.8 percent and expenses at 2.6–2.7 percent. A one percent difference in market share translated into $2.1 million dollars, positive or negative, as seen in Figure 18–1. Managed care was managing reimbursements, and hospitals were required to

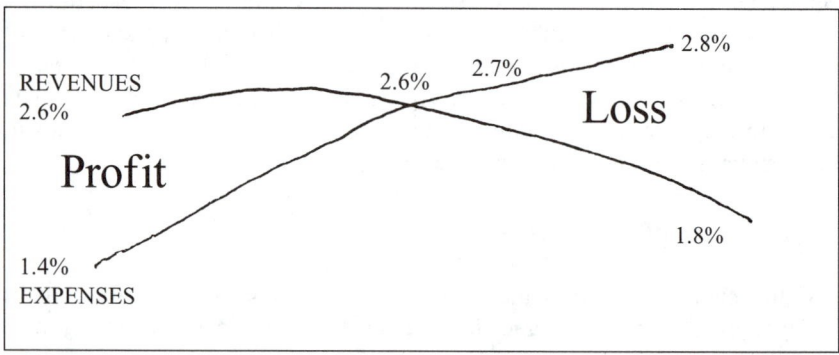

Figure 18–1 Projected Revenues Compared to Expenses (Five Years). *Source:* Courtesy of Mission Hospital Regional Medical Center, Mission Viejo, California.

manage costs. The one positive factor with the onset of managed care was an increased emphasis on quality differentiation and measuring outcomes.[4]

MHRMC is one of 11 hospitals within the St. Joseph Health System. This system, as well as its sponsor, the Sisters of St. Joseph of Orange, is a mission- and values-driven organization. Professional activities designed and implemented would ensure consistency of the values of dignity, excellence, service, and justice, as follows:

- The value of dignity emphasizes the commitment to share information with providers, clients, and employees.
- Excellence emphasizes the importance of working together as team members and being responsible stewards of resources.
- Service holds employees accountable to meet the needs of those served.
- Justice discerns how the good of the whole is best served.

As MHRMC embarked on the process of practice change, existing programs were examined and "best practices" were researched. To increase the likelihood of success, the approach selected was based on the strengths of the organization: a strong clinical focus with variety in range of services and a reputation as a leader in the community. The development of an outcomes management program was a step necessary to achieve redesign of patient care delivery. The goal for the organization was to identify the process to improve patient care. Everyone in the organization required knowledge about the change; individual accountability, clinical and financial, for care given; and an awareness of the results or outcomes of delivered care. Based on the strategic objectives of the institution, the approach targeted services across the continuum of care. A crucial aspect was the integration of the clinical and financial services—a key to the organizational strategy.

The goals identified to drive service changes included the following:

- Decrease fragmentation.
- Decrease inappropriate utilization of resources and services.
- Increase satisfaction.
- Increase market share/service base.

Through existing sources, clients consistently noted difficulties in the continuity of care across departments and the continuum. A well-designed process would improve the coordination of services. Decreasing the demand for services and/or ensuring improved access to service would result in overall decreased costs of providing care. Based on payer mix, impact on the bottom line would be significant. It was believed that as services, access, and appropriate utilization improved, satisfaction of patients, providers, and payers would occur. Ultimately, a better operating system would attract more contracts and thus more members.

MHRMC approached the redesign process so as to use its existing strengths. Key patient populations were identified through a variety of sources and included

- internal clinical leaders
- top hospital diagnosis-related groups (DRGs)
- outlier populations
- capitated payers
- Medicare top DRGs

A team of internal clinical leaders was established and charged with identifying high-risk populations, that is, patients who were complex, unpredictable, and hard to manage, such as trauma patients. Reviewing charges and volume, the hospital identified its top DRGs as defined by highest charges or highest numbers of admissions. Those with extended lengths of stay and high resource use were identified as outliers.

MHRMC had signed its first capitated agreement in 1993, and it collaborated with this payer group to identify outliers and high-risk enrollees. The senior population (Medicare patients) always presented opportunities for improving services and is a significant component of the overall population.

Finally, MHRMC wanted to experience a high degree of success. If an individual physician or group was interested in a defined population, the diagnosis was included. Five service lines evolved from this process by grouping similar populations: cardiovascular, surgical, neurovascular, women and children, and general medicine.

The administrative staff took an active role in planning change for the organization. Communication and resource allocation were some of the critical responsibilities assumed. MHRMC historically had a philosophy of physician-led and -driven processes. To effect change, the model selected would need to maximize this approach. Physicians would be at the helm to drive the process, and administration's role would be one of facilitator, supporter, and integrator of disciplines and services. Therefore, a clinical model was developed (see Exhibit 18–1) to facilitate the change process for both hospital staff and physicians. Physicians are scientifically trained professionals who are data driven and thrive on using a research approach. This profile would move care toward the discovery of best practice. The model focused on the potential benefit for the patient and the established program goals. CNSs were chosen to lead the efforts because they were hands-on clinical experts and credibly established with staff and physicians. They understood pathophysiology and issues related to a patient's disease pro-

Exhibit 18–1 Clinical Model Approach

- Research-based scientific approach toward the discovery of best practice
- Physician driven
- Patient centered
- Across the continuum
- Clinical experts
- Not financially focused

Source: Courtesy of Mission Hospital Regional Medical Center, Mission Viejo, California.

cess. It was determined that the emphasis would not be on controlling or authorizing care. The CNSs would not have discharge planning or utilization review responsibilities. Through effective design, the emphasis was placed on clinical care improvement resulting in cost reduction. The hospital would distance itself from the physician if the driving force were cost reduction.

Using existing roles, the hospital restructured, redesigned, and developed new roles for this effort. Unit-based educators, clinicians, and CNSs were centralized to two departments. Traditional educators were assigned to the education department with little change in focus but a widened scope of responsibilities. A new department, outcomes management, was created based on the five identified service lines. From the department's inception, the institution used existing full-time employees, and no new positions were added. The clinicians over each service line were titled outcomes managers (OMs) and had responsibility for a defined service.

The CNS or advanced practice nurse was the expert to facilitate the delivery of quality care. The OMs are master's prepared in nursing or an allied health field or are currently enrolled in a master's program. They are assigned by patient populations and have at least two years' experience in a specialized area.

Outcomes management would differ from case management in several ways. Case management focuses on managing the care of individual patients. Outcomes management focuses on patient occurrences as an aggregate population, the experience of a defined population as a whole, which allows research-based decisions to enhance patient care. The role of OM incorporated the traditional role of the CNS as clinical practitioner, consultant, educator, and researcher and added the role of financial analyst.[5]

As a clinical practitioner, the outcomes manager supports the bedside staff to care for patients using the changes in care recommended by the multidisciplinary team. The practitioner may case manage high-risk patients requiring complex care, such as those who need multiple specialty consults, are psychologically or functionally challenged, or have an unusual or unfamiliar diagnosis. The OM as a consultant identifies areas for patient care improvement, monitors and evaluates patient care, and recommends changes to patient care in collaboration with a multidisciplinary team. The OM's educator role is to share knowledge and apply educational concepts to design patient and family teaching standards to prevent disease complications. The OM's researcher role incorporates the research process to develop an understanding of the patient population, clearly define variances associated with routinely delivered cases, establish an accurate and reliable basis for clinical decision making, and identify opportunities for improvement. The measurement of care effectiveness is managed through the data-analysis process. The outcomes manager as a financial analyst uses knowledge and understanding of patient care to improve cost outcomes across the continuum of care, facilitates a systems approach for the appropriate utilization of health care resources, and is accountable to meet targeted financial outcomes.

An additional aspect of the OM role was that of change agent. Personal traits and characteristics of leadership—being politically astute, a master of change, and a risk taker—were evaluated and considered in selecting individuals. A director for the department was selected by the clinical and financial leaders of the organization. Organization of the approach was clinical, reporting to the vice president of patient care services, with strong links to information systems, financial services, and managed care within the organization. The department also had a link to all clinical and ancillary services of the hospital and the medical department committees. Once the OMs were hired, an extensive orientation was conducted to develop, guide, and mentor the staff in their new roles. A mission and values statement for the department was developed in alignment with the hospital's mission and values.

IMPLEMENTATION OF OUTCOMES MANAGEMENT PROCESS

Once the outcomes management department was developed, a task force of clinical directors established its mission, process, and key definitions. This task force eventually became the outcomes management steering committee. The purpose of the steering committee was to provide guidance and direction to the OMs on proposed diagnoses, suggestions for multidisciplinary team members, and other outcomes projects, as well as insight to data analysis. The committee is composed of directors from the cardiovascular service line, patient and family services, business development, and managed care; the quality management coordinator; information systems clinical analyst; all outcomes managers; the chief financial officer; and the vice president of patient care services.

The definition for outcomes management at MHRMC is a multidisciplinary health care delivery process designed to integrate all clinical services, clinical and financial, while maintaining or increasing quality throughout the continuum of care. The multidisciplinary health care delivery process is intended to facilitate interdepartmental collaboration, which would positively affect patients. The service representatives bring problems in patient care to the multidisciplinary team, and together team members seek to improve patient care for a given population. Through this process the multidisciplinary team becomes interdisciplinary and integrated in the care for a given population. The team agrees on clinical and financial indicators that serve to measure patient care outcomes. Clinical and financial indicators monitor the effectiveness and efficiency of patient care. The clinical indicators measure quality of care. The purpose of outcomes management is to coordinate services, provide cost-effective and cost-efficient care, and increase or maintain quality of care. Financial indicators measure efficiency of care and consumption of resources used in patient care.

The goals of clinical outcomes are as follows:

- Prevent illness or hospitalization.
- Increase the preparedness for admission and/or discharge.
- Increase patient, family, physician, and payer satisfaction.
- Increase the coordination of services and providers throughout the patient and family's continuum of care.
- Decrease fragmentation and maximize continuity of care.
- Increase organizational efficiency and effectiveness.
- Decrease complications.
- Decrease mortality and morbidity.
- Increase the service base or market share through reported outcomes.
- Increase desired outcomes, thus increasing quality of care.

Clinical changes to the delivery of patient care are calculated in dollars. For example, if clinical changes are made to meet national standards in patient care, such as decreasing antibiotic administration from five days to two days, the dollars saved from delivering antibiotics for the three days is added and multiplied by the number of patients in the population. This amount becomes the targeted financial outcomes for a given patient population. The goals of financial outcomes are the following:

- Optimize use of resources.
- Decrease the inappropriate utilization of resources and procedures.
- Decrease cost per case.
- Decrease length of stay (LOS).
- Decrease readmissions.

Care "across the continuum of care" focuses on patient care in different disease phases. The Joint Commission on Accreditation of Healthcare Organizations (Joint Commission) defines continuum of care in the following phases: pre-entry, entry, within the organization, pre-exit, and exit. *Pre-entry* is the phase in which screening and prevention of illness takes place. Individuals do not have symptoms of disease or illness but seek strategies to promote health. The *entry phase* of disease is significant in that individuals experience symptoms and seek access to care. Care may be accessed in the emergency department, a physician's office, or an urgent care setting. *Within the organization* is the phase of hospitalization in an acute care setting. The *pre-exit phase* is the patient preparation activities necessary for impending discharge. It is the process of educating patients and families to prevent disease complications. Education elements include instructions on diet, activity level, and frequency of physician visits posthospitalization. The *exit phase* of illness is patient follow-up to monitor patient progress, understanding of instructions, and compliance with health care plans.[6]

The outcomes health care delivery model describes the dynamic process of patient care. The patient, population, or community is at the core or focus of the health care process. The key communicator is the health care team (HCT), which actively interacts with the patient and family during the five phases of the health care continuum. The results of those interactions help meet the clinical and financial outcomes. Critical in the evaluation of outcomes are the social, environmental, cultural, and spiritual dimensions of care that describe the uniqueness of a targeted population and affect the method in which information is exchanged.

The outcomes management process begins with submission of an application to the quality management steering committee to establish an organizational improvement team. Each proposed team is evaluated by defined criteria and must meet a specified number of points for approval. Teams are time limited to minimize the impact on hospital staff time away from patient care areas. Following approval, the outcomes management process is implemented in a series of steps, as follows:

1. Define the patient population and multidisciplinary team members (validate with physicians and payers).
2. Conduct a literature review (perform retrospective and concurrent chart review).

3. Compare practice with national, state, and local standards (benchmarking).
4. Develop clinical, charge, and patient and family education pathways (in collaboration with the multidisciplinary team).
5. Target clinical and financial outcomes to monitor quarterly (based on recommended changes to patient care).
6. Implement, evaluate, revise, validate, and reevaluate (predict changes to aggregate population).[7]

The first step is to decide on a patient population. This is defined from a list of high-risk diagnoses. High-risk diagnoses are defined as high-volume, high-LOS, or high-charge diagnoses. Also part of this step is the selection of team members. Typical team members for the multidisciplinary team include the following department representatives: nursing, physicians, utilization review or discharge planning, pharmacy, pastoral care, laboratory, dietary, materials management, rehabilitation, respiratory care, imaging, and cardiology (as appropriate). A minimum of three physicians representing three different group practices are invited as members of the team. Each team member is aware of the time commitment. There is a maximum of three meetings, each lasting one hour. Subgroup task force meetings serve to accomplish the specified tasks, and their findings are presented at regular team meetings.

The second step in the outcomes process is to conduct a literature review to identify national patient care standards. Published medical care guidelines are available from the Agency for Health Care Policy and Research (AHCPR)[8] and can be found in many medical libraries. Additional pertinent information may be found in a risk-adjusted diagnosis database currently available in most organizations. Chart review notes past practices and recent changes in practice and becomes the foundation for the development of the clinical pathway.

Comparisons of the organization's volume, charges, LOS, and outliers can be achieved with national, state, and local standards in the third step of the process. A baseline benchmark report affords insight into progress on the clinical and financial outcomes for subsequent quarterly reports.

The fourth step is the development of pathways. The purpose of clinical pathway development is to specify actions or interventions that will take place with the patient and family to achieve desired outcomes. The use of clinical pathways achieves collaborative communication between disciplines, appropriate bedside care, positive clinical outcomes, and decreased resource consumption. A clinical pathway is to be used as a guideline only in the plan of care. Physicians have the right to deviate from the plan when the condition of the patient warrants. Charge pathways are developed for several reasons. They are used to determine total charges incurred per day and charges for each cost center. They identify opportunities to decrease resource consumption and determine appropriate LOS. They validate frequency of test or medication orders to be added to the clinical pathway. Patient and family education pathways communicate the expectations of the patient care plan. Pre- and posthospitalization pathways match the plan of care (clinical pathway) and LOS.

The next step in the outcomes process is the identification of recommended outcomes to be reported quarterly. The clinical outcomes represent key variances to care that affect patient recovery and LOS. Clinical outcomes are unique to a patient population. They are listed as clinical variances on the clinical pathway, and the nurse caring for the patient evaluates patient care based on the variances. Financial outcomes to be reported are the targeted charge savings per patient population. Each change in current practice has a resultant financial dollar impact. Therefore, all charges are summed to reflect an aggregate dollar savings for the population, based on volume per year and per quarter.

The physicians on the multidisciplinary team present the clinical pathway, physician orders, and patient and family education pathways to the appropriate medical committee(s) for approval. The chair of the medical department presents the information to the medical executive and medical affairs committees and the board of trustees. The preprinted physician orders are presented by the pharmacist team member to the pharmacy and therapeutics committee for review. The OM presents the same information to the clinical practice, management practice, and administrative nursing councils of the hospital and to the quality management committee. This committee oversees improving organizational performance activities for the organization to meet Joint Commission standards. Finally, all printed materials are presented to the forms committee, which reviews them for compliance with institutional form guidelines.

Quarterly, the OMs receive their data from the established database used in collaboration with the hospital information system. The benchmarking report provides clinical and financial outcomes and demographic data on each diagnosis. Outcomes are compared to baseline. This is prepared and submitted to the quality management committee with the improving organizational performance (IOP) quarterly summary data analysis report. Clinical and financial outcomes are communicated to the respective nursing units and medical staff. If a clinical variance occurs in greater than 20 percent of the population, the multidisciplinary teams are reconvened for the reevaluation and revision process.

Reports are generated on clinical and financial outcomes and compliance to the clinical pathway. These reports include comparisons to baseline measures. By year's end, the outcomes management department will be able to report on actual resource reduction through a decision support system. Reviewing these measures has proven successful with the payers. They have a vested interest in reducing unnecessary resource consumption that does not affect the quality of care. Historically, with other pathways, this information has been appreciated by payers, and goals to enhance care have been identified. Reports are separately prepared so that they contain only a payer's own patients.

CASE EXAMPLE

Using the FOCUS PDCA[9] (Find, Organize, Clarify, Understand, Select; Plan, Do, Check, Act) model, which is integral to the quality management program, a coordinated outcomes management project began in 1996 to examine major orthopaedic procedures. The process began with a review of severity-adjusted data that identified total hip replacement, total knee replacement, and open reduction and internal fixation (ORIF) of the hip to be among the three highest volume and highest charge procedures performed at the institution. Following an extensive review of the literature, many clinical, quality, and financial issues arose, and the direction for an IOP team came into focus.

The outcomes management IOP team began by conducting a review of current issues and research, the results of which were then presented to a multidisciplinary team (Exhibit 18–2). Topics were reviewed and action plans developed. Clinical and quality topics included anticoagulation standards, morbidities, health promotion and disease prevention program development, preoperative class attendance issues, and the possibility of a comprehensive patient education handbook for total joint replacement. Satisfaction issues addressed patients, payers, and providers. Targeted for clinical improvement were pain control recommendations (based on AHCPR guidelines), supplemental educational materials, blood utilization (intraoperative autotransfusion versus autologous and donor directed), prosthesis selection criteria, and LOS. Exhibit 18–2 represents the FOCUS PDCA model for collaborative patient care management in patients undergoing major orthopaedic procedures. Changes in clinical issues affect resource consumption and define financial outcomes.

The IOP teams recommended three major changes to begin process improvement: development of a comprehensive clinical pathway across the continuum of care, educational materials for patients and family, and development of health promotion and disease prevention programs.

Clinical Pathways

Clinical pathways were drafted for the following procedures: total hip replacement, total knee replacement, and ORIF of the hip. They were drafted based on current and best practices and had accompanying preprinted postoperative physician's orders. Pathways for each procedure were developed to include an acute care phase (days one through three), followed seamlessly by the transitional

Exhibit 18–2 Collaborative Patient Care Management for Patients Undergoing Total Hip Replacement

---

Mission Hospital Orthopedic IOP

Find a Process

Use the outcomes management approach to improve the quality and efficiency of care given to patients undergoing total hip replacement throughout the continuum of care.

Organize a Team

- Orthopaedic surgeons
- Physiatrist
- Occupational therapist
- Physical therapist
- Clinical educator
- Materials management
- Operating room staff

- Laboratory services
- Discharge planner
- Home health
- Surgical staff nurse
- Rehabilitation unit personnel
- Epidemiology coordinator

- Blood bank manager
- Pastoral care
- Quality improvement coordinator
- Nutritional care services

Clarify Current Process

Data of 1995 baseline clinical outcomes were collected and analyzed:

- Charges greater than California average
- LOS less than California average
- Limited educational materials available
- Lack of health promotion and prevention programs
- Preoperative class attendance at 70 percent

Understand the Variation

- Data indicate a large variation in charges and LOS for hip population.
- Physician variation existed in patient management, based on medical record review (i.e., Coumadin regimen).
- Educational materials, preoperative class attendance, and health promotion/ disease prevention programs were not adequately developed to support optimal outcomes.

---

continues

Exhibit 18–2 continued

Select a Process for Improvement

Improve the management of the patient undergoing a total hip replacement across the continuum.

Plan

Total hip replacement across the continuum:

Pre-Entry   Entry   Within Organization   Pre-Exit   Exit

Do

- Clinical pathway
- Education
- Health promotion and disease prevention programs

Check

- Clinical outcomes
- Patient satisfaction
- Variation in patient management
- Class attendance
- Resource utilization
- Compliance with clinical pathway

Act

Evaluate results

Source: Courtesy of Mission Hospital Regional Medical Center, Mission Viejo, California.

or acute rehabilitation stay (days four through seven). Additionally, the operating room (OR) nurse on the team developed a pathway to be used by the OR staff.

Implementation of the pathways began with a housewide introduction through various nursing and medical committees. The clinical pathways (already used for various surgical procedures) were well received. A significant amount of time was saved. The pathways detail daily expected interventions and outcomes and serve uniquely as a nursing progress record allowing charting by exception. With this approach, a significant amount of nursing time is saved. Therefore, pathway compliance for all three surgical procedures is total hip, 100 percent; total knee, 96 percent; and ORIF, 79 percent. Use of the preprinted postoperative physician orders is at 70 percent.

The hospital opened a transitional care unit in 1996. In the team evaluation of open reduction and internal fixation of the hip, it was determined that a large number of patients were transferred from acute care to a skilled facility or the acute rehabilitation unit prior to home discharge. Physician orders and a clinical pathway were written to track clinical outcomes from this setting. The pathway was initiated in 1996. One of the problems encountered was that pathways were developed to be used by the bedside nurse in an exception by documentation approach. There was no accommodation for ancillary staff documentation. In the acute rehabilitation and transitional care settings, all ancillary staff and bedside nurses document on the same progress record. Therefore, this pathway was revised to allow for multidisciplinary charting by exception. The intent is to expand multidisciplinary documentation to all other pathways.

Patient and Family Education

Comprehensive educational booklets for joint replacement were developed as well as teaching plans and patient educational materials for Coumadin therapy and fall prevention. A preadmission, preoperative joint replacement class was established. This class is conducted by an OR nurse, discharge planner, physical therapist, and dietitian. Initially it was not mandatory, and attendance was at 70 percent. Therefore, the attendance problem was brought to the team, and approval from the orthopaedic executive committee was obtained to make the class mandatory. A form letter, signed by the chairman of orthopaedics, was developed to request a response from the surgeon with an explanation for why a patient did not attend the class. Since implementation of the mandatory class, attendance has only risen by 10 percent. Upon review, this was found to result from a percentage of patients who simply could not attend due to severe physical limitations. Therefore, a process was established to mail the handbook to the patient's home if the patient was physically unable to attend class. Otherwise, patient books are distributed to every patient during the class.

Coumadin dosing recommendations were developed and approved to allow "dosing per pharmacist" with a physician's order at the physician's discretion. This resulted in better timeliness of dosing and consistent early morning follow-up of values.

A fall-risk reduction patient education guideline was developed by the acute care physical therapist. The guideline is reviewed with the patient by the physical therapy department during therapy in the hospital. The guideline includes a checklist to assess the home environment prior to patient discharge.

Health Promotion and Disease Prevention

Prosthesis usage was examined to ensure the right prosthesis for the right patient based on patient activity level and manufacturer utilization and prosthesis grade. The original goal had been set to achieve 80 percent commitment to three prosthesis vendors. Prosthesis grade was evaluated prospectively over a six-month period using selection criteria approved by vendors and the orthopaedic department. Information regarding physical status, age, and activity was collected on 50 total knee and hip patients to determine if the appropriate grade of prosthesis was used (high, medium, or low demand). A 98 percent agreement with the criteria was found. Further negotiation also led to the establishment of a ceiling price for any hip and knee prosthesis used.

A fall-risk reduction program was organized as well as an osteoporosis exercise clinic. These initiatives were developed to address the needs in the community across the continuum. The physical therapist participating on the orthopaedic IOP team was interested in decreasing the number of elderly people who entered the hospital with a broken hip. Therefore, the therapist established a fall-risk reduction program in collaboration with the acute rehabilitation medical director. The program started in 1996 with the purpose of addressing balance, flexibility, and movement. Participants are instructed in exercises to improve general endurance and functional awareness. Balance training addresses dynamic challenges of stepping and reaching. One of the outcomes measures collected in this population is the Sharpened Romberg Test, which is a static standing balance test. The average baseline balance time prior to initiation of the program was 11 seconds. Postprogram average balance time was 32.3 seconds, indicating an increase in balance time by 21.3 seconds, 194 percent improvement from baseline. To date, 100 senior citizens have enrolled in the program. Functional outcomes are reported quarterly from the physical therapy department.

Clinical and Financial Outcomes

The clinical indicators collected on these patients are

- body temperature >101°
- pain >5 on pain scale
- activity intolerance (based on today's expected activity outcome)
- nausea/emesis

- inability to void after catheter removal
- urinary catheter in >48 hrs

None of the variances to this pathway affected greater than 20 percent of the population. Table 18–1 compares baseline (before clinical changes) and fiscal year 1998 average LOS results. Target cost savings estimated for all orthopaedic diagnoses are $200,456 per year. Average cost savings for fiscal year 1998, resulting from the clinical changes in practice, were $201,095, slightly higher than the targeted amount. In the future, compliance with pathway utilization will be reported from the transitional care unit and acute rehabilitation units.

OUTCOMES MANAGEMENT, 1998

The outcomes management department started with four OMs in September 1995. The initial diagnoses that were evaluated by the outcomes department were pneumonia, laparoscopic cholecystectomy, lumbar laminectomy, and hysterectomy. The first financial reports for all diagnoses were available in January 1996, and the first clinical reports were presented in July 1996. To date, there are 10 diagnoses and three additional outcomes projects reported on a quarterly basis. Fiscal year 1998 (ending June 30, 1998) reported total charge savings of $3.1 million and cost savings of $1.3 million. The actual cost savings exceeded the targeted cost savings of $1 million by 27 percent. Six out of 30 (20 percent) clinical indicators affected greater than or equal to 20 percent of the population. Two of these have been addressed in subsequent multidisciplinary team meetings, and new interventions have been recommended.

It is the intent of the outcomes department to not evaluate all diagnoses but to prioritize the original intent of the high-risk diagnoses only. The department has nearly completed this goal. Future direction is to expand evaluation of the popu-

---

Table 18–1 Average LOS Comparisons

	Baseline 1996	1998	Change
Total Hip	4.43	4.31	– 3%
Total Knee	4.38	4.0	– 9%
ORIF	4.15	4.16	–19%
TOTAL	4.65	4.16	–11%

Source: Courtesy of Mission Hospital Regional Medical Center, Mission Viejo, California.

lation to completely provide services across the continuum of care, such as that seen with the orthopaedic case example.

The outcomes management department is visible in the organization and has grown in the past three years. Some of the evolving changes to the scope of the department included the following:

- Since reported financial savings have consistently exceeded the target, the outcomes management department is held accountable for a yearly contribution of at least $500,000 in cost savings. Outcomes are itemized in the yearly proposed hospital financial fiscal year budget.
- An oncology OM was added to the department in 1996 at the request of the cancer committee, a hospital medical committee. The committee's goal was to track, trend, and report outcomes for the cancer program and provide consistency in patient care.
- A clinical research department was added to the outcomes management department in 1996 to support the efforts of providing the research tools needed to make research-based changes to clinical practice. Two outcomes managers are principal investigators in research studies. One of these studies is on pain perception. The interest in researching pain at MHRMC was fostered after determining that pain variances from clinical pathways occurred in greater than 20 percent of the population. Pain management was determined to be a hospitalwide problem, and efforts to collect additional information on pain were supported by the organization.
- Clinical pathways were initiated with contracted home health agencies. The form is sent to the agencies, and the home health nurse uses the pathway during the home visit and mails a copy of the form to the respective OM to track clinical outcomes. These outcomes are reported with other patient population outcomes to the quality management committee quarterly.
- The collection of patient functional outcomes started in July 1998. These outcomes are collected in the congestive heart failure (CHF) patient population. This allows functional outcomes on patients to be linked with the severity of illness score or acuity index measure (AIM) category. Patients admitted with CHF are asked to complete a health survey during hospitalization. This is considered the baseline functional score. Patients are called at home at 30, 60, and 90 days and one year postdischarge and given the same health survey. The scores are compared to baseline scores to determine functional outcomes. The intent is to collect additional functional outcomes in other patient populations in the future.

CONCLUSION

The outcomes management department at Mission Hospital Regional Medical Center was established to change the process of patient care delivery. This change was designed to decrease fragmentation of services, decrease resource utilization, increase satisfaction, and increase market share. The reengineering process leaders throughout the organization were clinical nurse specialists, now transitioned to OMs. The outcomes management process is a clinically driven process designed to positively affect the hospital financially. The outcomes process is a population-defined, outcomes measurement–based, team planning process. The communication of the outcomes process took place at team meetings, where different service disciplines were active participants in setting clinical and financial goals for specific patient populations. Hospital staff integrated the new approach in their respective departments and incorporated it as part of their care delivery. The OMs consult as needed to assist staff in determining outcomes and outcomes collection methods. From the initial four diagnoses evaluated in the outcomes management process, the scope has expanded to include 10 completed diagnoses. The department continues to report clinical and financial outcomes quarterly and, through the three years, has maintained a positive impact financially for the organization. The steps taken to change care delivery were deliberate, planned, and successful for the organization. As health care facilities struggle with changes in care to deliver cost-effective care, outcomes management is a positive alternative without forced downsizing.

REFERENCES

1. Bennefield RL. *Health Insurance Coverage, 1996.* Washington D.C.: U.S. Dept. of Commerce, Economics and Statistics Administration, Census Bureau; 1996.
2. Bureau of Labor Statistics: *Civilian Labor Forces;* 1995. Table 3.
3. California Health Facilities Commission. *Aggregate Hospital Discharge Data for California.* Sacramento, CA: State of California; 1996.
4. Mission Hospital Regional Medical Center. *Market Share Patient Base.* Mission Viejo, CA: Mission Hospital Regional Medical Center; 1995.
5. Gibson SJ, Martin SM, Johnson MB, Blue R, Miller DS. CNS directed case management. *J Nurs Adm.* 1994; 24:45–51.
6. Joint Commission on Accreditation of Healthcare Organizations. *1996 Comprehensive Accreditation Manual for Hospitals.* Oakbrook Terrace, IL: Joint Commission; 1996:225–238.
7. Windle PE, Houston S. Comit—Improving patient outcomes. *Nurs Management.* 1995; 26(6):64AA–64HH.
8. Agency for Health Care Policy and Research. *Clinical Practice Guidelines.* Silver Spring, MD: AHCPR Publication Clearinghouse; 1994.
9. Swanson RC. *The Quality Improvement Handbook.* Del Ray Beach, FL: St. Lucia Press; 1995.

CHAPTER 19

Home Health Care Documentation: Process Reengineering through Information Systems

Rella Adams, PhD, RN, CNAA
Maia Baker, MSN, RN
Lisa Freed, MSHA, RN
Karen Vest, BSN, RN

Over the years, the health care environment has undergone dramatic changes, and the rate at which these changes have occurred is unprecedented. There is no such thing as business as usual. To survive, organizations are finding new and innovative ways to provide lower cost, higher quality services to their customers. Reengineering has become a way of life. According to Hammer, after reengineering takes place within an organization, the organization will naturally become process centered.[1] This chapter describes the reengineering and process-centered strategies for patient care documentation for Valley Baptist Medical Center's Home Health Agency (VBMC Home Health).

Valley Baptist Medical Center (VBMC) is a 588-bed tertiary care, nonprofit hospital located in Harlingen, Texas. It offers a broad spectrum of services from acute care to skilled care to community health. VBMC is rapidly growing into a full-service integrated delivery system encompassing the full continuum of care, including rural health clinics, home health and hospice agencies, a durable medical equipment company, and various outpatient specialty clinics. Thus, one of VBMC's primary process-centered strategies was to develop a seamless continuum of care for its customer base.

Like many organizations, VBMC has reengineered and restructured the way it delivers care in order to meet the changing health care environment. The advent of the computer age and advances in information technology (IT) have played an increasingly important role in meeting the demands and pressures of the health care environment. Information is the key to success and the infrastructure from which an organization must operate. Flow of information is vital to an integrated health care delivery system and the continuum of care.

In response to this challenge of survival, VBMC's Strategic Healthcare Information Resource Initiative (SHIRI)[2] was born. This strategic information management plan was designed to ensure timely data collection and retrieval, ease of use, improved accessibility, and ultimately an integrated patient medical record across the continuum. The goal is to have all patient information, clinical and financial, easily accessible whenever and wherever it is needed. If the goal is met, efficiency and productivity are improved, patient care is improved, and customer satisfaction, external and internal, is improved as well.

As part of the initiative to entirely overhaul its methods and tools for total information management and meet the desired goals, VBMC had to consider the framework upon which to realize its new strategies. This framework addressed multiple information technologies on various, and often disparate, operating platforms, while allowing its system components to perform as a seamless system for all users. Many new technologies have evolved, thus forming the framework for operationalizing VBMC's IT strategic plan, SHIRI. One of the components of VBMC's Project SHIRI outlined in this case study is the implementation of a computerized documentation system for VBMC's Home Health.

THE HOME HEALTH ENVIRONMENT

Home care services are rapidly moving from the periphery to the center of health care delivery. This means that health care delivery has come full circle, moving closer to the home as the primary site of care and the family as the primary care providers as it was 100 years ago. The major difference with the current model is the type of treatments and medical technology now used in the home environment. Central lines, ventilators, intravenous antibiotics requiring dosage titration, and dobutamine therapy are examples of home care treatments that have, until recently, been used only in controlled hospital environments. The key to providing this level of intervention—and doing so in a safe, efficient, cost-effective manner—is access to information for the home care nurse at the point of care. This includes patient information such as lab results as well as resource information such as policies, procedures, and patient teaching tools. The home care nurse does not have a coworker down the hall to provide help when a problem arises.

Information is the key to delivering quality care. Access to information is essential, and access to information at the point of care is the ideal. Home care presents several unique issues for a point-of-care system. Portability of the hardware is critical. Home care nurses often need to carry supplies and equipment into the home. Hardware, therefore, needs to be compact and physically manageable. It must be able to withstand a variety of environmental conditions, including extreme temperatures and being constantly moved, turned off, and restarted. It also needs to be powerful enough to sustain all the applications, including the interfaces from the hospital or a physician's office, for example. In addition, the screen needs to be large enough so that the user does not have to scroll constantly to obtain or input information, and it must be readable in less than ideal lighting conditions. Remote access in home care means multiple providers in multiple environments. Every home presents an uncontrolled environment, especially as compared to the hospital setting. Security issues and lack of backup systems such as phone lines and even electricity are hallmarks of home care. Portability increases the risk of the terminal being lost or stolen, which in turn leads to issues on security of information. The balance between security of information and user-friendly access is fragile. Information needs to be adequately protected in case of loss or theft, yet the nurse cannot spend unreasonable lengths of time going through layers of security checks at each home. Secure access is required, but access must not be so cumbersome that paper becomes more efficient or functional to the nurse. Nurses tend to be efficiency experts by nature and will take the path of least resistance to get the job done.

HOME HEALTH INFORMATION SYSTEM REQUIREMENTS

The primary requirement of home care software is to reduce and streamline the inordinate amount of documentation required of the home care nurse. Initial assessments—including patient consents, home safety assessments, time sheets, supply sheets, visit notes, the plan of care (the 485 form), and financial authorization—must all be complete, correct, and consistent. This not only is extremely time consuming for the nurse but also requires several manual audits. The home care information system needs to provide automated checks and balances to decrease the amount of auditing required. For example, a common problem occurs when patient acuity requires a change in visit frequency from the initial plan of care that reflects physician orders. The nurse can easily overlook revising the plan of care to reflect the change in frequency. This can result in delays in processing the visit, including billing, as the orders and visit notes do not match. The ideal software system should not allow any documentation for a visit that does not match the frequency of visits on the plan of care. Along with direct patient care documentation requirements, the system must also support operational and management processes. If the home care nurse is able to download visit information via modem from home, traveling to the home care office to drop off paperwork can be avoided, thus reducing costs. An automated scheduling system is also critical in home care where matching available nurses to competency to geographic location of the patient can be challenging at best.

Although the concept of an automated information system is ideal, reality presents a never-ending abundance of challenges. The major ongoing challenge is change in mind-set at the staff nurse level. The project team knew that the nurses needed to be involved in design of the system, but most of the nurses had limited, if any, computer experience. The team realized that the nurses would experience fear of the unknown as well as a reluctance to break away from the security of their strong and lifelong bond with pen and paper. Thus, a learning environment related to the project needed to be conceived and nurtured. Hammer describes the learning process as composed of two subprocesses, the first being exploration.[1] Hammer contends that an organization needs information that comes from out of the box if that organization is to realize the limitations of the box. Hammer's second learning subprocess is interpretation, in which the information is analyzed and decisions can be made to redesign processes.[1]

To maximize the potential for successful transition, a home care nurse was chosen as the project coordinator. Exploration and interpretation of all home care documentation and processes was her first task. Her firsthand experience and the nurses' ability to identify with her made her the perfect choice for "process owner" or "process leader" of this reengineering effort. The following is her account of the VBMC Home Health reengineering experience.

BACKGROUND: VBMC HOME HEALTH

VBMC Home Health is a hospital-based home health agency that serves a three-county area covering approximately a 100-mile radius of mostly rural south Texas. The agency serves all ages of clientele and provides all services, including neonatal care, home infusion therapy, and home ventilator cases. VBMC Home Health employs 30 full-time nurses, five full-time rehabilitation therapists, five full-time home health aides, and a relief staff of seven nurses. In fiscal year 1997, the agency provided 37,234 home health visits for an average of 3,100 visits per month. From an operations management perspective, VBMC Home Health is a service operation whose goal is to deliver a wide range of home health services to a large and varied customer base. Home health care involves high customer interaction and is a highly customized product in which the capability for flexibility within the system is key. Challenges for the agency include management of volume demand, scheduling, and managing growth. Other challenges for VBMC Home Health are hiring, training, and retention of staff; compliance issues; reporting to various regulatory agencies as mandated by law; and continuous performance improvement.

The automated documentation system for home health at VBMC is a part of the master plan for reengineering information management to support clinical functions at the medical center. Above and beyond the information management needs for the medical center, the changing environment in which home health agencies function dictates the need for changes in the way agencies do business if they are to survive. For example, one of the latest challenges to home health agencies that accept Medicare payment is the new Conditions of Participation (COPs) that mandate the use of the Outcome and Assessment Information Set (OASIS).[3] OASIS is a 79-item data set that must be collected at specified points during a patient's tenure with a home health agency. The data collected from the OASIS tool will be used by the Health Care Financing Administration (HCFA) to determine further restructuring of the reimbursement system to home health agencies across the country. The documentation requirements have become increasingly challenging for the agency from a cost perspective in times of decreasing reimbursement, as well as from a quality perspective in terms of remaining in compliance with various and increasing regulatory requirements. Finally, from a clinical perspective, the nurse at the bedside is doubly challenged by ever-changing documentation requirements along with an increasingly acute patient caseload.

Hammer contends that the needs of a changing business environment necessitate a process-centering focus for organizations to survive in the new age of business.[1] Process centering in the post-reengineering era is well established in the manufacturing sector. The service sector has yet to fully realize the potential of process centering as a powerful strategy for realigning the way business is done in the health care industry, but this trend is slowing changing. At VBMC Home Health, the process-centering efforts are evolving as a natural progression from the implementation of the automated documentation system. The software exists on a hand-held device that fits into a lab coat pocket. The goal is for the staff to "chart" at the point of care using a database that contains all of the organization's current assessment tools, teaching flowsheets, and the OASIS data set. Staff will also be able to receive information on new or added patients without a trip to the office. The automated documentation system communicates with the database via a modem, and staff can call up new or additional electronic records as needed from the field. At the end of the day, the staff will connect the hand-held device to their home phone line, and their daily documentation will be downloaded from home via a modem. Achieving a successful implementation and making clinical documentation at the point of care a reality is a complex task. A solid foundation for the core development process is key. VBMC Home Health adopted Hammer's concept[1] for creating a process-centered organization in order to operationalize its goals and sustain its vision.

PROCESS CENTERING AT VBMC HOME HEALTH

The concept of process centering as presented by Hammer[1] is a tool for businesses to diagnose those tasks they must perform to create value for the customer. Hammer also contends that before process centering can occur, a business must recognize and define its strategic service vision.[1] The strategic service vision of an organization shapes and defines the services to be delivered and is related directly to the mission statement of the organization that defines the overall goals of the organization.[4]

The mission statement of VBMC describes a multipurpose organization dedicated to providing quality health care and organized to promote health, religious, charitable, scientific, literary, and educational programs. At VBMC Home Health, defining the strategic service vision comes from the agency philosophy that includes a commitment to continually seek opportunities for improvement in both organizational and clinical functions that will maintain the highest level of quality service at the most efficient cost. Promoting individual and process improvement to continuously improve the quality and value of services provided to patients and the community is an important component directly related to the clinical informatics project.

To apply the concept of a strategic service vision, VBMC Home Health needed to define its internal and external customers and determine what value means to them and if they perceive the agency's product as valuable. External customers of VBMC Home Health consist of the patients it serves and outside referral sources such as physician offices, hospitals, outside agencies, and third-party payers. The product the agency wants to supply for its external customers is quality home health care, an easy and hassle-free referral process, and an accurate and reliable precertification process. Internal customers include the staff and support departments such as billing, medical records, and the home infusion pharmacy. The product the agency wants to supply to internal customers is a work environment that is user-friendly and enhances their ability to perform at their very best.

In the case of clinical staff, we would venture to say that the majority went into health care because of the challenges and rewards of patient care, not to collect data for HCFA. External and internal agency customers value competency, safety, security, responsiveness, accuracy, speed, flexibility, and cost-effectiveness. Agency customers will rank certain elements of the value equation over others based on their frame of reference. Once the agency has identified a target market, the service concept, and the elements of value that are important to customers, it can then refine and position its product to create value that will exceed customers' expectations. Process centering is a method to enhance value for our customers.

THE REENGINEERING EXPERIENCE

This case study focuses on the reengineering process for patient documentation that will enhance the value for the agency's primary internal customer, its staff. It is widely known in service operations that the most valuable and expensive capital investment is the human resource. As recruitment and retention of professionals are costly and time consuming, morale of staff is crucial. Home health is labor intensive with a high degree of customer involvement, and staff are being asked to handle more and more paper. The agency wants to improve the effectiveness and efficiency of staff at all levels so that they may excel at those tasks where the "magic moment" occurs—with the customer at the bedside, the taking of a referral, or the precertification process for insurance or Medicaid reimbursement. Some of the benefits expected from the new system are lowering costs, improving the productivity of staff, giving staff immediate access to the decision-making information they need, and the capability to pull out performance improvement data with the ease of running a report. The design of the hand-held device itself with its compact shape, miniaturized features, and audio alerts has had an unexpected effect of boosting staff morale. Comments about the device, such as its being "neat" or "cool," welcomed the agency to the cutting-edge of clinical documentation.

At the inception of the automated documentation project, key players were identified from both clinical and information services support staff. A project team was formed that included a project coordinator and a medical informatics specialist. The implementation team was charged with preparation of the software database, training of staff, and oversight of multiple other processes to ensure the agency met its "go-live" target date. The team also worked with an account manager and a nurse from the vendor supplying the software program.

The software chosen for the automated documentation system is flexible. The ability to customize the software was a primary consideration. Customization allows the agency to set up the database to meet documentation needs rather than asking the staff to conform to a hard-coded system. This also provided the opportunity for the staff to contribute to the setup of the screens. The flexibility of the software also allows the agency to respond rapidly to the regulatory changes affecting documentation requirements, which occurs frequently in home care, and thus to avoid possible delays while waiting for a vendor to change a hard-coded system.

The first few months of the implementation involved going over every form and documentation requirement presently in use and configuring the software accordingly. The next phase consisted of upgrading and adding to all the hardware in the home health office as well as testing the software on the hand-held devices. A careful review of the agency's current processes in preparation for the process changes that will be necessitated by the implementation of the automated documentation system was also completed. The third phase was the go-live phase. Go-live involves training staff to use the software and hardware. Although many of the nurses had never used a computer before, the initial response to the hand-held device was very positive. The staff document using a stylet and tap on a series of knowledge branches. The branches lead staff through a selection of item choices that allow them to create a note, generate an order, develop a care plan, or process any other required data.

The fourth and final phase entailed the upgrading of the current billing software and automation of the current manual scheduling process. The new billing and scheduling system was chosen for its ability to interface with the agency's clinical documentation system. Phase 4 also includes the integration of an interface with the main hospital's clinical documentation system, which will provide automated access to referral and clinical information on those patients coming to the agency from the medical center. The agency also will be adding extensive use of a report writing program that will allow the agency to customize and then extract performance improvement, auditing, and payroll information from the database as needed.

Four Steps to Process Centering

Step 1: Name the Process

Hammer states that there are four steps to process centering, the first of which is naming the process.[1] VBMC Home Health named its process the "clinical documentation process." The clinical documentation process for VBMC Home Health begins when a request for services is received (referral) and ends with the generation of a bill. The current process is represented in Figure 19–1. There are many subprocesses involved, including medical records, data entry, billing, supply inventory management, clinical audit, and, most important, collection of clinical data at the bedside by the nurse. These subprocesses all receive information from or add information to the clinical documentation process. This case study focuses on the processing of the patient care plan (485 forms) and the patient visit note. The timely and accurate processing of the 485 forms and visit notes is crucial to the agency because they contain the required physician's orders and clinical data that are used for reimbursement purposes. The 485 forms and clinical note also demonstrate agency compliance with various regulatory requirements and are used by various accrediting organizations as a measure of the agency's overall performance and outcomes measures.

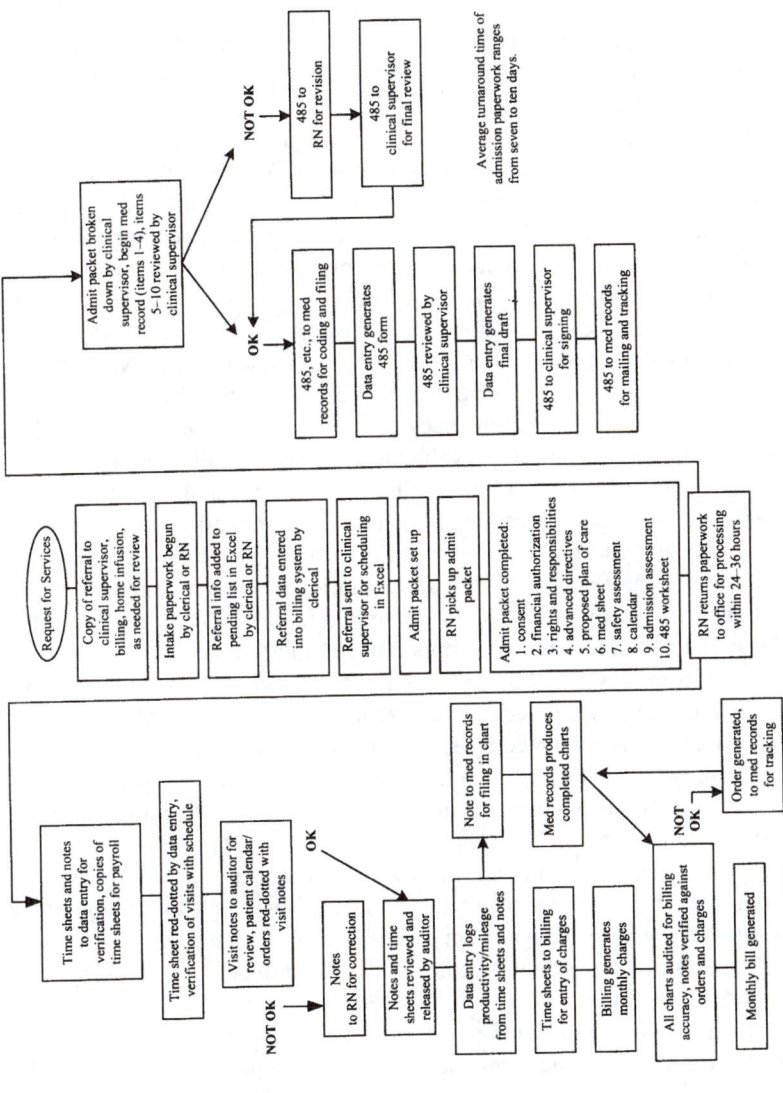

Figure 19–1 Clinical Documentation Process Preautomation

Step 2: Process Awareness

Mapping the current clinical documentation process in the form of a flowchart was essential to get an overview of all the steps involved in processing the 485 form and the visit note. During implementation planning, the agency's current process flowchart was analyzed to identify areas of non–value-added but necessary steps. Hammer describes non–value-added but necessary steps as those that do not contribute to the end product directly but are necessary for the successful processing of documentation.[1] Examples of non–value-added but necessary steps in the agency's current process included staff coming into the office to pick up or drop off clinical documents, manual coding of ICD-9 diagnostic codes by medical records, and data entry of the 485 forms. Several areas of waste work were also identified within the current process. Waste work is defined by Hammer as that which contributes nothing to the final product and in fact decreases one's ability to deliver quality service.[1] Inspection time, transportation time, and waiting time are categories of waste work. Examples of inspection time waste work inherent to the agency's current process were the review of the 485 by the clinical supervisor, the front-end audit process, and the back-end billing audit. Transportation time waste was evidenced by the staff traveling to and from the office to pick up and drop off paperwork. An example of waiting time waste was the 24- to 36-hour period allowed for current processing of admission paperwork.

The implementation team was well aware of the importance of identifying current processes and areas of non–value-added but necessary steps and waste work as it proceeded. As the success of the implementation project required a multidisciplinary team effort, it was imperative to include medical records, billing, home infusion, inventory management, rehab services, clerical, data entry, nursing, and information services in the process awareness phase. The concept of process awareness, as presented by Hammer,[1] was new to many people on the interdisciplinary team. The implementation team enlarged the flowchart and projected it on an overhead screen, analyzing it step-by-step to allow everyone involved to speak to his or her "step" in the process. Next, the team took the current process apart, mapping out the new clinical documentation process and integrating the automated documentation system. This was a turning point for many of the staff who had never seen a graphic representation of all the things that are done to process a clinical note. The revised documentation process is represented in Figure 19–2.

With the initial implementation of the automated system, most of the process changes were realized on the front end with the initial processing of the HCFA 485. Medical records no longer has to code because the ICD-9 codes are assigned automatically by the database software. Data entry no longer generates a 485 form. It is created by a report-writing program that interfaces with the

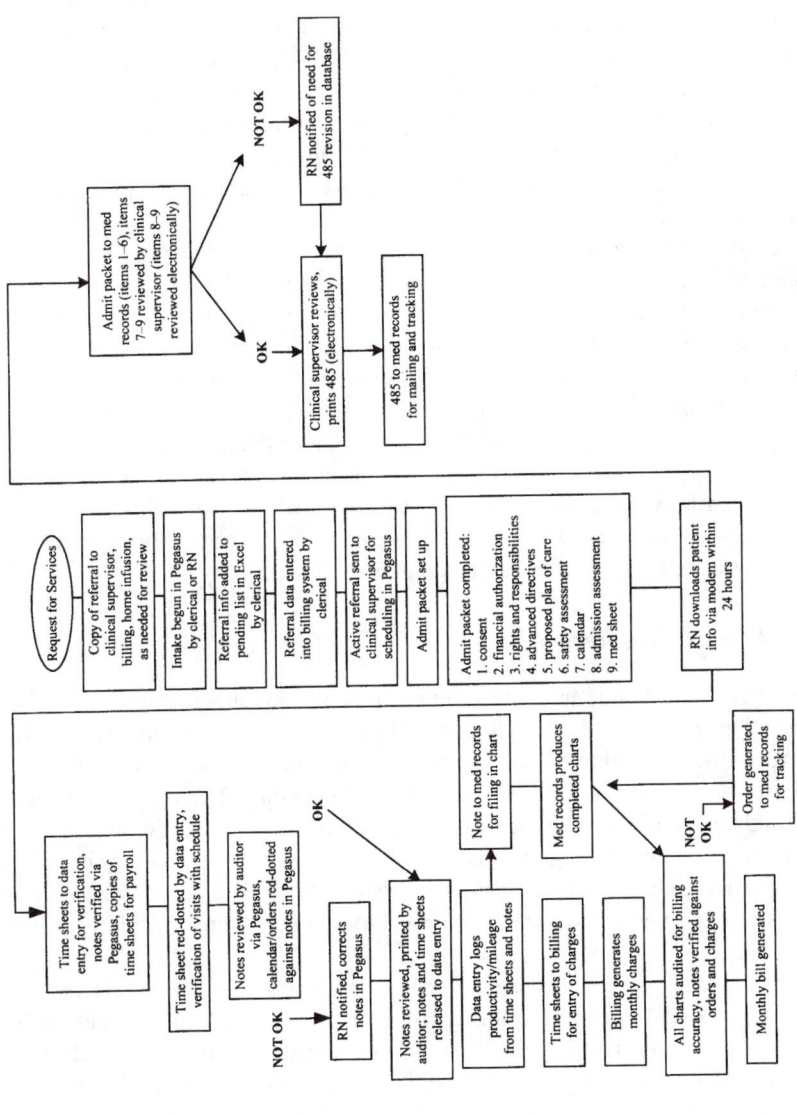

Figure 19–2 Clinical Documentation Process with Automation of Clinical Documentation Only

database to collect the required information. The agency thus will eliminate many of the pieces of paper that are required to be filled out, passed around, and filed by staff.

An example of elimination of actual paper is seen with the agency's intake/referral form, which will now be entered directly into the database as the referral information is received. Rather than copying the intake form to the receiving nursing team, it is now possible to view the information electronically. The elimination of physical paper is repeated throughout the process flow because patient documentation is no longer physically passed through the office but rather is viewed and reviewed electronically to the point where a hard copy is provided for signatures.

An example of combining and eliminating steps is seen with the processing of the admission documentation, in which the physical paper—including consents, financial authorization, the proposed plan of care, and all other forms requiring patient signature—can be turned in directly to medical records for filing. The software system will have signature recognition in the near future, and the intent is to allow the patients or responsible parties to sign their consents with the stylet directly onto the hand-held screen. This will eliminate the need for signing multiple documents. The clinical documentation needs to be reviewed for completeness and can be viewed electronically and corrected electronically if needed. Automation will allow the agency to review and print electronically, eliminating four process steps currently being handled by three data entry staff.

Step 3: Process Measurement

Hammer claims that if an organization is to be serious about its processes, the organization must know how well it is performing.[1] The implementation of the automated documentation system prompted the agency to look at the big picture in relation to its current clinical information processing. The agency initiated front- and back-end audits to measure the accuracy and quality of clinical documentation, and it now has a good measure of the timeliness and accuracy of those processes. The ultimate goal is a paperless system. Above and beyond a paperless system, current process measurements reveal room for refinement within current operations.

An example of performance improvement via process refinement exists in the front- and back-end audit systems. Because the clinical document is a legal document from which services are billed as well as evidence of compliance with state and federal law, front- and back-end audits are accepted as standard operating procedure for most home health agencies. Note that the audit processes represented in Figures 19–1 and 19–2 are minimally reduced by the automation of documentation. Volumes of data reflecting areas for revision are collected via these audits. Clinical documents deficient in critical areas are held until corrections can be made, thus delaying the billing process. A process-centered approach to the necessary but non–value-added audit entails extensive training of staff to do it right the first time and transforms the accepted practice of correcting deficiencies to one of professional development by proactive performance. Doing it right the first time invalidates the need for the "review, generate variance report, revise, and clear" cycle that had become a full-time job for the audit nurse. The effectiveness of the agency's process-centering efforts is reflected in a decrease in the number of variances reported as well as a decrease in the number of claims held. Thus, a measurable decrease in the overall length of the billing cycle is realized.

Step 4: Process Management/Process Owners

Process management, according to Hammer, is the fourth step an organization must take if continuous process and performance improvement is to be realized.[1] Process management calls for the constant attending to an organization's processes. An organization must ensure that it is performing up to its potential and must continue to look for opportunities to make itself better. The concept of process management necessitates the existence of a process manager to ensure the success of the project. Hammer states that all those performing a process have some ownership of that process but that a "process owner" assumes overall responsibility for the design, coaching, and advocacy of the process-centering movement.

For VBMC Home Health, the clinical documentation process owner is the project coordinator who has experienced the fundamental inefficiencies and duplication of effort inherent to the current processes. From the outset of the automated documentation project, the project coordinator worked continuously with the information services department and the vendor, identifying areas that could be automated, deleted, or combined. Taking a "what if" attitude, the process owner, with the help of the implementation team, identified any and all areas where paper and/or steps could be eliminated via the use of interfaces, linking, combining forms, and deleting duplicate items. Each step in Figure 19–1 was explored to verify if it was necessary, waste work, or value adding. Areas that could be automated or linked to other databases were then identified, leading to the design of the new process to grow beyond the clinical note and 485 form processing. The desire to eliminate as many non–value-added processes as possible eventually led to the decision to install new billing and scheduling software that would interface with the clinical documentation system. This decision demonstrates that the process-centering focus had expanded beyond the home health department. The process owner's ongoing responsibility will be to continually monitor and evaluate how the addition of each new automation piece affects the overall process performance.

Thinking Outside of the Box

The focus of this case study has been on the process changes that have occurred with the implementation of the automated documentation system. "Thinking outside the box" is a popular phrase and the topic of many seminars accompanying the reengineering trend since the late 1980s. At VBMC Home Health, documentation methods are radically changing, but it is recognized that health care workers are notoriously attached to their paper. Process centering also changes the way the agency does business and the roles of the people involved in the business. Teaching staff the new documentation process requires thinking outside the box, such as using a computer at the bedside to document and a modem to download paperwork. In addition to the process change of collecting patient information for the clinical document, the most radical role changes will be seen in the home health office. The data entry role will be all but eliminated, since clinical staff will now be creating the 485 form directly in the database from the patient information collected at the bedside. Clinical supervisors who now spend approximately 50 percent of their time scheduling will see time spent in that role dramatically reduced by the addition of the scheduling program. Plans have been made to transition the soon-to-be-idle data entry clerk into the role of scheduler, thus transitioning the clinical supervisors from their data entry role to a management role—a more appropriate and cost-effective use of their time. One clinical supervisor has expressed concern that she will not have anything to do once the new system is in place! Thinking outside the box, the clinical supervisor will now have time to devote to clinical functions such as field visits with staff, teaching, follow-up calls to patients, and handling clinical issues.

Medical records is another area whose role will dramatically change. Medical records staff currently spend most of their time and space filing notes and creating the chart. At this time, a decision has been made to continue to print a hard copy of each chart. Thinking outside the box would allow medical records to forgo daily printing of the clinical document for filing, but, as mentioned above, health care workers have a love-hate relationship with paper. We complain about paperwork all the time but cannot imagine not having that paper chart in front of us. The hope is that, in time, the perceived need to print the chart will fade, and the agency will keep only hard copy forms that are from outside the system in the chart (i.e., orders from referring agencies, lab results from outside sources, etc.).

Medical records staff's role will be tracking of outstanding orders and auditing electronically for completeness. The filing and space required to store charts will be significantly reduced, which will be another cost-saving measure.

Thinking outside the box led to creating the process shown in Figure 19–3. Meeting the agency's goal of creating an interface for the billing, scheduling, and clinical documentation systems, along with the hospital clinical information system, will allow the agency to transform a 30-step clinical documentation process into a 20-step process. The process flow demonstrated in Figure 19–3 shows the reduction of process steps and a change toward each of these steps occurring primarily at the front end. The back-end audit still exists largely unchanged. The agency understands the need to be vigilant with staff in teaching them to do it right the first time. But it is also recognized that the human element can never be eliminated in a service operation. Automating the documentation process allows the agency to devote more time and energy to serving its customers: patients, referral sources, third-party payers, and staff. The automated clinical documentation system for VBMC Home Health allows staff to spend more time on value-added activities such as customer service follow-up calls and allows the agency to decrease operating costs, improve clinical data collection and reporting, streamline necessary but non–value-added audit functions for corporate compliance, and free staff from the voluminous paper that has always been the hallmark of health care. The goal of process centering is to streamline operations, eliminate inefficiencies and duplication, and allow a company to create maximum value for its customers. The clinical documentation system has been the driving force for process centering within the agency.

CONCLUSION

The reengineering of the clinical nursing documentation system at VBMC Home Health is ongoing. Through a careful and thorough assessment and evaluation of previous processes and ongoing monitoring of the changing processes, the project has been enlightening and is continually evolving. The implementation of the home health computerized documentation system is another step toward operationalizing the master strategic information management plan, SHIRI. Although the reengineering effort described involved only the home health agency, the impact is felt throughout the system and represents another link in the strategic plan for a seamless flow of information across the continuum of the integrated health care system.

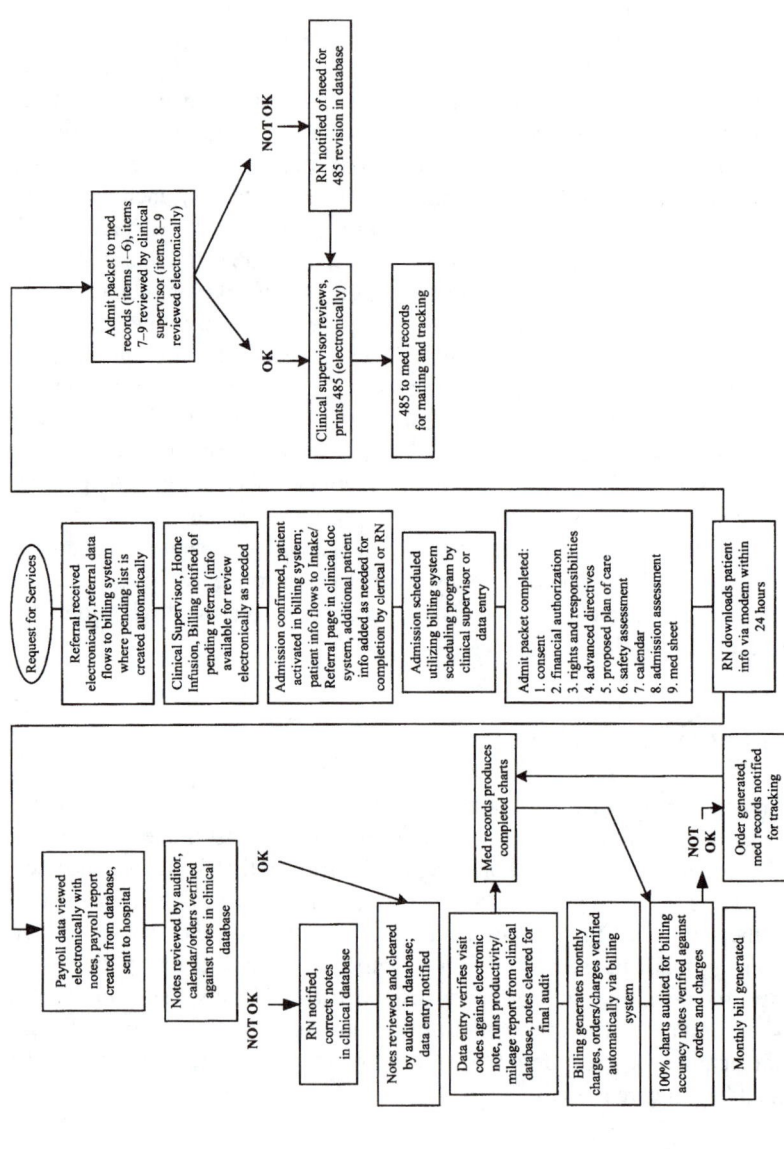

Figure 19–3 Clinical Documentation Process with Complete Automation and Integration of Clinical, Billing, and Scheduling

REFERENCES

1. Hammer M. *Beyond Reengineering: How the Process-Centered Organization Is Changing Our Work and Our Lives.* New York: Harper Business; 1996.
2. Adams R, Gray LE, Six E, Watkins TH. Reengineering information management to support clinical function. In: Blancett SS, Flarey DL, eds. *Reengineering Nursing and Health Care: The Handbook for Organizational Change.* Gaithersburg, MD: Aspen Publishers, Inc.; 1995:302–319.
3. Shaunessy PW, Crisler KS. *Outcome Based Quality Improvement.* Denver, CO: Colorado Center for Health Policy and Services Research; August 1995.
4. Heskett JL. *Managing in the Service Economy.* Cambridge, MA: Harvard Business School Press; 1986.

CHAPTER 20

Developing and Maintaining a Team-Based Organization as Processes Evolve

Jo Manion, MA, RN, CNAA, FAAN
Phyllis M. Watson, PhD, MEd, RN

Never has the health care environment changed at such a rapid pace. A key to dealing effectively with change is the development of resiliency, flexibility, and adaptability within health care organizations. The dangers of entering a new millennium with an organizational structure that is a relic of the past are becoming increasingly obvious. In 1987, during the strategic planning process at Lakeland Regional Medical Center (LRMC) it became clear that traditional productivity improvements and downsizing strategies were only short-lived solutions to the key issues the organization was facing. The executive team agreed to take a proactive stance. Examining all processes and rethinking the way patient care and services are delivered were the first steps. In effect, a complete restructuring, or reengineering, of the organization was planned.

This chapter explores one aspect of the reengineering work accomplished by LRMC: the development of a multidisciplinary team-based structure. The original pilot unit established a team-based structure to ensure continuity and accountability. However, the needs of the teams were not well understood, and teams were not proactively developed after they were established. Like all aspects of Lakeland's evolution, teams were on a journey. Thus began the evolution to a team-based structure.

HISTORY

The process began in January 1988 when LRMC and a major national consulting firm initiated jointly funded diagnostic analyses of how LRMC provided pa-

Source: Adapted from J. Manion and P. Watson, Developing Team-Based Patient Care through Reengineering in *Reengineering Nursing and Health Care: The Handbook for Organizational Transformation,* S. Smith Blancett and D. Flarey, eds. pp. 241–260, © 1995, Aspen Publishers, Inc.

tient care. The 1988 results of these data-based analyses included several startling findings[1]:

- Only 16 percent of the hospital's structure was spent delivering medical, technical, or clinical care.
- Documenting, scheduling, and coordinating were the primary operating functions of the hospital.
- "Ready-for-action" (structural idle time, waiting for something to happen) was the largest single consumer of hospital resources.
- As much time was spent in coordinating and scheduling activities and procedures as was spent in providing medical, technical, and clinical services.

Conclusions based on these analyses were that the true drivers of performance and cost included the organization's operating structure and approach, management processes, and deployment strategies.[2] Significant structural redesign was undertaken to position the organization for the future. In April 1989, the patient-focused model was initiated as a pilot project.

Intense scrutiny of all processes contributing to the delivery of patient care resulted in several new operating imperatives[2]:

- The patient care unit would be "decompartmentalized" to ensure that staff resources were better utilized and patient focused.
- Jobs on the unit would be structured for the greatest possible continuity of patient care, creating the need for employees to be cross trained to perform work outside their usual areas of functioning.
- Restructured jobs would increase the quality of work life and job satisfaction for health care workers and support staff.
- Patient outcomes (quality of care and satisfaction with care) would be measured at the staff level, and teams would be held accountable for these outcomes.
- The unit's operating approach would stress responsiveness to enhance quality of care for patients and support for physicians.
- The hospital would be separated into five operating centers, each managed as a unique entity with a patient-driven operations approach that emphasized accountability for the quality and cost of services provided.

The success of this pilot unit has been reported in many forums. Since that time, reengineering of the organization has continued at a steady and incremental pace. The senior and middle management at LRMC now recognizes that reengineering is a journey with no end, a continuous performance improvement process to be embedded in the organizational culture rather than a one-time event.

As the journey toward continual improvement through reengineering has progressed, the process has been guided by four principles:

1. Resources must be patient focused and fully utilized.
2. All operations must be responsive to patient and physician needs.
3. Individuals at all levels must be accountable and satisfied.
4. Patients must readily perceive value in their care.

These principles gradually evolved and are now used daily in problem solving and in planning solutions to the challenges faced in redefining what LRMC does, how it does it, and how well it does it.

Historically, the use of patient care teams in health care was significantly different from this current evolutionary step. Many people hear *teams* and think the concept of patient care teams is a reversion to a form of "team nursing," when in fact it is truly the next step in the evolution from primary nursing. The team, rather than an individual nurse, is fully accountable for the care of patients for whom the team has accepted responsibility. The team assesses needs and plans, implements, and evaluates the patient's care. This model is based on the recognition that the work of patient care is dependent on the contributions of more than one individual from one discipline. The teams are responsible for the continual reengineering of their work processes.

LRMC has adapted the definition of teams used by Katzenbach and Smith.[3] A team is a small, *consistent* group of people with a relevant shared purpose, common performance goals, complementary skills, and a common approach to its work. Team members hold themselves mutually accountable for the team's results and outcomes.

The goal at LRMC is for processes in the organization to be restructured so that the team caring for the patient provides 85 percent of all services and care required—a "whole piece of work" to the extent that is feasible in a complex institution driven by high-level technology. Consequently, cross training and redeployment of key services to the patient care unit are essential for the model to work effectively. Caregivers gather laboratory specimens and transport patients rather than delegating such responsibilities to other health care workers. For the team to be accountable for the full scope of services required by the patient and family, team members must have the responsibility, knowledge, skills, and clear authority with which to carry out the services.

All professionals from radiology, laboratory, nursing, and support staff report to the patient care department leader and not to a central (tribal) leader. Ownership for the "full piece of work" includes full accountability for personnel, leadership, management, quality of work, expenses, revenue, and costs. This concept alone may seem contradictory to the conventional wisdom that the professional nurse should be fully utilized for the advanced professional skills he or she brings to the patient and should not be "bogged" down in responsibilities that can be delegated to other, less professionally prepared workers. However, from the patient's perspective, that conventional wisdom results in more and more "faces in the parade" and increased fragmentation of care.

Fragmentation of care reduces the quality of care because it is in the transfer of responsibility between caregivers and between departments that errors are more likely made. Recent approaches to patient care delivery, such as the partnership model, are based on the recognition that in today's complex environment it takes more than one person to be effectively accountable for patient care; it takes a team.

Staff at LRMC quickly learned that there are at least two major aspects to building effective patient care teams. The first is designing the structure. How many team members are needed for this patient population? What complementary skills need to be represented? The second aspect is the cultural change needed, not only by team members but throughout the entire organization. How will team members share the work? How will they accomplish the work? How do they make the transition from an individual-based practice to a team-based practice? Over time, LRMC has also learned that professional groups will seek out ways to return to like tribes, regardless of the structure.

TEAM STRUCTURAL DESIGN

A successful team design depends on the careful analysis of patient care needs. If people are arbitrarily placed together on a team because of previous assignment patterns or schedules, the model is not patient focused but instead is determined by convenience or by existing patterns and structures. Analysis of patient care needs is based on review of historical data that reflect the full spectrum of self-care assistance (patterns of care) and services needed by the patient. Services include the assessment, diagnosis, and prescription expertise of each professional, in addition to testing and treatment services, which include laboratory and radiological examinations and treatments and procedures ordered, as well as the pharmacological needs and the workload required for care of the patients. At LRMC, decisions are always based on data, not on intuition or perception of past experience.

Patients are regrouped (or reaggregated) on the basis of analyses of similarity of the patterns of care and services required. Team structures are then designed specifically to meet the needs of the patient in each of the populations. The workload requirements of the patient population drive the team structure. In addition, team structures may be different based on the length of stay of the patient population. For example, in the emergency services care team design (Figure 20–1), the length of stay of patients is in minutes or hours, not days. Consequently, care team designs are specific to shift and the needs of the patient population. (Teams seldom pass off their patients to another team.)

The care team designs for the adult and geriatric patients are different from those for the pediatric patients. Further, care team design is affected by the level of acuity of the patients within those groups. For example, as depicted in Figure 20–1, pediatric type 1 and 2 patients (e.g., a child with acute respiratory distress) would be cared for by a registered nurse and a registered respiratory therapist who are working in a pair on that shift. Patients would be assigned to the pair on the pediatric team by the gatekeeper (a person expert in both triage and resource management) on the basis of the patient's identified needs at triage. The quad team (four individuals: two unlicensed staff, one registered respiratory therapist, and one licensed caregiver, probably a licensed practical nurse), would receive pediatric patients in less acute, stable condition, with no medical complications (types 3 and 4). Other members of team I are the physician and physician extender, who work with both the quad and the pair to meet the needs of pediatric patients in either highly acute or less acute conditions.

In contrast, team II would receive adult and geriatric patients in highly acute conditions. For example, one triad of registered nurses in team II would receive adult patients experiencing mild cardiac infarction, while the other triad of registered nurses would receive geriatric patients experiencing mild cardiac infarction. Subteams of team II are composed of a greater number of licensed individuals, and team II is designed specifically to meet the needs of the adult or geriatric patient in a highly acute condition. Team III is specifically designed to meet the needs of the adult or geriatric patient in a less acute condition. These team designs were the product of 16 months of work by staff and physician project team members—expert emergency department (ED) practitioners—in cooperation with the consultants. The team composition and work capacity were designed so that patients in highly acute conditions would never wait for care and patients in less acute conditions seldom experience a wait for care. Consequently, resources were shifted to professional personnel to meet the medical, technical, and clinical needs of patients as they became well understood after the months of workload quantification and data analysis. Since the organized design described was implemented, the ED patient population has grown to nearly 100,000 visits annually. Consequently, LRMC added space and redesigned processes and team structures.

In contrast, in a patient population such as the mother-baby population, the length of stay is 24 hours to several days. Therefore, teams surround patients and cross shifts so that total patient continuity can be attained. Examples of the care

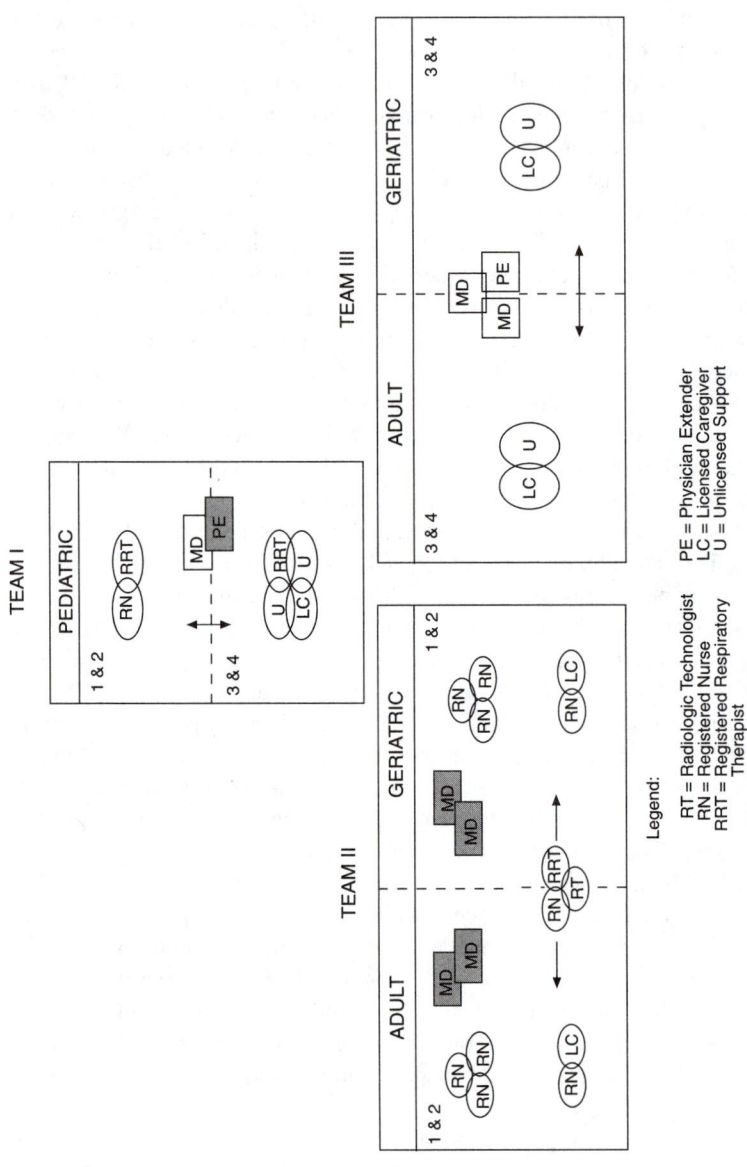

Figure 20–1 Care Team Design for Emergency Services (Day Shift). *Source:* Courtesy of Lakeland Regional Medical Center, Lakeland, Florida.

teams and support teams designed for the labor/delivery/recovery/postpartum (LDRP) unit are depicted in Figure 20–2. As illustrated in Figure 20–2, the teams in LDRP were designed to meet all the needs of the mother-baby populace and their extended families, including labor, delivery (including Caesarean section), postpartum care of the mother, bonding of the mother and the infant, and infant care. Consequently, these teams are staffed by registered nurses and operating room technicians 24 hours a day, seven days a week.

Individual care teams, such as care team I and care team II, care for their patients from admission through discharge and seldom pass them off to another team. Care team III has more personnel on the day shift because they will be assigned the patient population with elective Caesarean section (C-section). Consequently, this team's workload will be higher on the day shift than on other shifts. Again, staff and physician teams worked for over one year to analyze the needs of the patient population, including patient admission patterns by hour and day, predictability and variability in workload, and variations and complexity of patient needs. Eleven separate patient types were identified, and the workload of each patient type was quantified. Teams were designed so that patient needs could be met during both high- and low-workload periods. The patient-focused development team at LRMC provided the analytic support to the project team's workload quantification and care team design.

Annually, department leaders, operations resource managers, the physicians, and the teams themselves work to improve team effectiveness and efficiency. Numerous factors are considered, including changes in the patient population; patient, physician, and staff perceptions and satisfaction levels; the external market; payer forces; and facility constraints. All of these factors have come into play in LRMC's current review of the structure of services and team design in all of perinatal services, including the LDRP teams. Group B strep has dramatically changed the needs of newborns, and a significant increase in the volume of births has stretched the teams and challenged the units of the facility. Consequently, service processes have been reorganized to better utilize staff and the facility. This will drive new team designs and clinical processes.

Within a year following implementation, patient volumes had grown, federal mandates increased length of stay, teams were fully utilized, and space was inadequate. These changes required a complete review of processes. Elective C-sections have been moved out of the LDRP teams, and a triage function is being implemented in the labor and delivery teams. Restructuring is a journey, not a destination!

In the past, many health care organizations used shift-based patient care teams. In such teams, caregivers on one shift form a team and assume responsibility for certain patients. Membership of the team may or may not be consistent from day to day. There were teams on each shift, and patients could be assigned to two or

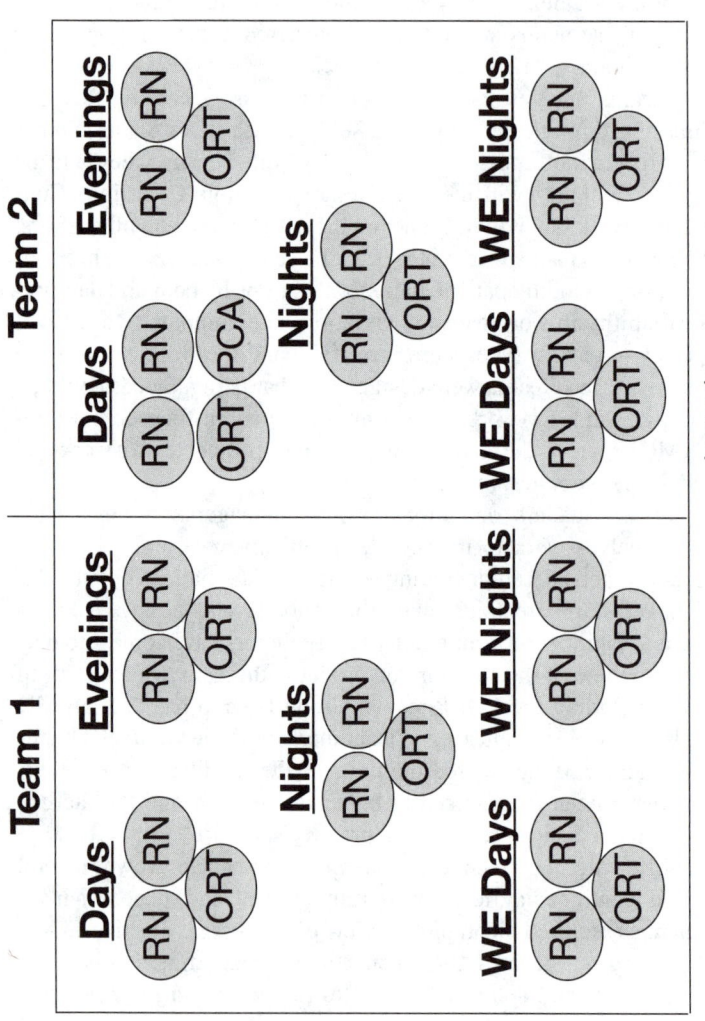

Figure 20–2 Care Team Design for LDRP. *Source:* Courtesy of Lakeland Regional Medical Center, Lakeland, Florida.

three different teams during a 24-hour day and even to teams with different members the following day. In the patient-focused care team, most teams consist of the caregivers across all shifts. The members of the team are consistent from day to day and even on weekends, using weekend staff. Figure 20–3 depicts these differences.

ASSIGNMENT OF PATIENTS TO TEAMS

With a fixed-team organizational structure, patients are assigned to teams rather than staff being assigned to patients. This is a very different concept from determining the patient's needs and then assigning the patient to a staff member or partners on a shift-by-shift basis. Traditionally, data on the acuteness of the patient's condition are obtained and then used to quantify workload and the number of caregivers needed, whether the caregivers work individually, in partnerships, or as teams. In the patient-focused approach at LRMC, the fixed-team structure is designed around the predetermined and predicted needs of the patient population. Teams are established, and patients are then assigned to (put into) teams, like

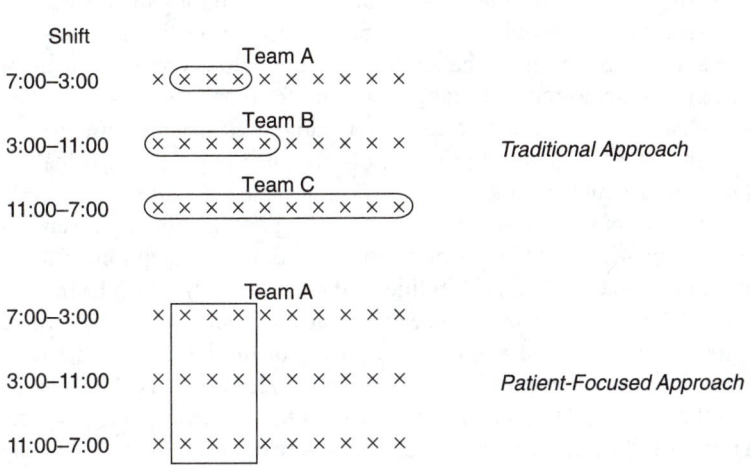

Note: X represents a patient.

Figure 20–3 Team Approaches. *Source:* Courtesy of Lakeland Regional Medical Center, Lakeland, Florida.

adding a cup of water to a pitcher. When the pitcher is full, the next cup is put in another pitcher. Thus, patients are assigned to a team for their full length of stay. Teams are fully utilized but not overloaded. The economic pressures of managed care demand that each team work effectively to carry a heavy load. Less time is available to develop the team, yet highly developed teams are essential to meet the demands of managed care. This feels like a "Catch 22" and stresses both staff and managers.

DEVELOPING "TEAMNESS"—THE CULTURAL CHANGE

Simply structuring people into teams was not enough to ensure that they would provide patient care as a team at LRMC. Few of us have had experience truly working as a team in the workplace. We may have been a part of an effective work group in which we coordinated our efforts and communicated to others what we had done. Being part of a team, however, implies joint problem solving and planning and working at all times to improve the results of the team. There is a process to building effective teams, and if the teams are not committed to the process, they will not become high-performing teams capable of self-direction.

Teams were not part of the original design for the patient-focused model but, in fact, developed as a result of evaluation of the operational effectiveness of the model. For caregivers to be accountable as fully as possible for patient care outcomes, their span of responsibility needed to be increased, as well as their level of control over as many aspects of the patient's care as possible. A consistent team of caregivers can be empowered at a higher level and for more responsibility than can an individual. Thus, it became clear that a team-based structure was necessary to meet the intent of the third principle of reengineering, that individuals at all levels must be accountable and satisfied. Therefore, the evolution of the early teams to truly functioning teams was slow. In the beginning, the teams were responsible for patient care outcomes and self-scheduling. Assumption of additional traditional managerial responsibilities did not come until much later.

After several years' experience, it became clear that teams would not evolve without expert leadership and a specific approach or discipline to assist their development. Recently, this approach has been formalized and is used for groups coming together as teams. The major components of this process—team purpose, roles and responsibilities, and performance goals—are discussed in the following sections.

Team Purpose

Individuals will not form a team unless they have a clear, identified purpose that is relevant to them. For patient care teams, the purpose may appear very clear. However, the team members must do the work of identifying their purpose or there will not be the same commitment as when the purpose is established by a higher authority. An example of a team purpose statement is the following:

> Together with your physician, we pledge to provide quality and continuity of services to the patients and families entrusted to our care by meeting their physical, emotional, educational, and spiritual needs. We strive to support and help each other, learn from each other, and be a role model for others.

The team does not develop this purpose in isolation. In the early stages of team formation, strong and supportive outside leadership is critical. Identifying individual and team values is an important part of this work. The team members discuss their stated values and what they mean. They also evaluate gaps between their desired values and their daily experience as a team. The team's values can be included in its purpose statement. An example of an actual team's value statement is the following:

As a Team We Value:

- *Teamwork*—working synergistically together and cooperatively working with others toward a common goal
- *Competence*—being good at what we do and being capable and effective
- *Integrity and honesty*—acting in line with our beliefs, "walking our talk," and being sincere and truthful with ourselves and others
- *Communication*—communicating through open dialogue and the exchange of views and by open and honest dealings with each other and those with whom we come in contact
- *Creativity*—finding new ways to do things and developing innovative solutions to issues and problems

During their discussion of gaps between values and experience, the members of this team identified competence, integrity, and honesty as essential values they had to live by. They also discovered that during times of stress, their value of creativity was the first to go.

Each patient care team works on its purpose and values during a team retreat day. Some teams even develop descriptive slogans, a coat of arms, and stationery. When new teams form now, this is the first work they do together as a team. Ongoing teams are reminded to evaluate and revisit their purpose on an annual basis.

Team Roles and Responsibilities

Empowerment and acceptance of responsibility cannot occur if there is confusion about roles and responsibilities. This major issue arises early in the formation of multidisciplinary teams. Team members work together and gradually reach agreement on how they will deliver patient care. Sharing responsibilities begins to occur in their daily practice.

However, the team must consider not only its functional work (patient care) but also its operational work (becoming a team and accomplishing team roles). Who will be responsible for collecting quality data, for scheduling, for education, and for coordination with other teams? At LRMC, an approach was adapted from Wellins and colleagues[4]—the team 101 concept (Figure 20–4). Basically, the team decides what responsibilities it has for team operations and how to share the

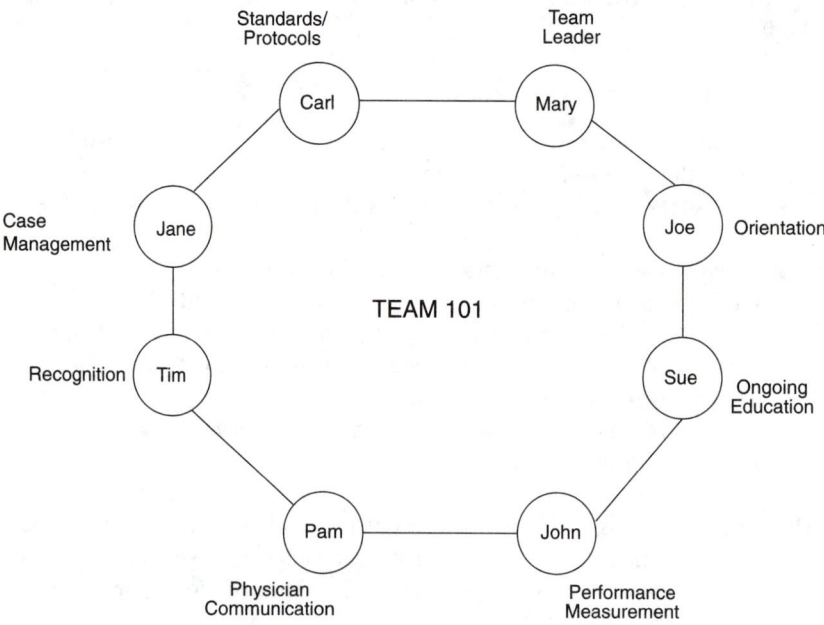

Figure 20–4 Team 101—Assignment of Responsibility within the Team. *Source:* Courtesy of Lakeland Regional Medical Center, Lakeland, Florida.

responsibilities. Team members accept these responsibilities for varying periods of time. Team members also agree on a common approach for the team's work. How will team members communicate with each other? When and where will team meetings be held? Will an agenda be used, and who will prepare it? These are some of the areas in which agreement is needed. Team consideration of these questions helps to clarify team roles and structure and helps teams to function more effectively.

In the original design of the patient care team, the need for complementary professional skills is considered. As the team comes together and begins its work, the emphasis switches to the interpersonal skills of the team members. During the team's development, there are cases in which additional skills are needed within the team, and arrangements are made to obtain those skills. For example, during the early formative stages of a team, a member may leave and need to be replaced. The team may not have been taught interviewing and selection skills. For the team to accept the responsibility of selecting a new team member, members will need to develop these additional skills.

Performance Goals

Specific performance goals are needed for the team to continually improve and develop. Goals are developed and shared with the department leader(s). The team is responsible for developing action plans to implement and reach the goals. Well-written performance goals that challenge the team result in a sense of synergy that is extremely powerful. Typically, it has taken much longer for teams to gain skill and competence in writing and achieving performance goals than might be expected. The explanation for this phenomenon may be that goal setting is a higher-level skill than simply writing the goal correctly in an appropriate format. This skill also includes being future oriented and proactive, as well as having the ability to sort through a variety of possible actions and using judgment to choose a specific action. Well-delineated performance goals and quality measurements are essential for team accountability. The following example illustrates a specific team goal and appropriate action steps:

Goal: Identify the education needs of the team by June 15.

1. Draft a needs assessment survey by March 15.
2. Ensure that all team members complete the survey by April 15.
3. Tabulate results and discuss at the May team meeting.

4. Identify the three top team priorities and develop action plans for meeting these educational needs by June 15.
5. Ensure that individual team members have identified a personal educational action plan by June 15.

Working to clarify these issues of purposes, roles, and responsibilities and a common approach to the team's work form the foundation for good team development. Other issues also arise and must be addressed, but if the team has done this work, it is more likely to evolve successfully. Other key issues that must be considered are the role of organizational leadership in relation to the team, the need for team education, and how to maintain the link to the caregiver's professional discipline.

ADDITIONAL KEY ISSUES

Leadership

The nature of reengineering teams, especially self-directed work teams, implies a very different relationship to management and leadership than that in traditional structuring.[5] Responsibility, power, and decision-making authority must be transferred to the team; otherwise, the group does not evolve and develop as a team. Managers become coaches and leaders. In the beginning, coaching the team takes a significant portion of the manager's time. In fact, simple managerial tasks that previously were accomplished in very little time can take two or three times longer during transition. Time is involved as the manager teaches the team to take on new responsibilities. In addition, tasks completed by the team members require more time in the beginning because they are at the novice skill level. It is critical that supervision of the team and its members is not removed before the staff/team is ready. If this happens, anarchy occurs and staff lose direction and purpose.

The role of leadership for teams is paradoxical and difficult for many managers to grasp. It can be frightening for a manager to teach the team to do things for which the manager has been responsible in the past. Managers gradually begin to see that they now are expected to use their time differently. They begin to focus on coordinative efforts within the organization as a whole, such as strategic planning, coaching, and developing the team.

Managers need to learn the process of coaching and appropriate ways to develop teams. Some managers will simply turn responsibilities over to the team with little or no guidance, a "sink-or-swim" approach. Others will provide resources such as educational opportunities but will relinquish their responsibility for team development to the educator or consultant. Managers must feel ownership of the process of team development or progress will be slow or nonexistent.

Managing teams is very different from managing individuals and is a difficult distinction for many managers to make. If there are 70 employees and seven teams in the department, the manager will often focus on managing the 70 employees. In a team-based approach, the manager focuses on the seven teams, developing a department "leadership team" consisting of the manager and the "in-team" leaders. The manager coaches the in-team leader, who then coaches the team. At times, the manager may be involved in coaching the entire team. Other issues faced by the manager in a team-based patient care unit include the following:

- how to build and maintain the vision of the unit as a whole
- how to prevent teams from becoming isolated
- how to help teams to work together
- how to recognize when teams are dysfunctional and intervention is needed
- how to recognize teams that are exceptional
- how to assess the teams accurately and determine their level of development
- how to avoid holding back exceptional teams, since not all teams are at the same degree of development
- how to coach teams for continual development and improvement

Another dilemma for the manager stems from the growing competence of teams. As teams grow and become more competent in their roles, they take on some of the most satisfying management functions. For example, as teams solve and/or prevent problems, the manager has to give up the role of "unit/department savior." The tricks of salvation previously gave traditional managers a great deal of recognition and satisfaction. An example relates to clinical leadership and relationships with physicians. In a fixed-team structure with the manager as leader, physicians relate primarily to the teams and do not expect managers to solve problems. This transition is difficult for both the manager, who previously received a great deal of recognition from the physician and satisfaction from that recognition, and for the physician, who begins to question, "Who's in charge? Who's the captain of the ship?" Some physicians feel that their authority is diminished in this flattened structure because they relate directly with "staff level" personnel rather than management and administration. It takes time for the physicians to see that their bonding and input to the team structure is actually much greater and has a more significant impact on patient care than it did in a traditional structure.

In the same way, the manager/leader has to give up the role of "clinical expert" and "patient savior." Over time, as managers change roles and become leaders, their satisfaction comes from seeing the staff become clinical leaders who make a major difference in patient outcomes by teaming with the physicians and really focusing on changing practices that can have a dramatic effect on patient outcomes. The managers realize satisfaction by developing people and leading teams of people.

Education

The transition from working independently to working as part of a consistent team is difficult for many health care employees. At LRMC, patient care teams require not only increased technical competency in a wider range of skills but also greater ability to facilitate interpersonal relationships than before. Developing competency in multiple clinical skills was a key focus in the early years of this conversion: This continues to be a major challenge after years of effort. There was also an appreciation of the need for interpersonal and team-building skills. However, in more recent years, leaders have realized the critical need for an educational process that teaches team members how to do the work of becoming a team. This education must be ongoing for each team and must occur "just in time" for movement to higher levels of development. The formal education must be followed at each step with new expectations, mentoring, and support. The provision of education is a shared responsibility of team members, the manager, and the central education department. Education is like planting a seed. If the ground is not watered and fertilized, the flower will never bloom. This describes the nature of the relationship between education and leadership. Education can plant the seeds, but they will not bear fruit unless coaches and leaders are there to nurture and nourish the team and provide competent, caring, and consistent guidance as the team accomplishes its work.

Governance Structure

The impact of tribal behavior on multidisciplinary team formation is significant. Peg Neuhauser, describing tribal life in organizations, points out that we are all members of a tribe.[6] Some of us belong to a professional tribe, and others belong to a departmental tribe. At issue is how to move the organization from being tribal within single disciplines to being tribal as teams, without losing the value of the professional tribe.

Tribal barriers are broken when multidisciplinary teams begin to form. Members of the different disciplines get to know each other and learn each other's language and values. As the team goes through its early formation and attachments, it becomes important for team members to focus on their similarities rather than their differences. Consequently, they may choose to ignore their differences. As an example, during the first year of multidisciplinary patient care teams at LRMC, the nurses in the teams decided they did not want to celebrate national Nurses Week unless "everyone" could celebrate Nurses Week. They were deemphasizing their uniqueness. This issue was confronted immediately as being potentially destructive in the long run. It is the very differences and pride in the uniqueness of each person and profession that makes the team effective. The differences are to be recognized and celebrated rather than deemphasized.

The redeployment of professionals from the pharmacy, the laboratory, social services, dietary services, and physical therapy, as well as the integration of radiologic technologists and respiratory therapists into the care teams, raised the need for a structure that keeps professionals closely connected to their specific discipline. A governance structure for each profession has evolved to ensure continued involvement in professional standard setting, issues relating to scope of practice and professional ethics. A professional governance structure is far more than a committee structure for participative management. It is the discipline that assumes responsibility for determining appropriate professional standards and practices. The practice councils also represent the important values of the profession and may set policy and procedure for professional practice.

BARRIERS TO TEAM-BASED STRUCTURE

There are significant barriers to implementation of a team-based structure. Culturally, we are inclined to value independence and individualistic thinking and behavior. Working in partnerships and on teams requires people to function differently, and this can be difficult. In addition, there is a tendency to return to previous and comfortable ways of working together, as well as a tendency to confuse team structure with a bureaucratic structure. The continual evolution of teams is a challenge to people's need for stability and closure. In addition, there are many system issues that create difficulties for teams. Under the stress of continual changes in health care, staff want to return to the comfort of older and more traditional structures, and leaders are worn down into accepting rationale to dissolve multidisciplinary teams.

System Issues

The typical bureaucratic organization is full of barriers and roadblocks to the implementation of a team-based structure. Three of the most common issues have to do with team-based information reports, reward and recognition systems, and performance appraisal. These three examples are closely interrelated. Teams accepting additional responsibility, such as controlling expenses, maintaining a high level of patient satisfaction, or managing length of stay, need information to be reported on a team basis. In most organizations, patient satisfaction survey results and budgetary variance reporting is usually accomplished by a department rather than a team. Changing these traditional systems can take years in an organization.

Most reward and recognition systems are individually based rather than team based. Employee of the month programs allow no recognition for teams. It takes a conscious effort to build in ways to recognize team achievements. The performance appraisal system is one possible way to do this. Organizations committed to recognizing and rewarding team performance have tried basing a team member's annual salary increase, at least in part, on the performance of the team. To do this effectively, however, there must be team-based data, all team members must be evaluated at the same time, and outcome measures for evaluation of the team's performance must be developed.

The individualistic approach to performance evaluation was another barrier to team effectiveness. Individuals were evaluated based on the anniversary of their date of hire. Consequently, even if team outcomes were a part of the individual's performance standards, team members received different scores on the same standards because they were evaluated at different points in time. It was clear that this did not reinforce team behavior or team accountability. Consequently, Lakeland began converting its entire performance evaluation structure so that entire teams could be evaluated at the same time. Every team member received the same score on all team accountability items on an individual performance evaluation. This approach had a significant impact on reinforcing team authority, responsibility, and accountability. However, this effort was not successful at LRMC. Currently, the entire staff is evaluated during a two-month period each fall. Each person's evaluation includes a combination of department outcomes, team outcomes, and individual behaviors. The individual's performance score on this tool qualifies the employee for an annual incentive bonus. The bonus is based on center and hospital quality and financial outcomes.

Structure

When managers or teams are faced with difficulties or challenges, they tend to revert to previous structures with which they are familiar. Often, superimposing a bureaucratic structure on a team structure will stifle the resilience and flexibility that is a prime benefit of the team structure. Consider, for example, the team 101 concept previously described. It is an excellent method for clarifying and defining responsibility within the team. It provides much-needed structure for individuals who require structure to function comfortably. One consequence experienced, however, was that this then defined the committee structure within the unit. In other words, the team members from each team who were responsible for education became the department education committee. The same was true for areas such as performance measurement, standards/protocols, and recognition. Soon, important decisions on these elements were being made in the unit-based committees, in essence, replacing team-based decision making with a bureaucratic model. Some decisions are appropriate for a unit-based committee, but many need to be made within the teams. Guarding against this tendency to use traditional structure to solve operational problems requires continual vigilance on the part of leadership in a team-based organization.

Another issue that creates difficulty in any team-based organization is its leadership team structure. There remains always a hierarchy of teams, but the challenge for internal leaders is in getting these leadership teams to relate to other teams and function interdependently. It is often easier to revert to the individual hierarchical structure, asking a key individual executive for a decision or intervention or using a representative of one team to report or discuss an issue with another team. Absolute clarity in each leadership team's purpose and working approaches must be agreed upon and communicated to other leadership teams to avoid confusing overlapping of responsibility and unintentional problems with authority. Effective, true teams at the leadership level are a special challenge to form and maintain, but they are critical in modeling team behavior for the rest of the organization.

Reteaming

Another issue surfaces when there is a need to reform teams or to intervene when a team is dysfunctional. Once teams form, they tend to want to remain as teams. This tendency is in opposition to the philosophy of continual improvement. In some cases, teams are no longer appropriate, or the original design is not as effective as anticipated, and reteaming is necessary. An early example at LRMC was the original decision to pair caregivers. These caregivers formed extremely close partnerships but provided care on only one shift. When the need to enlarge the team to include caregivers across all shifts was identified, it was a struggle for these partnerships to become part of the larger team.

The impact of devolving a team was underestimated. When the group has become a fully functioning work team, members are completely committed and fully engaged in their work as well as their identity as a team. In the normal course of organizational life, and certainly when continual improvement and progress is an expected way of that life, there are times when it is appropriate to dissolve a team. Its work may be completed (e.g., the organization's development team) or the service may no longer be needed (e.g., an orthopaedic surgeon taking his or her practice elsewhere, resulting in the need to dissolve two patient care teams). However, team members grieve the loss of the team, and sometimes the impact can be felt throughout the organization. The depth of loss felt by members is difficult to anticipate, but it may be severe and actually result in a reluctance to commit as fully in the future. Assimilation into the next team can take longer. At LRMC, actual interventions were identified to assist with the devolution and reforming of teams.

MOVING BEYOND PATIENT CARE TEAMS

Implementation of a team-based structure proceeds differently in every organization.[7] In some instances, teams may be implemented throughout the organization, not just in the patient care units. At LRMC, the team-based structure began with patient care teams. Soon, it was obvious that this structure left out the support staff and the focused professionals (e.g., pharmacist, laboratory technician, social worker, and physical therapist) on the unit. A parallel structure has been developed, and these employees also work in teams. In addition, LRMC has used the team process to implement leadership and project teams within the organization. Figure 20–5 shows the current organizational chart. Figure 20–6 depicts the structure of an operating center. Both structures are based on work teams functioning as the structural component of the centers.

CONCLUSION

The implementation of team-based patient care through reengineering has improved the quality and cost-effectiveness of patient care significantly at LRMC. The process continues to unfold, with new lessons learned daily. The journey has been eventful. The experiences of the past years will be useful as the organization evolves in response to the needs of its community. Processes will continue to change, and teams and jobs must also change to efficiently manage the processes.

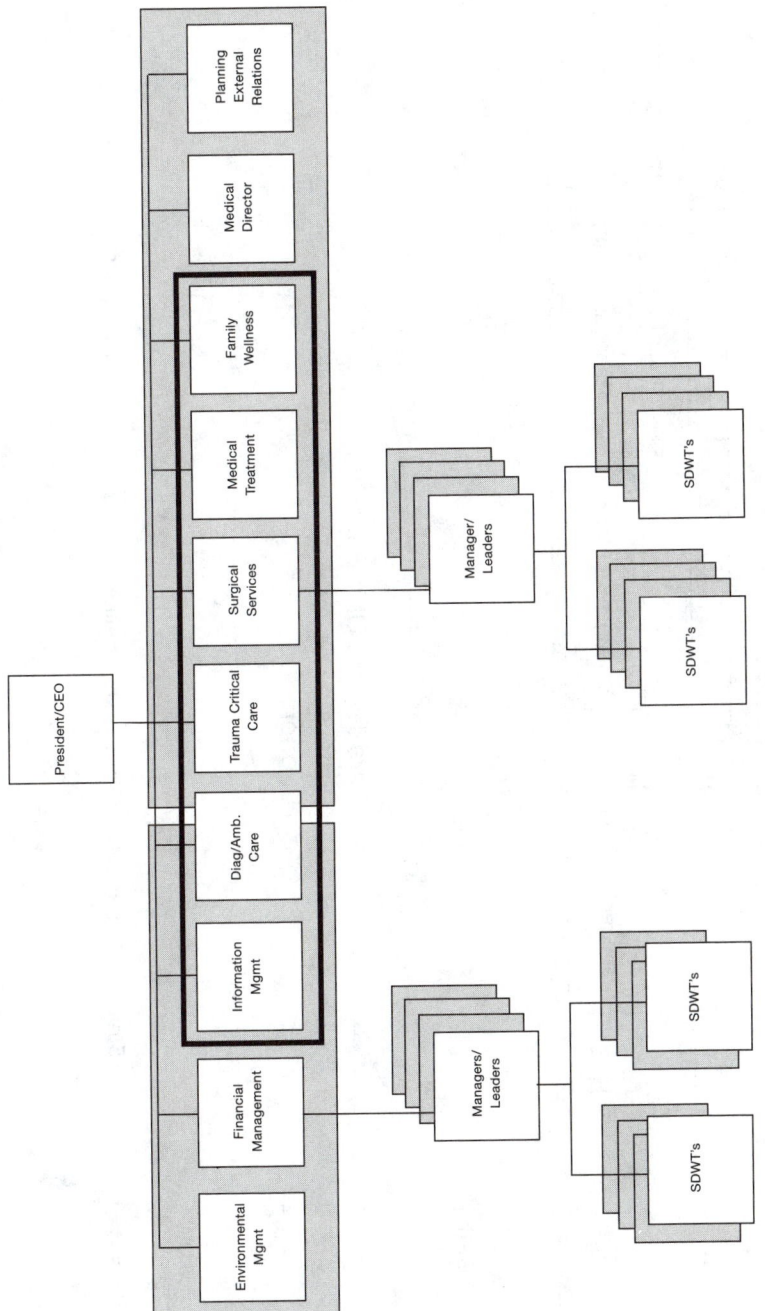

Figure 20–5 Organizational Chart. *Source:* Courtesy of Lakeland Regional Medical Center, Lakeland, Florida.

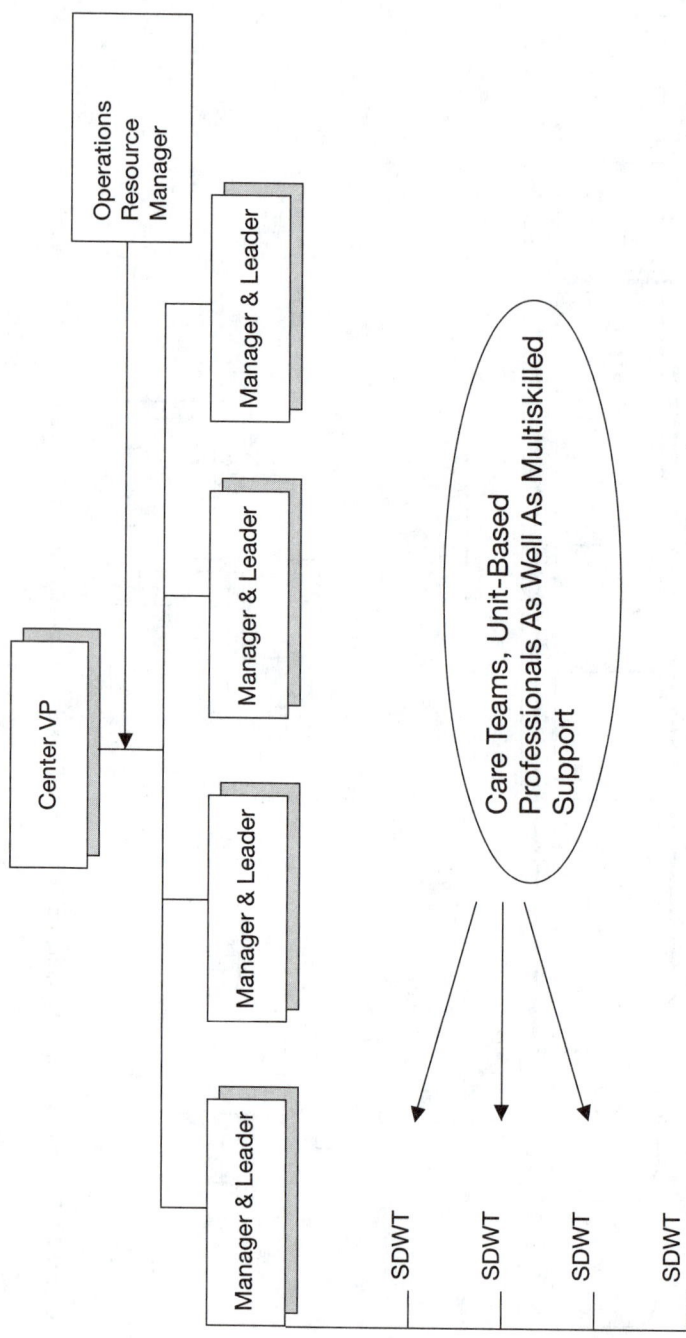

Figure 20–6 Organization Structure of an Operating Center. *Source:* Courtesy of Lakeland Regional Medical Center, Lakeland, Florida.

REFERENCES

1. Leander W, Shortridge DL Jr, Watson PM. *Patients First: Experiences of a Patient Focused Pioneer.* Chicago: Health Administration Press; 1996.
2. Watson PM, Shortridge DL Jr, Jones DT, Rees RT, Stephens JT. Operational restructuring: A patient-focused approach. *Nurs Adm Q.* 1991; 1(6):45–52.
3. Katzenbach JR, Smith DK. *The Wisdom of Teams: Creating the High-Performance Organization.* Boston: Harvard Business School Press; 1993.
4. Wellins RS, Byham WC, Wilson JM. *Empowered Teams: Creating Self-Directed Work Groups That Improve Quality, Productivity, and Participation.* San Francisco: Jossey-Bass; 1991.
5. Manion J. Teams 101: The manager's role. *Semin Nurse Managers.* 1997; 5(1):31–38.
6. Neuhauser P. *Tribal Warfare in Organizations.* Cambridge, MA: Ballinger; 1988.
7. Manion J, Lorimer W, Leander W. *Team-Based Health Care Organizations: Blueprint for Success.* Gaithersburg, MD: Aspen Publishers, Inc.; 1996.

CHAPTER 21

Pediatric Intravenous Medication Delivery: An Innovation Project

Maura MacPhee, MS, RN
Karen Terry, MS, RN

Hammer[1] describes the "business" of an organization as its processes. In the hospital, everything revolves around care delivery processes. The hospital is a "system" in which the people, their work, the linkages between them, and their values and beliefs must be attuned to the continuously changing needs of the clients they serve. This is how organizations, such as hospitals, will succeed now and in the future. The old ways of doing trend analyses and using business forecasts will not suffice in a world changing so quickly. Instead, the organization must track its clients' needs and be ready to adapt its processes to meet those needs on an everyday, every-moment basis.

Many hospitals, including the authors' hospital, went through a reengineering phase to prepare for rapid change and customer demands. The hospital restructured and downsized, but that was not enough. Instead, the hospital's focus has turned to continuous quality improvement (CQI) of the processes that serve its clients. As a central operating philosophy, CQI has guided hospitals through the transformation process, has helped them keep up with change, and has broadened professional attitudes and identities.[2] CQI was popularized almost a decade ago. Since then, organizations have discovered the finer, more complex manifestations of CQI. To make it work, there must be complete management commitment, and there must be systems mechanisms in place, such as communications networks, to ensure linkages among people.[1,3]

Organizations are discovering that relational systems, the way people connect and communicate, drive processes. The nuts and bolts of continuous evaluation and adjustment are necessary to keep the processes running smoothly, but people are the essential ingredients. People are also vital to the identification and promotion of new clinical processes that add the edge to success in this competitive world. This chapter, therefore, will provide a relational view of how one hospital's nursing staff used innovation to redesign a clinical care process—the delivery of intravenous medications.

THE BEGINNING

The Children's Hospital (TCH) is a 200-bed, pediatric, tertiary care hospital located in Denver, Colorado. It has a Trauma I designation and two intensive care units that serve the community, the state, and the 13 surrounding western states. It is affiliated with the University of Colorado Health Sciences Center (UCHSC). The affiliation process began about a decade ago with the transfer of all UCHSC pediatrics programs and personnel to the hospital. The affiliation forced TCH to make difficult decisions before the full momentum of managed care was under way. It prepared staff to look ahead, to expect the unexpected, and to adopt new paradigms about themselves and their clients.

Health care has historically been based on basic provider-patient relationships. In the present managed care environment, it has become population oriented, and the borders have blurred among the complex array of care delivery services. Professional roles have also blurred.[4] TCH staff wrestled with these realities during affiliation negotiations. They learned how to consolidate two complex systems with a large cast of characters and diverse motives. They grew wiser through the experience and stronger through the addition of so much human resource potential. This helped the organization throw out old paradigms and eased it into a new paradigm. In this new paradigm, multiple systems interact, and multiple opportunities exist to provide creative, meaningful service. This new paradigm became the foundation for reinvestment in the organization's mission statement: "To improve the health of children in Denver, Colorado, and the region, through the provision of high quality, coordinated programs of patient care, education, research, and advocacy."

THEORY TO PRACTICE

After the affiliation, population-based service provision became a top priority. Managed care was also demanding provider accountability. The organization's leaders had to design a new system with a flatter organizational structure, as well as a new culture based on the hospital's mission statement. They recognized that their chief competitive advantage was their diverse employee population, their human resource potential. Early in the planning and design phases, a great deal of decision-making authority and control was transferred to the professional staff. Interdisciplinary groups were charged with establishing integrated patient care delivery systems. These working groups created client-focused care paths that promoted professional collaboration and communication.[5]

The division of nursing charged the nursing departments to design shared governance models suited to their needs. Shared governance is a type of partnership between nurse employees and their organization.[6] Nurses are given professional autonomy over nurse practice decisions. They have the authority to decide how they will deliver nursing care to clients. They are responsible for determining what constitutes safe and effective care, and they are responsible for the delivery of quality care to the clients.

Shared governance is a change process that requires professional role and function redesign.[7] Research on shared governance models has shown that there is no "best" way. Models can vary between units in the same institution. Nurses on different units share common ground rules, but there is considerable variability in model design and role interpretation. Shared governance is positively related to general job satisfaction and perceived level of professional responsibility.[8]

At this hospital, each nursing unit has designed and implemented its own version of shared governance within the legal boundaries of the profession and the contractual boundaries of the hospital. The division of nursing and the human resources department are in the process of evaluating shared governance via employee satisfaction surveys.

THE NEW PARADIGM

Reengineering creates new paradigms, or new perspectives on the world.[9] Employees are no longer at work to do a job and fulfill an obligation to the organization for pay and benefits. Rather, the professional's sense of accountability and obligation "are embedded in the professional role."[10(p.42)] This is a significant transformation in thinking for organizations and employees. Organizations have to trust that a sense of professional responsibility will enhance quality of care, and professionals have to trust that, through their efforts, they can make a difference in client outcomes. Hospital leaders become facilitators, providing support via information and material resources to affect the quality of service delivery.

In a reengineered paradigm, traditional values and assumptions are transformed. Nurses become partners with clients and other health care professionals. "As the process of patient care incorporates more critical thinking, negotiation, and creativity, authority for decision-making must rest with the clinical practitioners in partnership with the patient."[11(pp.101–102)] The nurse becomes responsible for planning care with the client. The nurse is in collaborative practice with other professionals and health care providers. Collaborative practice, another example of reengineering, describes the professional relationships that arise within and outside the organization to meet the needs of clients.[11] Nurses, therefore, engage in multiple relationships, depending on the needs of their clients.

Hammer's perspective of professionals is significant.[1] Professionals must know how to apply the major concepts in their field. This does not mean the status quo or "business as usual." It requires a special perspective—the willingness to think beyond typical situations and to search for the "what-ifs." Hammer refers to this as "value-added" knowledge. A professional must really care about what he or she is doing. To rise to the challenge of change, nurses must be willing to go beyond standards and routines.[11]

Despite the best efforts of reengineered health care organizations, many nurses (and other professionals) stay focused on "surface system" issues. According to Hammer, organizations have surface systems and deep systems.[1] The surface system is composed of the organization's processes, the structures that support these operational processes, linkages and communication systems, and the values and mission of the organization. The deep system is responsible for "sleuthing." The deep system drives the surface system by scoping the environment for external changes and priming the surface system to change accordingly. "Everyone . . . must live simultaneously in the surface and deep systems, simultaneously performing today's work and reflecting on it."[1(p.217)]

In today's health care environment, nurses are at the heart of hospitals' core processes, such as care and therapeutics and diagnostics.[12] They are poised to be an organization's "essential innovators."[13] In the surface system, authority has been ceded to nurses through mechanisms, such as shared governance, to directly address their professional responsibilities to clients' care. In addition, nurses are being encouraged to join the deep system—to reflect on what they are doing and to innovate care delivery. Successful reengineering depends on the integration of both systems, surface and deep.

A paradigm shift, therefore, has critically positioned nurses to go beyond their traditional roles and workplace obligations. There is an opportunity to take direct responsibility for clients' care outcomes (surface system) and to dynamically contribute to the future of health care delivery (deep system).

ESSENTIAL INNOVATORS

Post uses an energy model to describe how innovation can be cultivated.[14] Post's framework has also been used for managing organizational change. Innovation may be the catalyst for systems integration. The first phase, preparation, is the foundation of the whole process. The organization's leaders must communicate their message of innovation—what it means and how it will affect nursing roles and responsibilities. Resources must also be allocated to support innovative behavior. This includes mentors to assist nursing staff with issue identification and problem solving. In many instances, mentors are also needed to enhance group work and team building.[13,14]

The second phase, movement, encompasses a structural plan for supporting nursing innovation. The structural plan includes approval guidelines and funds for allocation. Although nurse leaders and executives create a master plan of nursing care delivery and goals for the division of nursing, each nursing unit may operationalize the goals in different ways (as with shared governance). This phase also hinges on mentoring support, and, in the case study reported here, many of the hospital's nurses have received mentoring on business nuts and bolts. Depending on the nature of a proposed innovation, nursing may collaborate across disciplines and departments, such as marketing and public relations.[13] During this phase, people may become discouraged by the amount of time and energy it takes to be innovative. And innovations are not always successful. "There must be support, not just tolerance, for ambiguity, making mistakes, and plan revision."[13(p.174)] The hospital leaders in this case study continuously demonstrate their support toward innovation.

Team creativity describes the third phase, in which nurses operationalize their plan. Potential projects are prioritized on the basis of available resources, and project assignments are determined among staff members. A leader or project coordinator helps facilitate communication among team members and, in many cases, intradepartmentally and interdepartmentally. "Access to specialists in other departments is important. Members of the project teams may need training in practical creativity techniques, such as game playing, brainstorming, mind mapping, story boards and attribute analysis."[13(p.176)]

It may take a long time to produce actual results from an innovation project. Innovation leaders have to pay attention to the waxing and waning of group energy. The fourth phase, the new reality phase, is a time to reflect on what has been accomplished and to pause, perhaps to regroup and to reenergize. Although intrinsic rewards, such as personal satisfaction from new skill development, may sustain team members, external rewards help solidify the reality of what has been accomplished. Celebration ceremonies, newsletters, and even monetary rewards are mechanisms for acknowledging and rewarding innovation efforts.[13]

The final phase is integration/closure. The project coordinator summarizes what has been learned and accomplished through the innovation activity. This helps individual group members identify what they have gained through the experience—whether or not the project has succeeded. This is also a good time for the project coordinator to point out the paradigm differences that have occurred, that is, how the nursing staff have taken a professional step forward.[13]

It is apparent that there are some key ingredients to innovation, such as teamwork and leadership. Underlying the whole innovation process is evaluation. There must be objective, measurable parameters of successful innovation.[13,15] In addition to broad-based process outcomes discussed by Hammer,[1] "critical indicators" or short-term goals should be measured frequently to ensure that the innovation process is on track. In the nursing literature, these short-term goals are typically set at three- or six-month intervals.[16,17] Staff or team members should participate in identifying and tracking objective, measurable outcome indicators of short-term goals and final project goals.[16] This requires a paradigm shift, too. When designating outcome indicators, it is important to constantly reframe the project objectives in terms of professional obligations to the client(s). It is easy to fall back on the traditional habit of dividing a job or duty into specific tasks and collecting data on whether the task has been accomplished or not. In the new paradigm, innovation is a complex process that may cross disciplinary boundaries across the organization. All the stakeholders in the process, therefore, should determine and frequently discuss whether the project is accomplishing its goal(s).[1,9] In health care, the ultimate goal is quality health care delivery to clients. In a reengineered organization, any change or any innovation that connects the organization's surface systems and deep systems is an inclusive process that depends on professional contributions from all its players. The following discussion examines how the nurses at TCH made this happen.

INNOVATION AT WORK

In addition to the new emphasis on the hospital's mission statement, the board of directors and senior management identified four key values to help recognize and reward employee contributions: quality client care, employee excellence, teamwork, and innovation. To facilitate innovation, the hospital leaders created an innovation program similar to Post's model.[14] This program, the quality initiative (QI) program, was simultaneously initiated hospitalwide and at the unit level. The program was introduced to employees after the successful completion of one change process, the establishment of the shared governance model for the nursing staff. Staff members were encouraged to look for opportunities in the environment to positively affect client care delivery. During the preparation phase, there was a hospitalwide push to immerse everyone in this new concept of creative change.

At the unit level, nursing directors and their staffs began discussing the QI program's implications for professional practice. Each nursing unit has a nursing director with a direct line of communication to hospital administration. The nursing director is usually the communication liaison of the nursing unit, with access to information and resources, and has the management skills to mentor and support staff. In the beginning, the nursing directors played a key role in facilitating innovation, although they were visibly supported by higher administration. It was not surprising to see the director of nursing services visiting the units and talking with staff.

During the movement or planning phase, the hospital leaders solicited, selected, and developed employees' ideas as hospitalwide innovations. At the unit level, nursing directors and their staffs established similar guidelines for approving nursing unit innovation projects, allocating budgetary and management support, and empowering staff to assume project responsibilities. The necessity for short-term and long-term goals was also addressed.

Planning for innovation also includes planning for staff access to resources. The hospital provides a library with support staff, an intranet for internal communications, an Internet site for communications with other health care institutions and providers, and a nursing education department with nurse clinical specialists available to facilitate staff development. The nursing directors are especially helpful when unit projects cross departmental/disciplinary boundaries. They serve as liaisons and mentors for staff on interdisciplinary/interdepartmental working groups.

The development of project proposals is a systematic process that begins with the identification of an opportunity for innovation. There are business models that detail the process of localizing the nature and scope of an innovation and bringing it to reality. Hammer discusses the importance of analyzing processes systematically, especially in terms of value to the customer.[1] In the health care setting, many nursing innovations focus on clinical care processes.[16] In general, the rationale for the innovation, the pros and cons, needs to be explicitly defined. Project selection criteria mirror project development criteria. Innovation proposals are more competitive if they have been carefully researched and developed.[16] In the case study hospital, a project proposal at either organizational level must contain data that explicitly describe the need for the innovation. There must be measurable goals or evaluation outcomes to demonstrate quality improvement and/or cost-effectiveness. The project must be congruent with the hospital's mission of client-focused quality care delivery, and proposed improvement opportunities should be presented from the client's point of view, as well as the staff's and hospital's perspectives. The creativity phase is actual implementation. Due to the complexity of today's health care environments, systematically staying with a plan can be especially labor intensive. "The issues of priority setting, climate developing, coordination, cooperation, team building and networking, and internal communications must be considered. Each of these issues is an important key, and lack of attention to any one will result in a system out of balance."[13(p.175)]

A hospitalwide incentive system is in place at the organization to maintain a climate of innovation (a new reality). This incentive system includes a recognition wall in the lobby where award recipients' pictures are displayed. Quarterly awards include a monetary bonus and a wristwatch with the hospital's logo presented in person by the hospital's chief executive officer. In addition, the hospital publishes a monthly newsletter with updates on creative staff ideas. Each nursing unit also has its own mechanism for rewarding staff participation. One nursing unit votes for an "employee of the quarter" and distributes movie passes as awards. There is a bulletin board in the nursing lounge where space is shared between professional literature articles and miniposters of innovation projects. On a larger scale, the hospital hosts an annual quality fair where departments' employees display posters of their innovation projects.

The integration phase includes evaluation. Improved client outcomes and client satisfaction are ultimate goals, although these need to be operationalized. Professional nurses know how to identify client-specific, objective, measurable outcomes. Many hospitals also evaluate other dimensions of client care, such as staff satisfaction, nurse/physician collaboration, and physicians' perceptions of the quality of nursing care.[17] A better appreciation of innovation can be gained by assessing all the stakeholders' perspectives on process outcomes.[9]

At TCH, nursing directors assist staff with identifying the key evaluation indicators for unit projects, and most units discuss their goals and outcomes measures at monthly staff meetings. Evaluation data are also posted in unit notebooks and on bulletin boards to share with everyone. Unit staff retreats and casual, spontaneous get-togethers are arranged by staff to celebrate the victories (and failures) at the closure phase, although most nursing units are discovering that innovation is more of a cyclical process than a linear one, since one issue or idea feeds into other issues and ideas. Innovation work is hard work, and nursing management, in particular, should stay alert to signs of excess workload and burnout. An open environment to air concerns, such as focus group forums, and socialization strategies during and after work send signals of respect and concern.[18]

The following example synthesizes the innovation process. It illustrates the components of a nursing unit's structural plan for innovation. It also illustrates how a unit project can stretch across many organizational boundaries and disciplines. In addition, this example demonstrates that nurses can take control (surface systems) of professional practice issues, and how deep systems processing (looking for improvement potential) is the impetus for surface system change. Perhaps most importantly, this example validates the relational nature of any innovation or change. Effective communications and teamwork are paramount to success.

CLINICAL CARE PROCESS INNOVATION—INTRAVENOUS MEDICATION ADMINISTRATION

An Opportunity for Innovation

Pediatric intravenous (IV) medication administration warrants special considerations. The pharmacokinetic properties of drugs are different for children than for adults, and these properties change as children grow and mature.[19] The hospital purchased and customized a commercially available formulary to provide safe dosing guidelines.[20] In the formulary, there is a description of each medication's mechanism of action, pharmacokinetics, adverse reactions including food and drug interactions, usual dosage for different developmental groups by age and weight, overdosage indicators, patient teaching information, and nursing implications. This formulary was adapted by an interdisciplinary committee, and it is updated regularly. The medical and nursing staff are required to use this formulary because its information is based on the most current research and clinical expertise.

The nursing implications section for each medication details what the nurse should do to provide the safest and most effective administration of the medication to the client. In the case of IV vancomycin delivery, the nursing implications state: "Peaks are drawn 30 minutes after the completion of a 1-hour infusion; troughs are obtained just before the next dose. Administer vancomycin by IV intermittent infusion over 60 minutes at a final concentration not to exceed 5 milligrams per milliliter of IV solution diluent.[20(p.476)]

The hospital is a teaching facility where many nursing students from area universities do their pediatric practicums. Expert nurses serve as student preceptors, and nurse clinical specialists from the nursing education department frequently serve as clinical faculty, assisting staff with student teaching and acting as resources for staff and students. The students are expected to use the hospital formulary for medication delivery.

During a student rotation, a clinical faculty member and student were reviewing the safe dilution and delivery of IV vancomycin based on the hospital formulary recommendations. The student's preceptor, however, proceeded to show the student an alternate way to dilute and deliver the medication. The student queried the clinical faculty about the differences, and this prompted a discussion between the faculty member and the nurse preceptor. Several other nursing staff joined in the discussion, and it became apparent that staff were administering the same medication in several different ways. Every staff member was able to provide a reasonable rationale for his or her delivery method, but this situation raised concerns about the latitude allowed for professional judgment. Was there a possibility for clinical error? Was there a possibility that the outcomes of different IV delivery methods might affect client outcomes? Was there a straightforward way to explain the basic concepts of IV medication delivery to students given the obvious variability among nursing staff?

Developing an Innovation Proposal

A clinical specialist from nursing education talked to staff on different units and reviewed patient charts to identify the range of nursing care delivery methods for IV vancomycin. The most notable differences pertained to amount of dilution and length of administration time. Vancomycin was being administered over a range of 60 minutes to two hours. The nurses administering vancomycin over two hours were allowing extra time to avoid Red Man's Syndrome, a hypersensitivity reaction that occurs with too-rapid administration.[20] Dilution issues were also related to nurses' attempts to avoid hypersensitivity reactions. Nurses administering vancomycin over 60 minutes in minimal dilution amounts were basing their decision solely on the formulary recommendation.

Many nurses had plausible explanations for their clinical practice decisions, based on experience and concern for the well-being of the clients. The clinical specialist from nursing education, however, was concerned with how these nursing practice decisions would affect kinetics studies and subsequent client care therapies. Vancomycin is a drug with peak and trough serum levels that guide pharmacists' dosage recommendations and physicians' dosage orders. These concerns were relayed to the housewide nursing quality performance committee and policy and procedure committee. These committees have nursing representatives from each nursing unit. The committees discussed this issue, and committee members agreed that it was critical to determine whether there was a best way to deliver IV medications, such as vancomycin, to ensure efficacious client outcomes. To answer this question, the committee members delegated the following responsibilities: interviewing the pharmacy and medical staffs, interviewing nursing education clinical specialists at other pediatric hospitals about their policies and practices, and reviewing the literature.

After six months of inquiry and deliberations, the IV medication task force recommended that each nursing unit review the purposes and intentions of the medication formulary. It was believed that nursing professional practice discretion was reasonable as long as nurses were aware of the rationale for formulary guidelines. In cases such as vancomycin, it was understood that there might be variability in delivery time and dilution, but communication with physicians and pharmacy would be paramount to ensure appropriate collection and kinetics of serum levels. Based on staff interviews and input from nursing students' clinical faculty and nurse preceptors, the task force made another education recommendation. Pediatric IV medications are often diluted and delivered with special dilution chambers and IV tubing. There are ways to mathematically calculate where a medication is in the dilution chamber or tubing en route to the client. This is another area of IV medication delivery where expert nurses intuitively know the medication delivery process, but novice nurses or new learners must struggle through the realities of algebra. To assist all the nursing staff and students with this learning process, and provide an educational review of the medication formulary, each nursing unit was also asked to assist nursing education with devising ways to standardize and educate all nursing staff and students about IV medication delivery through the dilution chamber and tubing.

Actual Implementation

During nursing unit staff meetings, the nursing directors and members from the task force talked with staff to gain their support and assistance. Each unit agreed that IV medication delivery was an important issue for everybody, particularly in regard to the serious clinical implications for clients. An appointed representative from each unit worked with nursing education and task force members to create a written and visual procedure to educate staff about IV medication delivery. A standardized version for staff and students was approved by each nursing unit and was incorporated into the nursing IV medication administration procedure. In addition, feedback and suggestions were solicited from medicine and pharmacy before formalizing the procedure. Pharmacy developed worksheets to be used by nursing staff for recording the collection of serum levels for medications such as vancomycin.

On a nursing unit level, each unit devised ways to transmit this new information to nursing staff. One unit hosted a "math madness" night outside the hospital. On another unit, a staff member created a series of medication problems for staff to work on during down time on the unit. Nursing education developed a skills module and videotape on IV medication delivery and formulary use. Members of nursing education rotated responsibility for offering this module at housewide "skills days," which are offered six times annually, and nursing education also agreed to create and track clinical outcomes indicators for the nursing staff.

Integration

Evaluation is a key component of any clinical process change or innovation. In this instance, nursing units conducted informal surveys among their respective staff members to detect the need for additional education assistance and ongoing procedure revisions. Housewide, staff members were required to pass an IV medication administration test developed by nursing education. A passing score was 100 percent. The tests were scored by nursing education staff to identify any common error trends. In addition, nurse educators met one-on-one with individual nursing staff who did not score 100 percent.

This innovation project was a success. A deep system initiative by nursing became a housewide, improved practice reality. Intradisciplinary and interdisciplinary staff members were involved in the problem-solving process. Surface system change resulted in formal staff and education programs, and a clinical care procedure was formally revised after extensive networking within and outside the hospital. Each unit relied on its respective structural plans and reward mechanisms to help its staff integrate pertinent clinical information. Clinical outcome indicators were developed by the nurse educators to help staff track their comprehension of important clinical information, and each unit used other informal mechanisms to ensure staff comfort with change. Short-term goals included goals created by the task force to pace itself, and the goals of each unit to complete staff education before housewide testing.

The nursing staff were rewarded for their efforts. Pass rates for the staff are now at 100 percent, thanks to housewide educational activities and unit-based education programs. Perhaps this will become one of the hospital's "innovation awards."

CONCLUSION

Although this example may appear to be a routine policy and procedure review, it was really a housewide innovation. It probably would not have happened without a paradigm shift. It required deep systems operations to recognize the opportunity to improve and to change nursing professional practice. It required a systematic relay of information and a structural plan to instigate change on a hospitalwide basis (surface system). It required a system of intradisciplinary and interdisciplinary networks, and it involved unit-level commitment and creativity to assimilate practice change. Underlying the motive to change or innovate was the regard for client outcomes. This was perhaps the most significant factor because initially the staff nurses were satisfied with their explanation of dilution and delivery differences. One nurse, however, recognized that variability might affect the client, physicians, and pharmacists. This is an example, therefore, of systems integration, catalyzed by innovative thinking and action.

Reengineering is not a fad—it is a way of life in the managed care world. It matters when an institution is truly committed to the reengineering process and transmits this message through its leaders. These leaders, in turn, must find ways to model the change process and support other professionals as they learn to maneuver the change process, to be innovative. Professional and institutional success depend on adaptation to change, and this example is a testament to small beginnings and nurses' strong sense of professional accountability to themselves and their clients.

REFERENCES

1. Hammer, M. *Beyond Reengineering: How the Process-Centered Organization Is Changing Our Work and Our Lives.* New York: Harper Business; 1996.

2. Ummel S, Schaffner J, Smith B, Ludwig-Beymer P. Advancing the continuum of care: The Lutheran General health system experience. In: Blancett S, Flarey D, eds. *Reengineering Nursing and Health Care.* Gaithersburg, MD: Aspen Publishers, Inc.; 1995:261–281.

3. Shortell S, Gillies R, Anderson D, Mitchell J, Morgan K. Creating delivery systems: The barriers and facilitators. *Hosp Health Serv Adm.* 1993; 38(4):447–466.

4. Shine K. Challenges facing academic health centers and major teaching hospitals. *J Nurs Adm.* 1997; 27(4):21–26.

5. MacPhee M, Hedrick L, Todd J. Bronchiolitis: Improving outcomes in the pediatric population. In: Blancett S, Flarey D, eds. *Health Care Outcomes: Collaborative, Path-Based Approaches.* Gaithersburg, MD: Aspen Publishers, Inc.; 1998:132–138.

6. Maas M, Specht J. Shared governance in nursing: What is shared, who governs, and who benefits? In: McCloskey J, Grace H, eds. *Current Issues in Nursing.* Boston: Mosby; 1994:398–407.

7. Comack M, Brady J, Porter-O'Grady T. Professional practice: A framework for transition to a new culture. *J Nurs Adm.* 1997; 27(12):32–41.

8. Hastings C, Waltz C. Assessing the outcomes of professional practice redesign. *J Nurs Adm.* 1995; 25(3):34–42.

9. Blancett S, Flarey D. Changing paradigms: The impetus to reengineer health care. In: Blancett S, Flarey D, eds. *Reengineering Nursing and Health Care.* Gaithersburg, MD: Aspen Publishers, Inc.; 1995:3–14.

10. Porter-O'Grady T. Reengineering in a reformed health care system. In: Blancett S, Flarey D, eds. *Reengineering Nursing and Health Care.* Gaithersburg, MD: Aspen Publishers, Inc.; 1995:37–49.

11. Wolf G. Creating an environment for reengineering. In: Blancett S. Flarey D, eds. *Re-engineering Nursing and Health Care.* Gaithersburg, MD: Aspen Publishers, Inc.; 1995: 100–117.

12. Veihmeyer C. Business process reengineering: One health care system's experience. In: Blancett S, Flarey D, eds. *Reengineering Nursing and Health Care.* Gaithersburg, MD: Aspen Publishers, Inc.; 1995:282–301.

13. Manion J. Chaos or transformation? Managing innovation. In: Blancett S, Flarey D, eds. *Reengineering Nursing and Health Care.* Gaithersburg, MD: Aspen Publishers, Inc.; 1995:167–179.

14. Post N. *Working Balance: Energy Management for Personal and Professional Well-Being.* Philadelphia: Post Enterprises; 1989.

15. Flarey D, Blancett S. Reengineering: The road best traveled. In: Blancett S, Flarey D, eds. *Reengineering Nursing and Health Care.* Gaithersburg, MD: Aspen Publishers, Inc.; 1995:15–36.

16. Boylan C, Russell G. Beyond restructuring: Futuristic rapid-cycle change to improve patient care. *J Nurs Adm.* 1997; 27(10):13–20.

17. Kinneman M, Hitchings K, Bryan Y, Fox M, Young M. A pragmatic approach to measuring and evaluating hospital restructuring efforts. *J Nurs Adm.* 1997; 27(7/8):33–41.

18. Johnston B. Managing change in health care redesign: A model to assist staff in promoting healthy change. *Nurs Economic$.* 1998; 16(1):12–17.

19. Blaho K, Winbery S, Merigian K. Pharmacological considerations for the pediatric patient. *Optom Clin.* 1996; 5(2):61–90.

20. *Formulary and Drug Dosing Handbook: The Children's Hospital of Denver.* Hudson, OH: Lexi-Comp, Inc; 1996.

CHAPTER 22

Warfarin Management in an Ambulatory Clinic

Janet Teeters, MS, RPh
Julie Schaffner, MSN, RN
Mary Pubentz, PharmD, RPh

In 1995, Lutheran General Healthsystem (LGHS) and Evangelical Health System (EHS) merged to form Advocate Health Care. Advocate Health Care, based in Oak Brook, Illinois, is one of the 10 largest health care systems in the country, providing services at more than 180 sites of care throughout metropolitan Chicago. In addition to eight hospitals, this integrated system includes home health care, extended care facilities, retirement complexes, hospice care, physician health organizations, and affiliated medical groups.

Almost 3,800 physicians are affiliated with the system, with 1,800 of them belonging to physician hospital organizations (PHOs) at Advocate hospitals. Also affiliated with the system are the Advocate Medical Group (AMG), a 260-member physician practice owned by Advocate; the Dreyer Medical Clinic, a 100-member physician group owned by Advocate that serves the far western suburbs; and the Advocate Health Clinics, which include 165 physicians. Lutheran General Hospital (LGH), one of the eight hospitals, is a 600-bed, tertiary care community teaching hospital with more than 800 physicians. Within the health plan associated with LGH PHO, there are 40,000 enrolled capitated patients.

ANTICOAGULATION THERAPY INITIATIVE

A number of collaborative efforts between the PHO and the hospital-based pharmacy have proven successful in improving medication use for the PHO patients. Redesigning the care of patients requiring anticoagulation therapy in an ambulatory setting is one such collaborative initiative.

Anticoagulants decrease the clotting ability of the blood, thereby helping to prevent formation of clots in the blood vessels. Coumadin, a brand-name form of the anticoagulant warfarin, is prescribed as prophylaxis or treatment for several diagnoses, including deep vein thrombosis (DVT), pulmonary embolus, atrial fibrillation, and certain other forms of heart disease. Warfarin is a high-risk medication with a narrow therapeutic index, meaning there is little room between efficacy and toxicity. Warfarin dose requirements are patient-specific and require close monitoring to ensure that patients receive the proper amount of medication. Warfarin therapy must be prescribed carefully to prevent the patient from experiencing serious side effects, manifested as external or internal bleeding, yet must be maintained in the therapeutic range to prevent clots from forming that could result in reoccurring DVTs or strokes. In either case, the result can be life threatening. Because other medications, comorbidities, and diet can have a significant impact on the effectiveness of the drug, patient education and monitoring are crucial.

Anticoagulation levels of patients on warfarin are monitored by measuring the amount of time required for a patient's blood to clot. If a blood test shows that a patient's blood-clotting time is not in a therapeutic range, a physician must determine an appropriate course of action, taking into account the complex set of factors that influence how a patient may respond to warfarin therapy.

An opportunity to improve the management of orally anticoagulated patients was identified in 1992 by a health plan internal audit. A 44 percent complication rate was identified (bleeding or disease recurrence warranting medical attention among patients receiving warfarin therapy [$n = 23$ patients]). Seventeen percent of these patients required admission to the hospital for warfarin-related complications. In addition to the high level of emergency department visits and hospital admissions related to anticoagulant therapy, the audit identified inconsistencies in oral anticoagulant management and a lack of documentation of patient education and compliance with the prescribed treatment plan.

These initial findings led to the formation of a continuous quality improvement (CQI) team focused on improving the warfarin management process within LGHS. The team believed that the enhancement of existing processes would improve the quality of care to patients on warfarin. An interdisciplinary team was assembled to represent all departments involved in the anticoagulation management process. The team consisted of representatives from the hospital (pharmacy, laboratory, nursing, quality assurance), the medical group (internal medicine, cardiology, family practice), and the health plan (quality assurance, medical administrator). The team focused on guideline development and education, with the premise that standardization of clinical practice would address the variation in practice and result in improved outcomes.

The team focused on all the processes involved in monitoring warfarin anticoagulation therapy and looked for opportunities to improve the system to reduce complications for patients receiving warfarin. Key quality indicators were identified that would help determine whether there was improvement in the process as changes were implemented. These indicators included appropriate monitoring, INRs (International Normalized Ratios) in therapeutic ranges, the incidence of hospitalizations related to complications, and documentation of treatment plan, patient education, and patient compliance.

WARFARIN PROTOCOL DEVELOPMENT

To provide a structured reference for anticoagulation management, the CQI team developed and implemented a systemwide guideline for warfarin use in October 1992. The guideline was a comprehensive document that included information on warfarin pharmacology, dosing recommendations, a main treatment algorithm, and subalgorithms for evaluating and managing bleeding complications and treatment failures. The guideline was distributed to all physicians on staff at LGH, and an information sheet was developed for inclusion in the patient chart.

A major educational initiative was launched by the team to increase physicians' awareness of the guidelines. Inservices, newsletters, and announcements at all major medical meetings occurred. Each physician on staff received a copy of the guidelines and concerns that had been identified by the team.

Six months later, a follow-up review was conducted to evaluate the effectiveness of the warfarin guidelines ($n = 36$). This subsequent audit demonstrated improvement in certain areas: therapeutic levels improved from 44 percent within range to 67 percent, and documentation of patient education increased from 22 percent to 47 percent. The audit also highlighted opportunities for additional improvements: consistent monitoring of the therapeutic level, chart documentation of indications for warfarin, target range, and intended duration of therapy. Many cases still lacked documentation regarding patient education and compliance. This information is important in the outcomes analysis, since without documentation of these events one cannot be certain that improved outcomes are the direct result of process improvements and not other patient factors.

The team found implementation of the algorithm far more difficult than anticipated. Not only was it difficult for the team to educate a diverse population of physicians, but it was also challenging to change physician practice without having a system in place to reinforce those changes. The algorithm called for significant changes in practice that many busy physicians had little time to learn, and since the process took place in physicians' offices, the team had little power to influence the change.

The CQI team decided that reengineering the process was needed to optimize warfarin management and focused on development and implementation of an ambulatory anticoagulation clinic where the multiple variables could be controlled. The warfarin management team regrouped into the anticoagulation clinic team in 1993 and proceeded with the design and implementation of the anticoagulation clinic. It was determined that the use of the guideline and the educational focus would be incapable of delivering the desired performance. The clinic "solution" created a set of processes that were fundamentally and radically redesigned to add value to the customer. Every aspect of the warfarin management process was rethought. The traditional physician management, requiring several visits to the office over time, was determined to add little value to the patient. The pharmacist responsible for managing the clinic was identified as the process owner, and customer-driven performance requirements were identified. Two primary customers, the physician and the patient, were identified, and the team's focus centered on identifying, reengineering, and adding value to these customers. Old paradigms were challenged and discarded. The "rethinking" strategy focused on intensification—improving processes to serve customers better. An advocacy and strong sponsorship role was played by the director of pharmacy, who helped shape the vision, motivate the team, and procure funding to make the vision a reality. With a superior design, the right location, the right staff, and stellar processes, the clinic concept was destined to succeed.

DEVELOPING AND IMPLEMENTING THE AMBULATORY ANTICOAGULATION CLINIC

The anticoagulation clinic team consisted of all but three members from the original team and a pharmacist who was hired to work in the new clinic. To study the effectiveness of warfarin therapy managed in an ambulatory clinic, the hospital applied for a clinical research grant from DuPont Merck Pharmaceuticals. A specialist from the system-based research and education department joined the team to develop research protocols, and when the grant was awarded, the person responsible for data collection joined the team.

Determining Feasibility

A financial analysis of the proposed clinic was performed to determine economic feasibility of the project. The anticoagulation clinic project was presented as a program that would initially require funding but would be self-supportive once a minimum capacity was attained. A break-even analysis was conducted to determine at what patient visit volume (visits/month) revenue would offset expenses and subsidization would no longer be required. Projecting revenue required an estimation of the anticipated payer mix.

LGH serves a large Medicare population, and it was assumed that the anticoagulation clinic would serve a similar population. Other assumptions were a patient visit frequency of 1.6 per month, a net growth of 5 patients per month, a weekly maximum of 75 visits, and an average reimbursement of $20.00 per visit (based on the then-current Medicare fee schedule). These figures resulted in a projected financial break-even point occurring around 225–250 active patients in two years' time.

Anticoagulation Clinic Goals

In designing the anticoagulation clinic, the following goals were established by the CQI group: (1) to improve outcomes in orally anticoagulated patients, as measured by a reduction in bleeding and treatment failure rates; (2) to reduce the number of emergency department visits and hospitalizations resulting from oral anticoagulant-related complications; (3) to maximize satisfaction (for both patient and physician customers); and (4) to share the clinical, operational, administrative, and CQI experiences and findings with the health system and medical community. The proposed clinic would be a site where patients could receive education as well as have blood tested. A pharmacist would operate the clinic because of pharmacists' knowledge of the drug and its potential interactions. A point-of-care fingerstick blood test monitor would be used to allow for rapid interpretation of results and adjustments in therapy during the visit.

Administrative Support

Information about the audits, the anticoagulation clinic proposal, and the financial analysis and break-even point was presented to administrators of the hospital, medical group, and health plan. With managed care increasing in the Chicago market and the continuum of care concept at the top of the system's goals, all of the administrators agreed that investing in prevention and risk reduction would provide quality patient care and better position the health system in a managed care environment.

To help facilitate development of the clinic, each portion of the health system provided some level of support. The hospital had just completed an outpatient resource center, and space was allocated to the anticoagulation clinic. The hospital pharmacy department was responsible for hiring the pharmacist and for the overall administrative oversight of the clinic. The health plan provided funds to purchase the Coumatrak Protime Monitor® that was used to monitor prothrombin (clotting) times (PTs). The medical group provided the support for billing and collections and identified a physician to serve as the medical director of the clinic. Both the hospital medical staff and the health plan would become the primary referral base for the clinic. In addition, the hospital, health plan, and medical group agreed to offset the operating costs until the clinic became self-supporting.

Clinic Staffing

Initial staffing consisted of one pharmacist who was responsible for all anticoagulation clinic operations, including scheduling, patient visits, billing, policy and procedure development, and maintaining laboratory certification. The pharmacist was expected to manage 200–250 active patients (320–400 visits per month). Administrative oversight was provided by a physician medical director and the hospital's pharmacy director. With the continued growth of the clinic, the staffing in 1998 was 2.75 full-time equivalent pharmacists managing 600 active patients (1,200 visits per month). A training and credentialing process is in place to guarantee consistent management of the patients in the clinic.

Location and Access

The anticoagulation clinic resides in a single-story outpatient facility located in a strip-mall directly across the street from LGH. Parking is free; there is little congestion from hospital traffic; and street-level entry allows easy access for patients in wheelchairs and other special needs patients. In addition, outpatient laboratory, radiology, and senior service departments are located in the same building for patient convenience. This represented a significant departure from the hospital's strategy of placing services within the hospital structure.

The anticoagulation clinic is open five days per week (Monday, Wednesday, and Friday from 8:00 A.M. until 4:00 P.M. and Tuesday and Thursday from 7:00 A.M. until 7:00 P.M.). Patients must be referred by their physician and are seen by appointment only. During the off-hours, a voice mail system is available for patients to leave messages, but patients are instructed to contact their physicians directly in emergency situations when the clinic is closed. If levels are required on the weekend, as determined by the staff, the patient is scheduled to have the test in the inpatient pharmacy at the hospital, using the same fingerstick methodology. Select staff from the hospital cross-train at the clinic and are scheduled on the weekends to provide this service.

Patient Visits and Laboratory

Upon entering the outpatient clinic, anticoagulation clinic patients are greeted by a receptionist who notifies anticoagulation clinic personnel that the patient has arrived. Once in the anticoagulation clinic, the patient is interviewed by the pharmacist regarding the occurrence of bleeding and/or complications since the last visit, as well as changes in medications, diet, and compliance with his or her regimen. A fingerstick PT test is performed by the pharmacist. The rapid turn-around time of the test results allows the pharmacist to evaluate the need for further dose adjustments and to counsel the patient about any changes during each visit. To complete the visit, the pharmacist schedules a follow-up appointment and gives the patient a dosage/appointment card outlining the patient's weekly warfarin regimen and next appointment date.

The clinic pharmacist reviews the results with the patient and asks if he or she is experiencing any side effects. If a patient's INR test result is not in the therapeutic range for his or her diagnosis, the pharmacist asks about any relevant behavior, such as compliance, changes in diet, or new medications. The pharmacist then uses the warfarin management algorithm to determine if a dosage change is appropriate. The dose is then raised, lowered, or maintained, and the patient is informed of the change. The entire visit takes about 15 minutes.

In contrast, when a warfarin patient is monitored by his or her primary care physician, the patient must go to the physician's office for a scheduled appointment, go to the laboratory to have blood drawn from the arm, and then wait for as long as two days for the physician to call with results.

In addition to reducing turnaround time for test results, the new clinic allows time for anticoagulation clinic staff to become much more familiar with each patient. The closer interaction enhances the staff's ability to determine causes of variation in patient test results, and individualized education reduces the likelihood of noncompliance. The clinic also reduces variation in treatment practice, since the responsibility of monitoring INR levels has been transferred from multiple primary care physicians to the anticoagulation clinic staff. The anticoagulation clinic staff use control charts to map individual patient variation, which is shared with both the patient and physician.

Laboratory Testing

At each visit, the patient's INR is determined using the Coumatrak Protime Monitor®, which measures the PT from a fingerstick sample of blood and converts it into an INR. This procedure takes two to three minutes and negates the need for more-invasive venipuncture. The rapidity of this procedure allows the pharmacist to couple laboratory testing with patient counseling during each visit.

Protocols

The basis of patient management in the anticoagulation clinic is the warfarin usage guideline. This document was created to assist practitioners in the management of warfarin therapy. The guideline includes information pertaining to appropriate indications, warfarin pharmacology and dosing, algorithms for PT/INR results, treatment failures and bleeding complications, and guidelines for vitamin K administration. This guideline is reviewed yearly by members of the anticoagulation clinic team and additional physicians having expertise with patients requiring warfarin.

The treatment algorithm facilitates the evaluation and management of patient PT/INR values based on the test result and the patient's condition. Return visit intervals are also included in the algorithm and vary depending on whether a dose adjustment is made, necessitating more frequent follow-up. If, after review of the patient's INR results and the patient's condition, the pharmacist feels that a dose adjustment is necessary, the pharmacist instructs the patient about those changes at the time of the visit. Dose adjustments are made as a percentage change (typically 10–20 percent) in the patient's weekly warfarin dose, with the new dose distributed throughout the week as evenly as possible. All patient visit data are conveyed via facsimile to the referring physician the same day.

In the event of a complication (bleed or treatment failure), a component of the guideline assists the practitioner in determining the etiology of the event and what course of action (reversal of therapy, discontinuation of therapy, etc.) should be taken. At this point, the patient is considered off protocol, and the referring physician decides how to proceed with patient management. Once warfarin therapy has been resumed, the patient returns to the clinic and reenters the treatment algorithm at the point requiring frequent follow-up to ensure the therapy is stabilized.

Additionally, the clinic offers oral vitamin K administration and daily follow-up visits when levels warrant the need for oral vitamin K and the physician concurs with the therapy. This has helped reduce the need for patients to go to the emergency department for subcutaneous injections of vitamin K and maintains close management of these patients.

Clinic Referral

Patients must be referred to the anticoagulation clinic by the physician who will oversee therapy. The physician completes and returns an anticoagulation clinic referral form that provides information regarding the indication for therapy, intensity and duration of therapy, history of complications, starting date of anticoagulation therapy, and the INR/dosage history (Exhibit 22–1). The form was de-

Exhibit 22–1 Referral Form

Lutheran General Hospital
Anticoagulation Center

Referral Patient Information Sheet

From Dr. _____

I am referring patient _____,

phone number (___)____-____-_____, to the

Anticoagulation Center for warfarin monitoring

(includes, as needed, PT/INR testing).

Physician signature: _____ **(required)**

Physician office fax number: _____

RETURN FAX TRANSMITTAL

TO: **Anticoagulation Center**
       8820 Dempster St.
       Niles, IL 60714

FAX: **847-723-2328**

VOICE: 847-723-2345

Indication(s) for Anticoagulation

Atrial Fibrillation
- ☐ No heart disease, age >60
- ☐ Valvular disease
- ☐ Prosthetic valve
- ☐ New onset (for cardioversion)
- ☐ Paroxysmal

Transmural MI
- ☐ Severe LV dysfunction
- ☐ CHF
- ☐ LV aneurysm

- ☐ Dilated cardiomyopathy

Venous Thromboembolic Disease
- ☐ PE, first time
- ☐ PE, recurrent
- ☐ DVT, first time
- ☐ DVT, recurrent

Valve Position
- ☐ mitral
- ☐ aortic
- ☐ pulmonic

Prosthetic Valve Type
- ☐ Bjork-Shiley
- ☐ St. Jude
- ☐ Starr-Edwards
- ☐ porcine
- ☐ other

DVT Location

Side   R   L

Locus LE UE

other

_____

Therapy Plan

Date of event requiring anticoagulation

_____

Date started on anticoagulation

_____

Intended INR intensity of anticoagulation

- ☐ INR 2.5–3.5 (mechanical prosthetic valves)
- ☐ INR 2.0–3.0 (other indications)

Intended duration of anticoagulation (*circle one*)

3 months   6 months

long term   perioperative

Other

_____

Proximity (for LE DVT) (*circle one*)

proximal   distal

- ☐ Orthopaedic surgery, perioperative prophylaxis

procedure _____

- ☐ Cerebrovascular disease

description _____

_____

- ☐ Other (*please provide specifics*)

continues

Exhibit 22–1 continued

Recent Warfarin History

It will be very helpful to have results of your patient's most recent INRs.

Patient's current dose _____

Latest INR _____   Date _____

    Dose _____

Previous INR _____   Date _____

    Dose _____

Previous INR _____   Date _____

    Dose _____

Hx of Warfarin Complications

Any bleeding episodes?   Y   N
Please describe

Other anticoagulant-related complications/problems?

Source: Courtesy of Lutheran General Hospital, Park Ridge, Illinois.

---

signed using check boxes to facilitate completion of pertinent patient data. This form is kept on file in the patient's chart and serves as physician authorization to manage the patient according to clinic guidelines.

Patient Education

Patient education is a continuous process that is paramount to the success of the anticoagulation clinic. Once a referral is received by the clinic, a 30- to 60-minute clinical visit/consultation is scheduled for the patient with a clinic pharmacist. The purpose of this initial visit is to obtain significant past medical and medication history, explain the program and protocol, and provide extensive one-on-one patient education regarding warfarin therapy and the patient's disease state.

During the initial visit, information regarding the indication for warfarin, risks and benefits of therapy, explanations of PT/INR, dosages, missed doses, drug interactions, signs of bleeding or disease recurrence, and diet is discussed with the patient. Patients are given educational aids to take home, and supplementary audio and video materials are available for review at any time. A checklist of these items is completed and signed by the clinic pharmacist and kept in the patient's file; therefore, any areas not covered during the initial visit or that require ongoing reinforcement are easily identified.

An inpatient education program was implemented at the hospital to introduce patients to the topic of warfarin therapy prior to hospital discharge, whether or not they are to be followed as outpatients in the clinic. The hospital patient education pharmacist uses a checklist similar to that used in the anticoagulation clinic when talking with the patient. This completed list is faxed to the clinic for inclusion in the patient's outpatient record as documentation of initial education. Any information not discussed during the initial consultation or that the hospital pharmacist feels requires further review can be discussed at the initial clinic visit.

Communication to Physicians

Referring physicians are faxed a progress report the same day their patient is seen. This report includes the patient's current and past history of warfarin dose/INR, historical graph of INR results, current medications, signs/symptoms of adverse events, demographic data, and a summary note (Figure 22–1).

Although the anticoagulation clinic is located in a facility with other hospital outpatient services, the system does not have a centralized patient filing system at this time. Shadow files are maintained for each patient within the clinic, separate from the patient's main medical record, which is kept in the referring physician's office. The comprehensive patient report faxed to the physician after each visit is forwarded to the office patient medical record following physician review for the physician's office chart.

Billing and Reimbursement

Initially, the clinic was established under the direction of a physician medical director, and the physician's current procedural terminology (CPT) coding was used for billing. The two codes used to cover services are CPT code 99211 for an established patient, nonphysician Level I office visit (does not require the presence of a physician) and CPT code 85610 for a PT test. For each visit, the patient is charged for both the office visit and the PT.

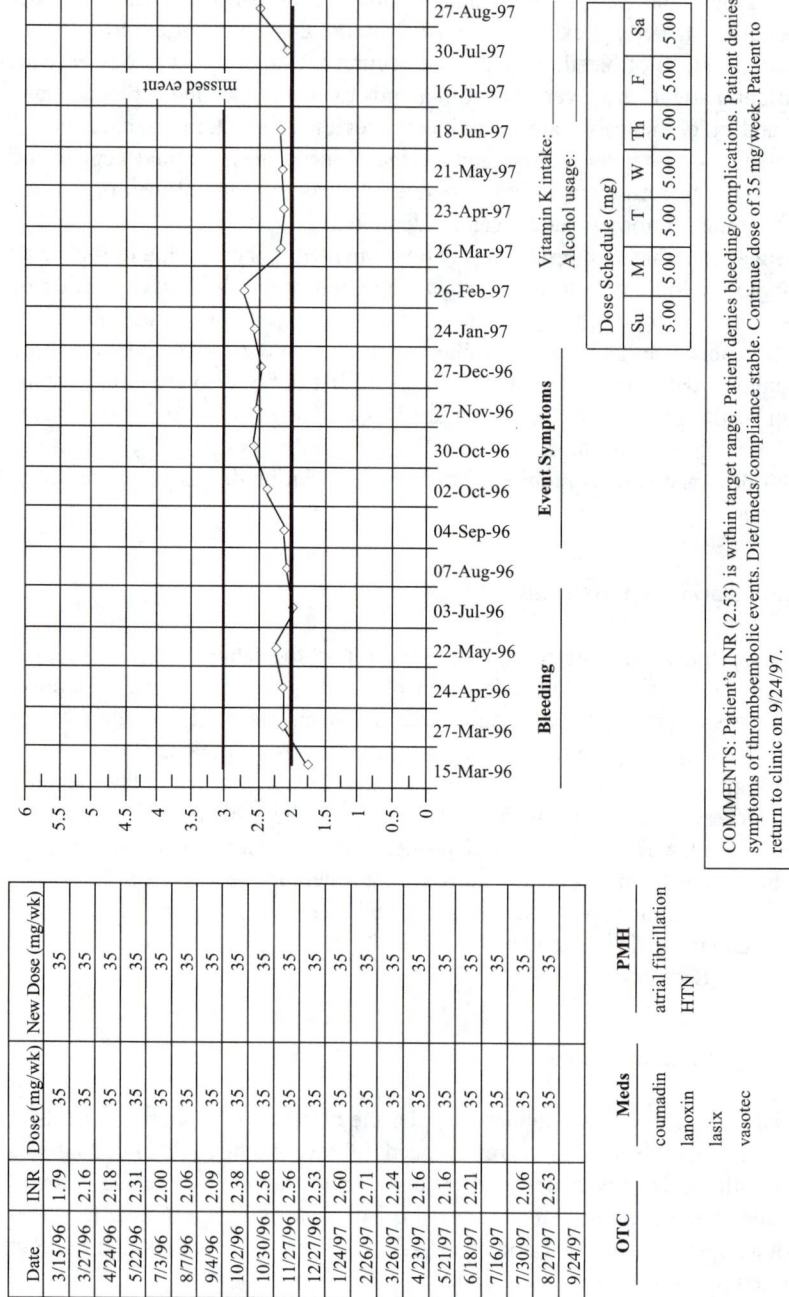

Figure 22–1 Sample Warfarin Monitoring Form. *Source:* Courtesy of Lutheran General Hospital, Park Ridge, Illinois.

Across all payer types, the anticoagulation clinic has averaged a 60 percent reimbursement rate for CPT code 99211 and 30 percent for CPT code 85610. Despite the continuous increase in enrollment and higher than expected patient volumes, the clinic has struggled to break even.

In early 1998, the decision was made to move the clinic from the physician medical group to the hospital, where the service will be billed as a hospital outpatient service. This was approved by the regional Medicare fiscal intermediary.

Performance Measures

Several performance measurements were evaluated to determine the success of each step of the implementation process. The improvements were compared to routine medical care and national benchmark data whenever possible. Performance measures included the following:

- warfarin management original quality indicators (monitoring consistent with guidelines, therapeutic INRs, documented treatment plan, patient education, compliance, and hospitalizations)
- complication rates (bleeds and reoccurrences)
- patient satisfaction
- average cost per patient treatment year

INRs

The current clinic population represents 1,008 patient years' experience (10/93 to 12/97) across all diagnostic groups. The clinic has been able to achieve an average therapeutic INR rate of 82 percent for all clinic patients, which is considerably higher than the 30–60 percent rate reported in the literature for routine physician management.[1] The 82 percent therapeutic INR rate from the Lutheran General Hospital anticoagulation clinic is consistent with reported results from other anticoagulation clinics.[2,3]

Warfarin Management Original Quality Indicators

The same indicators used for the initial 23 charts audited in 1992 were repeated after implementing standardization with INRs and guidelines (phase I—1993, $n = 32$) and then again after the anticoagulation clinic was implemented (phase II—1995, $n = 168$). Improvements were seen in all the areas after implementation of the anticoagulation clinic (Figure 22–2).

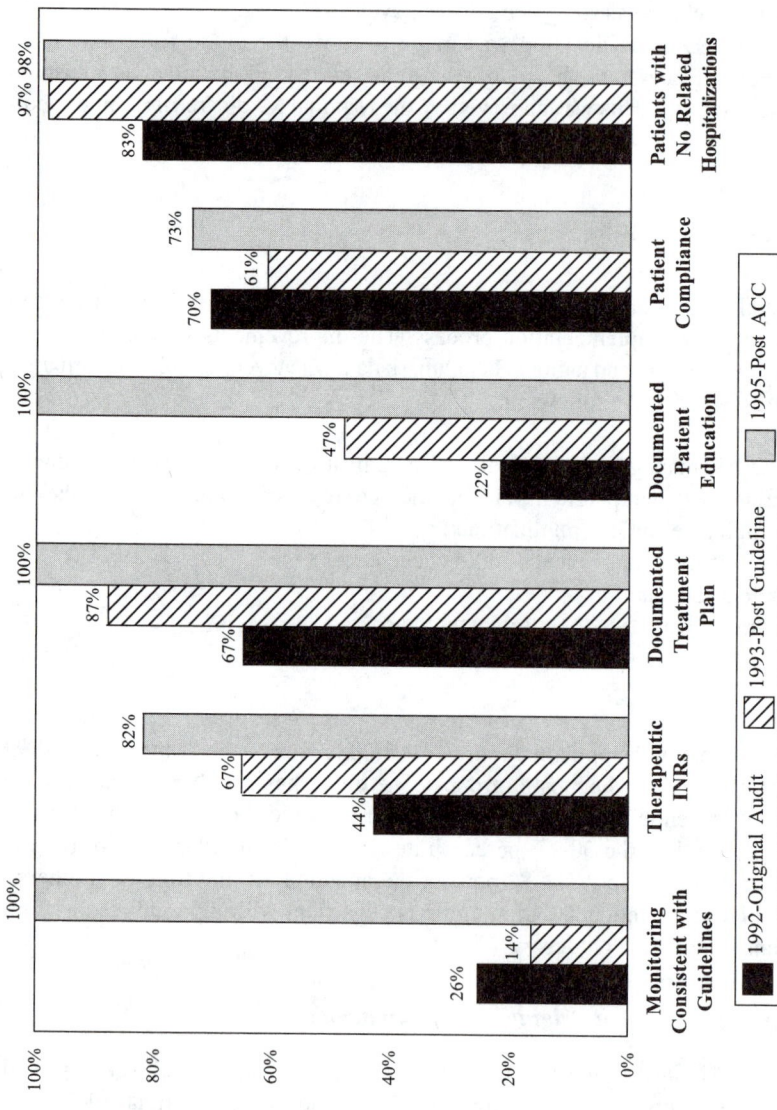

Figure 22–2 Warfarin Management—Quality Indicators. *Source:* Courtesy of Lutheran General Hospital, Park Ridge, Illinois.

Complication Rates

An audit was done of the medical group's practice concurrently with the anticoagulation clinic patients to see if there was a difference in complication rates. Patients reviewed included individuals who were on warfarin with atrial fibrillation (AF), DVT, pulmonary embolism (PE), and mechanical valves (MVs). To reliably compare complication rates internally and externally with national benchmark studies, the committee developed operational definitions for major and minor bleeds and symptom recurrence (thromboembolic events) that would be consistent with published studies. Bleeding and thromboembolic events were analyzed with units of percentage per patient year (number of events per one year of patient therapy), as is commonly reported in the anticoagulation literature. This review of patients occurred from October 1993 to July 1995. Four hundred sixty-six patient years occurred in the routine medical care group (LGH-routine medical care) and 151 patient years in the anticoagulation clinic group.

In the LGH-routine medical care, there was a 1.7 percent incidence of major and fatal bleeds, while the anticoagulation clinic group had no occurrences in this time period. Recurrent thromboembolic events occurred 4.3 percent of the time in the LGH-routine medical care and 2 percent of the time with the anticoagulation clinic group. The LGH-routine medical care group experienced 7.1 percent hospital admissions per patient year, while the anticoagulation clinic group experienced a 2 percent per patient year hospital admission rate. The anticoagulation clinic experienced more emergency department visits: 5.9 percent per patient year versus 0.9 percent with the LGH-routine medical care group. This was probably due to one patient being seen in the emergency department on three consecutive days for epistaxis. In addition, the anticoagulation clinic patients were aware of the seriousness of bleeding complications, readily reported them, and sought advice related to them (Table 22–1).

These results may be attributed to the fact that the anticoagulation clinic patients were more likely to have INRs in the therapeutic ranges, had their dose adjusted when outside the standard INR ranges, and averaged more INRs monitored per month than the LGH-routine medical care group.

Data collection in the anticoagulation clinic group is ongoing, and in four years' time there is now experience with 1,008 patient years of treatment. Major and fatal bleeds and recurrent thromboembolic events were also compared to national benchmarks. LGH-routine medical care had a 1.7 percent rate and the anticoagulation clinic had a 1.2 percent rate of major and fatal bleeds at the four-year mark, compared with benchmark data for routine medical care (4.3–8.5 percent).[3–5] National anticoagulation clinic data showed a 0.9 percent major and fatal bleed rate, while the LGH anticoagulation clinic had a 1.2 percent rate. This finding may be attributable to the fact that the clinic group covers 1,008 patient years and

Table 22–1 Complication Rates by Management Type

	Anticoagulation Center				LGH-Routine Medical Care			
	All	AF	MV	DVT	All	AF	MV	DVT
Number of patient years	**151**	58	49	44	**466**	233	179	54
Bleeding events (%/pt. year)*								
nuisance	**11.8**	10.3	14.3	11.4	**6.6**	6.9	7.8	1.9
minor	**2.0**	1.7	2.0	2.3	**3.4**	3.9	3.4	1.9
major	—	—	—	—	**1.3**	0.9	2.2	—
fatal	—	—	—	—	**0.4**	0.4	0.6	—
minor, major, and fatal	**2.0**	1.7	2.0	2.3	**5.1**	5.2	6.1	1.9
major and fatal	—	—	—	—	**1.7**	1.3	2.8	—
Thromboembolic events (%/pt. year)*								
nonfatal	**2.0**	1.7	—	4.5	**4.3**	3.9	3.4	5.6
fatal	—	—	—	—	**—**	—	—	—
total	**2.0**	1.7	—	4.5	**4.3**	3.9	3.4	5.6
ED visits (%/pt. year)*	**5.9**	10.3	6.1	—	**0.9**	0.9	1.1	—
Hospital admissions (%/pt. year)*	**2.0**	—	—	6.8	**7.1**	5.2	8.4	7.4

*Aggregate indices for complications were not amenable to statistical analysis because the rate represents the total number of complications divided by the total number of patient years of observation.

Source: Courtesy of Lutheran General Hospital, Park Ridge, Illinois.

---

the published study only covers 110 patient years. (At the clinic's 151-patient year mark it had a 0 percent rate.) See Figure 22–3.

Recurrent thromboembolic events occurred in 11.7 percent of routine medical care nationally, while LGH-routine medical care was at 4.3 percent and the anticoagulation clinic at four years' time is at 2.2 percent. The other benchmark anticoagulation clinic had a 3.6 percent recurrent thromboembolic event rate versus the LGH clinic rate of 2.2 percent.[3] See Figure 22–4.

Patient Satisfaction

A patient satisfaction survey was also conducted of anticoagulation clinic patients versus the LGH-routine medical care patients. Findings show that anticoagulation clinic patients were more often "very satisfied" with the process and their education than were routine medical care patients. In addition, a higher percentage of anticoagulation clinic patients "strongly agreed" with the statement that their overall care was excellent.[6]

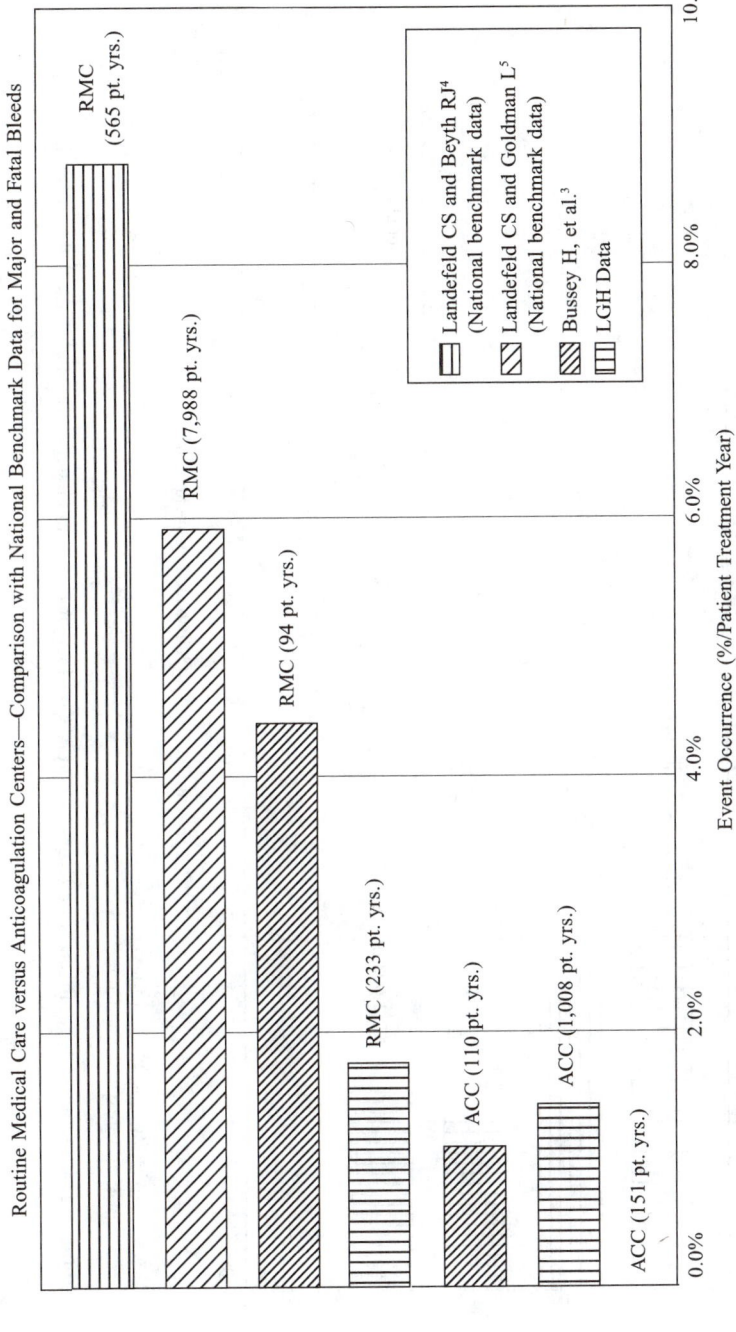

Routine Medical Care versus Anticoagulation Centers—Comparison with National Benchmark Data for Major and Fatal Bleeds

RMC (565 pt. yrs.)

RMC (7,988 pt. yrs.)

RMC (94 pt. yrs.)

RMC (233 pt. yrs.)

ACC (110 pt. yrs.)

ACC (1,008 pt. yrs.)

ACC (151 pt. yrs.)

Event Occurrence (%/Patient Treatment Year)

Landefeld CS and Beyth RJ[4] (National benchmark data)

Landefeld CS and Goldman L[5] (National benchmark data)

Bussey H, et al.[3]

LGH Data

Note: RMC = Routine Medical Care
ACC = Anticoagulation Clinic

Figure 22-3 Major and Fatal Bleed Rates. *Source:* Courtesy of Lutheran General Hospital, Park Ridge, Illinois.

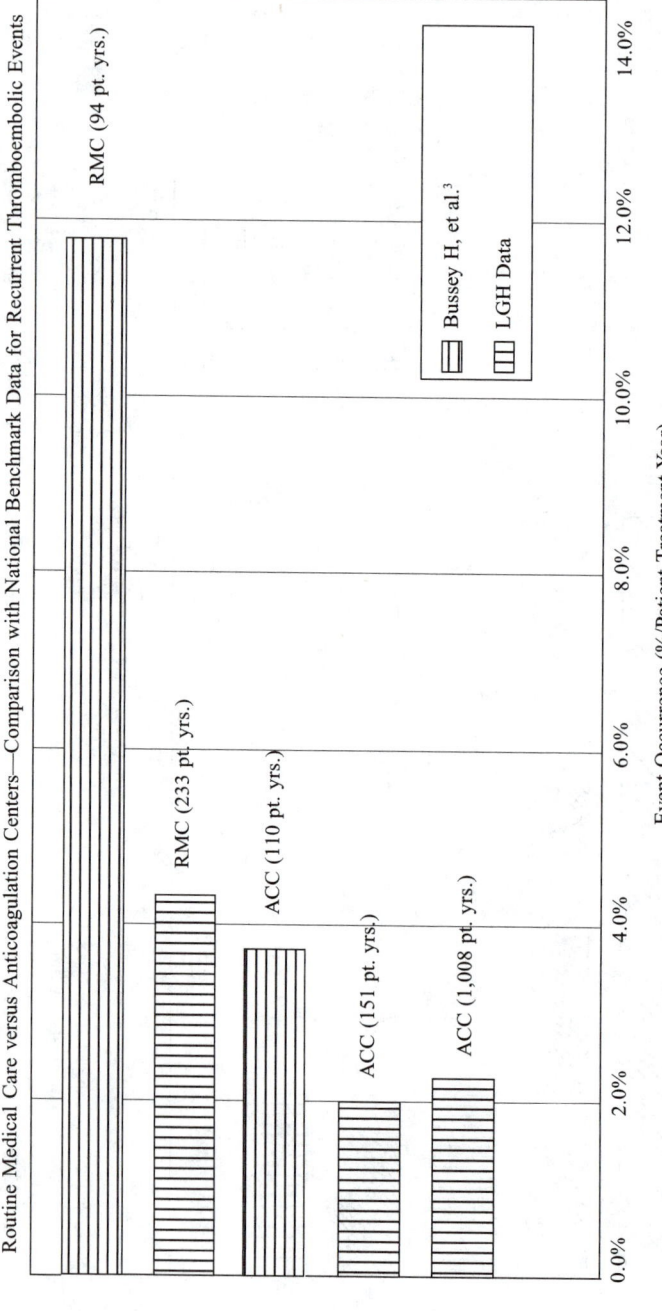

Figure 22–4 Recurrent Thromboembolic Events. *Source:* Courtesy of Lutheran General Hospital, Park Ridge, Illinois.

Average Cost per Patient Treatment Year

The average cost of a warfarin patient (monitoring and complications) was $245/patient year for an anticoagulation clinic patient versus $643/patient year for a routine medical care patient. The 600 patients managed by the anticoagulation clinic currently versus routine medical care showed a savings of approximately $238,800/year to the health system. Actual monitoring of the patients is slightly higher in the anticoagulation clinic group ($222/year for anticoagulation clinic versus $184/year in LGH-routine medical care); however, the overall savings result from fewer complications and treatment failures that result in expensive hospitalizations.

CHALLENGES

The first challenge was implementing a guideline pertaining to patient care that took place in the physician office rather than in the hospital. It was difficult for the CQI group to influence outpatient prescribing practices. The CQI group proposed an outpatient clinic that would be convenient for patients and physicians and would ensure appropriate following of the guidelines. In addition, due to the number of physicians and sites involved, the review of charts for data collection was difficult to obtain.

Another challenge to the program was the introduction of a pharmacist as the individual running the clinic and monitoring patients. Many physicians were more familiar with nurse practitioners and needed to gain trust with pharmacists in this new role. They soon learned to trust and respect the pharmacist running the clinic. As evidenced by their numerous calls to the clinic about potential drug interactions and the continued referral rate, the physicians have learned to rely on the anticoagulation clinic pharmacists.

Financial performance is an ongoing challenge. This program did not bring revenue to any of the supportive groups and barely broke even financially. In a totally capitated environment, this program would be a good investment, but managed care capitation did not spread as rapidly as predicted, and this program required justification each year. The hospital and health plan continued to provide financial support as the program continued to grow each year.

REPRODUCIBILITY

The information regarding the success of the clinic was shared throughout the Advocate system. In 1996, the team won the system award for excellence. A systemwide group began meeting to discuss implementation of anticoagulation clinics elsewhere in the system. In October 1997, an additional site opened at another hospital within the system. There is currently a plan to open an additional site at another medical group that is part of the system. The LGH anticoagulation clinic has expanded and added several staff members several times over its four-year history. During this growth, complication rates remain consistently lower than routine medical care. DuPont Merck Pharmaceuticals has engaged the anticoagulation clinic group to provide one-day workshops on implementing anticoagulation clinics to improve patient outcomes across the country. These workshops expand the experience beyond the system to have an even larger impact on patient populations receiving therapy. In addition, the lessons learned from this clinic are being used in the development of future clinics that encompass cardiac risk reduction and lipid management.

CONCLUSION

Due to its success, physicians continue to refer patients to the anticoagulation clinic. More than 600 patients are now enrolled in the clinic, resulting in more than 1,200 visits per month and more than 1,008 patient years of outcome experience. By implementing the guideline and standardization of INR reporting (phase I), LGH-routine medical care occurrence rates for major bleeds and thromboembolic events are lower than national benchmark data. As shown by the anticoagulation clinic patients at both the two-year and four-year mark, the anticoagulation clinic has been able to sustain recurrent thromboembolic event rates that are less than LGH-routine medical care and national benchmark data for routine medical care and other national anticoagulation clinics. Clinic patients have reduced major or fatal bleeding rates than LGH-routine medical care and national routine medical care benchmark data. By centering on the process, the group was able to redesign anticoagulation management in the system to improve the quality of care, reduce health care costs, and enhance patient satisfaction.

REFERENCES

1. Gray DR, Garabedian-Ruffalo SM, Chretien SD. Cost-justification of a clinical pharmacist-managed anticoagulation clinic. *Drug Intell Clin Pharm.* 1985; 19:575–580.
2. Garabedian-Ruffalo SM, Gray DR, Sax MJ, Ruffalo RL. Retrospective evaluation of a pharmacist-managed warfarin anticoagulation clinic. *Am J Hosp Pharm.* 1985; 42:304–308.
3. Bussey HI, Rospond RM, Quandt CM, Clark GM. The safety and efficacy of long-term warfarin therapy in an anticoagulation clinic. *Pharmacotherapy.*1989; 9(4):214–219.
4. Landefeld CS, Beyth RJ. Anticoagulant-related bleeding: Clinical epidemiology, prediction, and prevention. *Am J Med.* 1993; 95:315–328.

5. Landefeld CS, Goldman L. Major bleeding in outpatients treated with warfarin: Incidence and prediction by factors known at the start of outpatient therapy. *Am J Med.* 1989; 87: 144–152.

6. Calcagno DE, Pubentz MJ, Carey R. Improving patient satisfaction with warfarin management. *Am J Managed Care.* 1996; 2(7):804–810.

CHAPTER 23

Information Management: Supporting Process-Centered Work

Paula S. Forté, PhD, MSN, RN, CNAA

INFORMATION MANAGEMENT

One of the engines that drives the process-centered organization is information management. Werley et al. theorize that "with the rapid explosion of nursing knowledge worldwide, the amount of data nurses use and process in the delivery of care is extensive and . . . unmanageable."[1(p.421)] For nurses' care and management processes to be well monitored and managed, key information must be derived from the data that the processes themselves produce.

Data are not the same as information. Graves and Corcoran remind us that "data represent discrete entities . . . information represents data that are inter-preted."[2(p.227)] Many organizations keep data, horde data, even store data, but this is not the same as using data to generate information, and it is *information* that must be managed if the process-centered organization is to function effectively. How nurses interpret data is key to how they understand their processes and develop their capacity to improve them. This chapter presents an overview of information management along with short examples of how it can support process-centered work.

NURSING AND INFORMATION

Jones indicates that because little data exist that adequately describe the work of nursing, its processes, the interventions nurses perform, or the types of patient problems nurses address, nursing starts out in a compromised position.[3] This sense of starting out behind the eight ball is often the feeling nurses describe when they have to justify their work, explain their costs, or defend their practice. Proponents of the Nursing Minimum Data Set (NMDS) argue that when change occurs, nurses lack the essential data to demonstrate the value of their practice, the resulting patient outcomes, and the consequences or benefits of altering or restructuring practice.[4] Without this sort of information readily available, both the nursing profession and nurse executives are often in a poorly defensible position.

To take this a step further, work has been done to assemble a Nursing Management Minimum Data Set (NMMDS) that expands on matters of clinical practice and offers tools that executives can use to "respond to questions posed about costs and quality that challenge nursing's resource allocations."[5(p.44)] This data set will offer nurses, practitioners, and executives alike a marvelous tool for monitoring and managing their work. However, until such a data set is designed, developed, and installed in the thousands of settings where nursing is practiced, most nurses will have to survive with the information they have at hand.

One of the more common scenarios faced in creating the process-centered organization is coming to the realization that the many data sources (repositories) available to the administrator do not interface—they do not *speak* to each other. This lack of interactive capacity means that data that need to be integrated in the processes they represent are in actuality isolated. This isolation leads to difficulty in moving the organization toward becoming process centered. Two things are needed: the capacity to turn data into information, which depends on the ability to analyze those data, and the potential for connecting data sources so that they can rely on each other and thus produce more significant findings.

Since most people do not have the privilege of creating from scratch the organizations in which they wish to work, the reengineered organization will need some careful retooling of its information infrastructure to become a fully functional, process-centered corporation. This was made painfully clear when hospital executives, managed care executives, and physician group practice executives responded to a survey about the adequacy of information technology in their organizations. The study, reported in August 1998, indicated that of the three groups, hospital executives were least confident in their technological systems' performance. Across all three categories of respondents, clinical data sets—which create the capacity to measure outcomes and share patient information throughout the organization—were rated the lowest.[6]

DETERMINING INFORMATION MANAGEMENT NEEDS

Some parts of the retooling that health care systems require will be more costly than other parts. The well-advised administrator will begin with a thorough inventory of the data sources available and their output, utility, and unused capacity. This inventory allows much clearer decision making about the nature of the organization's needs for future data systems or sources. Exhibit 23–1 lists critical questions that must be answered to generate a meaningful assessment of the organization's capabilities and information management needs.

Exhibit 23–1 Key Questions for Informed Decision Making

- What data sources do I already have at my disposal?
- What data do they produce or are they capable of producing?
- Do the data have meaning, or do they merely represent frequencies rather than the relationship of one activity to another?
- At what frequency are reports generated, and is this the best schedule?
- Do the current data reports inform the work of departments?
- Do any of these data sources interact, or are they isolated?
- Who manages these data sources, and are these people thoughtful and analytical about the work of nursing and its information needs?
- What information do I need to "fine tune" the organization and refine its processes into efficient, effective tools that move the organization forward?

What Data Sources Do I Already Have at My Disposal? Most organizations generate mountains of data, and often these data are managed and maintained on a computer software program. Frequently, the data are not maintained by the department of nursing, and they may lead to useless, repetitious reports that add no value to decision making. Therefore, it is also important to ask which data sources are at the manager's disposal or are influenced by leadership. Whether the data sources are owned and operated by nursing or are provided through some other service department, the key is to know what is available and the manager's capacity to influence its use. The goal is for the data to serve the decision-making process.

The organization may have data repositories with information on internal nursing affairs such as

- staffing
- scheduling
- accumulated holiday/vacation time
- worker profiles

Other data repositories may provide access to information about major patient populations (demographic configurations and characteristics) that can offer insight into the department's major costs and opportunities, for example:

- diagnosis-related groups of significance
- characteristics of patient populations
- length of stay
- cost per case

Finally, there may be data sources that offer the opportunity to examine the work of nursing to measure its contributions and its costs. These data sources include databases that track

- patient acuity
- skill mix
- case mix
- census (not merely average daily census, but actual data that indicate variations)

Although these last data sources are more rare, they are occasionally found in organizations. Most systems that exist today were designed to assess the productive outcomes of medicine and finance, not nursing, and therefore these resources may need to be constructed.

What Data Do Data Sources Produce or Are They Capable of Producing? After noting what data are currently received from internal systems, it is wise to examine these data further and ask more questions. Is this useful information? Has it been sifted and analyzed, or is it raw and difficult to apply to the department's work?

EXAMPLE

It is not uncommon for inpatient facilities to measure their census activity at midnight. This may be a very reliable source of true information for some facilities, but for others, this single "head count" taken at a predetermined hour of the day does not represent the activity levels that the work and the workers must address. In one facility it became very clear, upon analyzing other, noncomputerized data, that for one in three patient beds, as many as three individuals may occupy the bed between midnight one day and midnight the next day. If the administrator were to fail to take into consideration the number of short-stay and transfer patients who were cared for within each 24-hour period, the calculations about staffing and other resource consumption expectations would be faulty.

Do the Data Have Meaning, or Do They Merely Represent Frequencies Rather Than the Relationship of One Activity to Another?

EXAMPLE

In one facility it was evident that the data were arranged to meet the needs of the infection control department but not the needs of the nurse managers on the patient care units, where the infectious transmission events occurred. The report did separate critical care units from medical-surgical units, but it did not distinguish between the surgical intensive care unit (ICU) and the medical ICU. As a result, the data report did not identify for the managers or the administrator where infection control processes worked and where they were lacking. It served the needs of the department that collected the data, but it failed to prove meaningful to the departments that could implement a practice change or make a significant difference.

Often, the data that managers receive do not constitute information but are presented as a simple spreadsheet of numbers that does not answer any questions or serve the manager's needs. It is essential to learn whether the reports being generated are all that the system is capable of producing or whether the manager *could* obtain the necessary information if he or she asked for it. All too often the lack of meaningful information stems from the lack of thoughtful requests on the part of the administrators. Ask for what you need—it increases the probability that you will get it!

EXAMPLE

One hospital administrator, when looking into the possibility of eliminating an in-house skilled nursing facility (SNF), posed the question, "What will happen to the patients we serve on this unit if we dismantle it?" The initial breakdown of patients showed a clear pattern: There were five identifiable populations of patients regularly served on the SNF. Two of the largest populations served were complex medical and orthopaedic cases. The initial assumption was that these two populations could be dispersed to the medical-surgical units without much difficulty. It was not until the reimbursement structures for these two patient populations were examined that it became clear that this was no easy decision. Within the two groups were subgroups of patients whose length of hospitalization would increase without the internal SNF. This increase would not be paid for beyond the specified length of stay. Within the subgroups were patients who were too sick to send home and too well to remain in acute care. They needed some ongoing, hospital-provided services, in this case, therapeutic radiology, but if the patients were outsourced to a community SNF, their transportation needs would not be reimbursed. The additional efforts to subdivide the major populations and test the initial assumptions led the administrator to a new set of questions and a new focus for his investigation.

At What Frequency Are Reports Generated, and Is This the Best Schedule? In many instances, data arrive a day late and a dollar short. Reports are often not timely and do not serve the manager's decision-making purposes. This is frequently the case when the data are derived from sources the manager does not control, such as finance, human resources, quality resources, etc. These departments often generate data on their own schedules to serve their own purposes, in which case, the data reports provide information about those departments, not information to enhance or improve nursing. It is imperative that such internal reporting systems work together, that they serve each others' purposes. If they do not, the process-centered organization cannot fully function, since it depends on a clear recognition of customer service, including internal customers.

EXAMPLE

One organization designed and installed new budget software in an effort to make calculating the annual departmental budgets easier and more standardized. The software was not delivered with much lead time for the managers to learn its full use. Once all the managers were minimally trained on the use of the software, the budgeting process began. The software was only available on a few computers throughout the organization. This required that the managers arrange to "borrow" time on a coworker's machine to access the software. Finally, managers took their hand-calculated resource needs and put them into the account categories delineated on the spreadsheet of the new software. To the managers' chagrin, the categories they were accustomed to using were not all present in the new software. They had to guess where they should load certain budget information. The tool designed to capture the number of full-time equivalents (FTEs) departments would require was not able to accept figures with decimal points. The result was that the software rounded all FTE counts up to the next whole number. This increased the counts overall. Finally, the instructions about calculating employee benefits changed three times over the course of the budgeting process, creating errors in the resulting documents. This required rework and correction after the fact.

If this describes your situation, it is critical that you negotiate for the data you need. Sometimes the data are easily available, but no one has informed the generating department of the deficiencies of its current processes. Sometimes it will not be available but *could* be generated if it were known that important decisions hang in the balance. All too often, it is simply a matter of failing to ask the right questions. As often said, "the quality of the answer is directly related to the quality of the question," so if managers ask poor questions, they will get poor information.

Unfortunately, the situation in most organizations is that data reports are generated for their own sake and at the convenience of the generator, not the end user. Managers who are end users need to make a compelling case for any changes required. Unfortunately, most data-generating departments are unaccustomed to talking with their customers to learn their needs or to receiving feedback from their customers regarding the utility or timeliness of their products.

Do the Current Data Reports Inform the Work of Departments? Data are not the same as information. Raw data may be useless to managers in their day-to-day operations. It is not uncommon for data reports to pile up in a corner of the office. They are unused, unread, and unscrutinized because the recipient does not understand the usefulness of the data. It can be very helpful to provide departments with a straightforward explanation of what the data are, why the data are being sent to them, and how they are to use and interpret the data in their daily activities.

EXAMPLE

Remember the organization with the new budget software? Feeling very proud of themselves for having mastered this daunting technological task, the managers set aside their calculations to see what the software would produce. They anticipated a better year than they had previously experienced because of their diligence in using the software. This was not the case. As the new budget year began, the monthly reports generated from the finance department did not represent the calculation expectations of the managers. Expenses intentionally spread over the year showed up as large quarterly bundles, as if significant errors in judgment had occurred. While managers had noticed the shift in categories early in their experience with the software, they expected that the new categories it offered would be the final categories that the finance department would use—not so. Monthly reports indicated that deficits existed in budget account categories where no monies had been budgeted. This was because the reported categories had not been available when the managers loaded the budget. In fact, they were surprised to see the new enlarged list of account categories. With the FTE calculations all rounded up, not one of the monthly report computations captured the true cost per FTE in a meaningful way.

Conversations between administrators and managers can serve two functions. They can be a useful management development tool, and they can serve to engage department leaders in dialogues that will ultimately improve the use and management of information. As department heads begin to see the relationships between the reports they receive and the work they do, their appreciation for and refinement of the data they have available will only improve.

Do Any of These Data Sources Interact, or Are They Isolated? Sometimes certain databases do interact and may be relational. Managers should exploit this situation fully. It is essential to know the extent to which different data repositories can serve integrated functions. Integration allows for a much fuller analysis of the data available. If cost can be seen in relation to expense, or if resource utilization can be represented in relation to certain diagnoses or populations, or if the volume of work can be reflected in terms of skill mix, this will greatly enhance the decision-making function.

These are the relationships that will answer age-old questions: What is the cost of nursing care? Why is it so expensive to serve the needs of certain patients? What is an appropriate assignment for staff members? Without solid data that are compiled in meaningful arrays, such questions remain in the domain of intuition, instinct, and guesswork.

When the available systems cannot do these correlations, it may be necessary for the manager to "connect the dots." This requires a level of analysis for which many managers are unprepared. Such a data analysis function may be available within the organization, but perhaps not within the nursing department. It is crucial that the administrator be able to explain the needs of nursing administration and translate the variables into meaningful language that the analyzing department will comprehend. A common expression in computer circles is "garbage in, garbage out." To avoid this sad situation, a skillful administrator will carefully consider the questions that must be asked and the answers that must be derived. As in any journey, real or invented, "if you don't know where you're going, you'll probably end up someplace else."

EXAMPLE

In most hospitals there is both urgency and dismay in trying to capture meaningful cost measures. Administrators and financial analysts usually want to know the cost per case. Because inpatient care, especially in a large or complex hospital, causes numerous internal transfers for patients, quantifying something like cost per case can be very elusive. One measurement variable related to cost of inpatient care, and decipherable by unit, is that of dollars per workload index. Workload index is a computation of the factors in the census and acuity of the patients and, when used as the denominator against labor dollars expended, gives the manager a fairly good picture of the cost of human resources used to render care. It can be generated by unit to provide a daily productivity measure for each day or each shift's work. This is not necessarily a well-understood calculation or one that administrators unfamiliar with inpatient care units would easily grasp. Unless the nurse executive can translate the meaning and the need for monitoring this variable into language that the data collectors can understand, obtaining clear, cogent results from such a monitoring effort may be very difficult. Without the ability to offer such a translation, the nurse executive may be coaxed to chase data that are far more complex to obtain and far less clear to report. Knowing the intended destination of the data search is essential for generating good questions and useful information.

Who Manages These Data Sources, and Are These People Thoughtful and Analytical about the Work of Nursing and Its Information Needs? Nursing is a complex business. Even within nursing circles, nurses spend a lot of time explaining their work and its implications to colleagues. Nurses need translators within the discipline to help them grasp the nature of nursing's various facets. Critical care nurses may fail to see the comprehensive nature of home care. Public health nurses may be totally disconcerted by the bustle of a large emergency department. Nurse educators may not recognize the subtle changes in the workplace for which they are preparing workers. Nurses often encounter these problems. And if these translation needs are so apparent to nurses, then the ones that exist between nursing and other departments or data analysts are even greater and worthy of more consideration and explanation.

The ability to communicate thoughtful and thorough explanations of nursing's needs, intentions, and vision in relation to the function of information management will become an increasingly important skill. Even if those who manipulate nursing-related data are from among our own ranks, there is ample opportunity for misunderstanding, mistake making, and cross-purposes. The administrator's willingness to explain what purpose the information must serve can only enhance the process by which the information is produced from the available data.

EXAMPLE

In putting the budget together for a large facility, there is often fragmentation of intent, especially if this work is initiated in a decentralized fashion. This was true of one organization in which the nurse executive had a goal of reducing the overall percentage of registered nurses (RNs) in the skill mix. This idea had been communicated in numerous meetings, especially meetings related to reducing the cost of care and inpatient lengths of stay. Somehow, the idea did not translate to every manager involved in the budgeting process. It seemed that each nurse manager had his or her own budget ideas. Even when the national benchmarking data were used as a guide, wide variation in budget planning seemed to prevail from unit to unit. Support personnel in finance did little to aid the end result because they too did not see the objective. Effective change in the first year of this effort was minimal. Difficulties in managing the budget in the subsequent year were equally challenging. In an effort to change this pattern, the nurse executive put in place a coordinator for "decision support," an overseer who could examine each budget and its contribution to the whole. This coordinator analyzed all the budgets as they were submitted, gleaned some perspective on the direction in which each manager was going, and held a personal conversation with the manager about the executive's goal, an RN skill-mix reduction. Some managers had misunderstood, believing the executive's goal had to be achieved on every unit rather than over the facility as a whole. Some managers had reduced their RN skill mix to very low levels, although this was not the executive's intent. Some had not altered their skill mix at all, thinking it was someone else's job. The goal was only achieved when the managers heard the goal regarding the change in RN skill mix in personal conversations about their budgets. The goal required three years and two complete budget cycles to achieve because managers did not understand the goal.

What Information Do I Need To "Fine Tune" the Organization and Refine Its Processes into Efficient, Effective Tools That Move the Organization Forward? It is of no benefit to managers or the organization to be inundated by useless data. An upfront investment in *thinking* about departmental needs is well worth the time and should always precede any request for assistance. What data and information do you need? Why do you need them? What purposes will such reports serve, and how will they improve the organization's functioning? Which processes are costly in terms of time, money, efficiency, and effectiveness? Where do staff "fall down on the job," miss the connections, fail to meet customer needs, lose time, increase costs, or simply wear themselves out?

EXAMPLE

In the ever-changing world of patient care, census and staffing are inevitably in conflict. Often this conflict leads to poor planning, staffing shortages, and the use of external staffing pool personnel. External staff are a very costly drain on staffing dollars. One facility tackled this problem head-on. The managers collected data on external pool use and its cost in real dollars. They analyzed absenteeism, learning that on some units a full 14 percent of staff were, at one time or another, not available to the unit. They examined other forms of nonproductive time and identified the number of FTEs required to have a full complement of staff available each day for each unit. From this calculation they enlarged their internal float pool by 32 FTEs and were able to reduce their external staffing costs 100 percent in the following year. Without the data and thoughtful analysis, the problem may have continued and grown for many years. A quarterly review is now in place that allows managers to monitor the process in real time and make adjustments as required.

CONCLUSION

Organizational processes are a window to the organization's effectiveness. If the processes do not work well, neither will the organization's staff. The systems that organizations create are perfectly crafted to get the results they already obtain. If we desire different results, we must create newer systems and processes that lead us to the end products we want.

REFERENCES

1. Werley H, Devine E, Zorn C, Ryan P, Westra B. The nursing minimum data set: Abstraction tool for standardized, comparable, essential data. *Am J Public Health*. 1991; 81(4):421–426.
2. Graves J, Corcoran S. The study of nursing informatics. *Image: J Nurs Scholarship*. 1989; 21(4):227–231.
3. Jones L. Building the information infrastructure required for managed care. *Image: J Nurs Scholarship*. 1997; 29(4):377–382.
4. Simpson RL. Ammunition in the boardroom: The clinical nursing data set. *Nurs Management*. 1995; 26(6):16–17.

5. Huber D, Schumacher L, Delaney C. Nursing management minimum data set (NMMDS). *J Nurs Adm*. 1997; 27(4):42–48.

6. Hospital & Health Networks leadership survey. *Hosp Health Networks*. 1998 (August); 72(15/16):40–43.

Index

About the Authors

Suzanne P. Smith, EdD, RN, FAAN, has been the Editor-in-Chief of the *Journal of Nursing Administration* and *Nurse Educator* since 1981. She is the author of two books that received Book-of-the-Year awards from the *American Journal of Nursing*; the founder of Nursing SCAN in Research: Application for Clinical Practice, which received two Sigma Theta Tau Media Awards; and the author of numerous articles. Writing under the name of Blancett, she is coauthor/editor, along with Dr. Flarey, of *Reengineering Nursing and Health Care: The Handbook for Organizational Transformation*; *Handbook of Nursing Case Management: Health Care Delivery in a World of Managed Care*; *Case Studies in Nursing Case Management: Health Care Delivery in a World of Managed Care; Health Care Outcomes: Collaborative, Path-Based Approaches*; and *Cardiovascular Outcomes: Collaborative, Path-Based Approaches,* all by Aspen Publishers, Inc.

A former baccalaureate faculty member and director of a federal manpower planning project, Dr. Smith earned her degrees from Simmons College and Boston University. She is a member of the American Organization of Nurse Executives, the National Advisory Board of the Center for Medical Ethics and Mediation, the American Academy of Nursing, the National League for Nursing, and the American Nurses' Association. Dr. Smith is a Sigma Theta Tau International Distinguished Lecturer and Distinguished Writer, Virginia Henderson Fellow, 1991–1995 member of the Board of Directors, and former chair of the Sigma Theta Tau Foundation.

Dr. Smith's public service has included serving as chair of a city board of health and as an elected member of a board of aldermen and a school board. She was also a member and president of a human services council.

Dominick L. Flarey, PhD, MBA, RN,CS, CNAA, FACHE, is President of Dominick L. Flarey & Associates, Inc., and the Center for Medical-Legal Consulting. He is also Editor-in-Chief of *JONA's Healthcare Law, Ethics & Regulation*. He holds a BSN, an MBA in health care administration, and doctorates in nursing administration and management. He has held positions as a certified nurse practitioner, associate administrator of patient services, chief operating officer, and administrator in acute care organizations. He is certified as an adult nurse practitioner and holds a certification in nursing administration from the American Nurses' Association Credentialing Center. He is also board certified as a health care executive and is a Fellow of the American College of Health Care Executives.

Dr. Flarey is the author/editor of *Redesigning Nursing Care Delivery: Transforming our Future*, published by Lippincott-Raven Publishers. He is coauthor/editor, along with Dr. Smith (formerly Blancett), of *Reengineering Nursing and Health Care: The Handbook for Organizational Transformation*, winner of a 1995 *American Journal of Nursing* Book-of-the-Year award; *Handbook of Nursing Case Management: Health Care Delivery in a World of Managed Care*; *Case Studies in Nursing Case Management: Health Care Delivery in a World of Managed Care*; *Health Care Outcomes: Collaborative Path-Based Approaches*; and *Cardiovascular Outcomes: Collaborative Path-Based Approaches*, all by Aspen Publishers, Inc.

Dr. Flarey is a member of the editorial boards of the *Journal of Nursing Administration, Seminars for Nurse Managers, Nursing Case Management*, and *Outcomes Management in Nursing Practice*. He speaks nationally on the topics of case management, reengineering, delivery systems redesign, organizational transformation, outcomes, and legal issues in health care delivery.

DEMCO 38-297